P9-DMX-506

Legacies in Law and Medicine

Legacies in Law and Medicine

Chester R. Burns

Editor

Science History Publications
New York · 1977

Science History Publications
a division of Neale Watson Academic Publications, Inc.
156 Fifth Avenue, New Yotk 10010

Library of Congress Cataloging in Publication Data
Main entry under title:

Legacies in law & medicine.

    Includes bibliographies.
    1. Medical laws and legislation--History--Addresses,
essays, lectures. 2. Medical jurisprudence--History--
Addresses, essays, lectures. 3. Public health laws--
History--Addresses, essays, lectures. I. Burns,
Chester R.
Law   344.04'1   76-29641
ISBN 0-88202-164-8

Contents

Introduction   1
     Chester R. Burns

LAWS ABOUT MEDICINE BEFORE 1500

Visigothic Medical Legislation   9
     Darrel W. Amundsen

The Court Mediciner and Medicine in the Laws of Wales   26
     John Cule

The Faculty of Medicine at Paris, Charlatanism, and Unlicensed
     Medical Practices in the Later Middle Ages   52
     Pearl Kibre

MEDICAL LICENSURE

A Seventeenth Century English Medical License   72
     John H. Raach

Liberty, Laissez-Faire and Licensure
     in Nineteenth Century Britain   79
     David L. Cowen

An Early New Jersey Medical License   90
     Josiah C. Trent

Early Medical Legislation in Louisiana
     and a State Medical Board Examination in 1816   93
     Charles I. Silin

MEDICAL MALPRACTICE

Malpractice Suits in American Medicine Before the Civil War   107
     Chester R. Burns

PUBLIC HEALTH LEGISLATION

The Parish Doctor: England's Poor Law Medical Officers
and Medical Reform, 1870-1900   123
  Jeanne L. Brand

Health and Politics: The British Physical
Deterioration Report of 1904   149
  Bentley B. Gilbert

Sanitary Reform in New York City: Stephen Smith
and the Passage of the Metropolitan Health Bill   160
  Gert H. Brieger

Government's Role in American Medicine:
A Brief Historical Survey   183
  Milton I. Roemer

Federal Public Health: A Reflection
of the Changing Constitution   204
  Morris Kagan

FORENSIC MEDICINE

✓ The Sarah Stout Murder Case: An Early Example
of the Doctor as an Expert Witness   228
  Albert Rosenberg

✓ An Historical View of the M'Naghten Trial   238
  Jacques M. Quen

GENERAL

Early History of Legal Medicine   247
  Erwin H. Ackerknecht

The Growth of Medicine and the Letter of the Law   270
  Benjamin Spector

Professional Ethics and the Development
of American Law as Applied to Medicine   297
  Chester R. Burns

Acknowledgements

We should like to express our appreciation to the following scholarly journals for granting us permission to reprint the following articles in this volume: *The Bulletin of the History of Medicine* (The Johns Hopkins University Press). "Visigothic Medical Legislation," *45*: 553-569, 1971, "The Faculty of Medicine at Paris," *27*: 1-20, 1953, "A Seventeenth Century English Medical License," *13*: 210-216, 1943, "Liberty, Laissez-Faire and Licensure in Nineteenth Century Britain," *43*: 30-40, 1969, "An Early New Jersey Medical License," *15*: 508-511, 1944, "Early Medical Legislation in Louisiana," *5*: 667-680, 1937, "Malpractice Suits in American Medicine before the Civil War," *43*: 41-56, 1969, "The Parish Doctor: England's Poor Law Medical Officers and Medical Reform, 1870-1900," *35*: 97-122, 1961, "Health and Politics: The British Physical Deterioration Report of 1904," *39*: 143-153, 1965, "Sanitary Reform in New York City," *40*: 407-429, 1966, "Government's Role in American Medicine," *18*: 146-168, 1945, "An Historical View of the M'Naghten Trial," *42*: 43-51, 1968, "The Growth of Medicine and the Letter of the Law," *26*: 499-525, 1952; *The Journal of the History of the History of Medicine and Allied Sciences*, "The Court Mediciner and Medicine in the Laws of Wales," *21*: 213-236, 1966, "Federal Public Health: A Reflection of the Changing Constitution," *16*: 256-279, 1961, "The Sarah Stout Murder Case: An Early Example of the Doctor as an Expert Witness," *12*: 61-70, 1957; *The Ciba Symposia*, "Early History of Legal Medicine," *11*: 1286-1304, 1313-1316, 1950-1951.

INTRODUCTION

CHESTER R. BURNS

This collection of essays is designed primarily for use in the classroom by teachers of history: general, legal, and medical. It is a convenient introduction to some principal legacies of law and medicine in the West, especially Anglo-American ones. Although these essays indicate the rather immature state of medico-legal historiography, an assessment of this predicament is *not* the intent of the compiler. The following comments serve only as guideposts to the essays that follow. (When referring to the essays included in this volume, I shall place the author's last name in parentheses. The numbers enclosed in parentheses refer to the references listed at the end of this introduction.)

Laws about Medicine before 1500

Remarkably little is known about medically related laws before 1500. Certainly they existed; most students of history would cite Hammurabi's Code enthusiastically and with justification (1). It listed specific fees for successful treatment and specific types of punishment or recompense for unsuccessful treatment. A practitioner's hands could be amputated if his patient died or lost his eyesight. If a dead patient had been a slave, a practitioner's slave could be given in exchange. If the treated slave lost an eye, the practitioner was assessed a fine. There were other types of punishment or penalty depending on the social status of the patient and the results of treatment. We have very little information, however, about the enforcement of these laws or about their impact on the behavior of Babylonian practitioners.

Ancient Greek practitioners did not have any anxieties about losing their hands as a consequence of state punishment for malpractice. The author of the Hippocratic treatise *Law* seemed to be distressed about the absence of state penalties for unethical practitioners, presumably those who were ignorant. The only penalty was dishonor. Consequently, the author claimed that the medical profession of his day was the least distinguished of all the arts.

The writer of *Law* implied that particular groups of practitioners could be distinguished primarily by societal evaluation. Since law was a principal mode of societal evaluation, its absence meant that there was no generally accepted standard of professional reputation in the Greek city-states. Even though specific laws about medical practice were absent, the author did imply that a state had a right to punish practitioners who did not adhere to its legal norms. If a community had procedures for enforcement, punishment would be avoided by those practitioners who obeyed existing legal rules; there is little evidence, however, that these procedures existed in ancient Greece.

Our meager information about the enforcement of medical laws in antiquity is of course no justification for considering them morally insignificant. Regard for Hammurabi's laws may have saved the hands of many practition-

1

ers. Dishonor may have deterred Graeco-Roman practitioners from engaging in bad practices. The legal situation changed during the Middle Ages: Medically relevant laws became morally significant *and* legally enforceable in the Latin West.

The *Lex Visigothorum* of the fifth and sixth centuries represents a blend of Roman law and Visigothic custom (Amundsen). Contrary to previous claims, these laws appear to have been designed to support the activities of competent practitioners and to protect patients from the errors of incompetent ones. Although bound to the practices and conditions of Visigothic Spain, these laws deal with some central physician-patient transactions that have timeless validity: The nature of contracts, consequences of a patient's death, heroic therapeutics, relationships to women patients, dispensing of drugs to prisoners, fees for apprentices, problems of abortion are all considered in these medieval codices.

The legal stipulations of kings ruling in tenth-century Wales offer another source of information about medieval laws relevant to the practice of medicine (Cule). As in ancient Babylonia, specific fees were itemized for different kinds of treatment. The relatives of a patient, moreover, were to assure the mediciner that he would not be harmed if his patient died; if the mediciner did not obtain this guarantee prior to treatment, he could be punished by the relatives of a patient who died under his care. Considerable attention was also given to the monetary worth of a mediciner's equipment and drugs. These laws, which also provided information about a medical practitioner's social status including his rights and privileges, were operative in Wales until displaced by English law in the mid-sixteenth century.

Licensure sanctions were not included in the laws of Visigothic Spain or tenth-century Wales. During antiquity and the early Middle Ages, most Western political authorities did not establish licensure policies. In view of the other laws enacted during these centuries, the absence of licensing laws is somewhat of a puzzle. Among possible explanations is the fact that there were no institutions to create and monitor professional standards. It does not seem to be merely coincidental that Frederick II's thirteenth-century licensure decree was issued after the medical curriculum at Salerno had been firmly established (2).

In Frederick II's Sicilian kingdom, he who wished to practice medicine was required to study logic for three years, medicine and surgery for five additional years, and was expected to serve another year as an apprentice. After his teachers had certified that he had satisfactorily completed his studies, the student was required to pass an examination administered by Frederick's officials. Upon satisfactory completion of that exam, the doctor was licensed to practice. Frederick's decree also included limitations on the number of daily visits to a patient and the amount of fees charged for services. Those practitioners who did not obey Frederick's laws could have their property confiscated and be imprisoned for up to a year.

During the later Middle Ages, other cities developed licensure policies. The licensing statutes of Bologna entrusted the obligations of examining candidates to a group of faculty and lay citizens. At Montpellier, licensure was a conjoint effort of the medical faculty and the ecclesiastical authorities. French kings began to issue decrees that supported the regulatory efforts of the medical faculty at the University of Paris. By the last quarter of the thirteenth century, this Paris faculty was responsible for approving those who would qualify for a license conferred by the chancellor of the Cathedral of Notre Dame (Kibre). Throughout the fourteenth century, the faculty's desire to supervise medical practice was supported by both popes and kings. In the early decades of that century, the Paris faculty claimed the right to prosecute persons who were illegally practicing medicine. Even though several individuals were found guilty of violating the law and were excommunicated, medical practices by unqualified persons continued. Although the regulations of the Paris faculty, eventually involving surgeons and apothecaries, did not altogether eliminate unqualified practitioners, they may have inhibited, as with Hammurabi's decrees, some unethical acts.

Medical Licensure

In London during the sixteenth century, the configuration of licensing authorities was not dissimilar to what had evolved in Paris. In 1512, Parliament created a medical licensing act which, with various revisions, functioned until 1858. This act entrusted evaluation of candidates to the medical faculties and to representatives of the Church. Although licenses existed for midwives (3), physicians (Raach), and even traveling mountebanks (4), possession of a license may not have mattered much in actual practice.

The principle underlying the British attitude was simple: Any person had the right to practice medicine, and a sick person had the right to seek medical attention from any other person. This regard for individual liberty remained predominant in the Medical Act of 1858 and subsequent British acts of the nineteenth century (Cowen). Under the Medical Act of 1858, a person professing to be a physician was expected to exhibit evidence of suitable qualification received from educational institutions and to have his or her name entered in a national register. Thereby, a lay person could distinguish a qualified practitioner from an unqualified one. Although minor disabilities were imposed on unregistered practitioners, they were neither restricted from practicing nor penalized for practicing without a license.

In contrast to their British forebears, North American colonials championed more restrictive forms of licensure legislation. In response to a petition of its medical society, New Jersey enacted a law on September 26, 1772 which restricted practice to those physicians who had been examined by members of the medical society and approved by judges of the colony's supreme court (Trent). Some 36 years later, the Legislature of the Territory of Orleans, five years after the Louisiana Purchase, passed another licensure act based on restrictive principles (Silin). But penalties for illegal behavior were not prescribed until a revised act was passed in 1816. The "Medical Committee" established in New Orleans to administer this act granted licenses to practice after careful examination of numerous individuals.

Were the New Jersey and Louisiana laws enforced? Although there are important studies of the history of medical licensure (5, 6), remarkably little is known about the enforcement of American licensure laws during the eighteenth and nineteenth centuries. It appears that these laws were seldom enforced, which suggests that the freedom of choice so dear to the hearts of British physicians and citizens was equally dear to their North American heirs.

Medical Malpractice

In the United States, licenses were badges made possible by legislated statutes. The absence of penalty clauses or enforcement measures between 1830 and 1870 did not mean that orthodox practitioners ceased to acquire licenses, nor did it mean that these licenses had no moral significance in the eyes of American citizens. Legislative edicts, moreover, contained in the licensing statutes were not the only ways in which citizens legally attempted to influence the medical profession. Far more important, at least before 1870, were common law decisions about medical malpractice.

Studies of trial court records are certainly needed and, if done, may alter generalizations that have been made from those cases appealed to state supreme courts. A study of twenty-seven malpractice suits in the latter group adjudicated before the Civil War (Burns) indicates that the state supreme court justices acknowledged, with few exceptions, the superiority of an orthodox medical education. These same justices also declared important precedents about medical malpractice that are still fundamentally valid today. Other legal opinions were added during the latter part of the nineteenth century (7). The paucity of studies in the history of medical malpractice should suggest many possibilities for historians, who will undoubtedly realize that other relationships between medicine and the Anglo-American common law tradition need exploration (8).

Public Health Legislation

During the seventeenth and eighteenth centuries several German states developed a concept of police that would, as a theory of administration, help in the attainment of their mercantilist objectives. The political and economic welfare of the state was supreme, and politically secure and economically prosperous states required healthy and productive citizens. During the latter half of the eighteenth century, various physicians responded to these governmental ideals by adapting the concept of police to medical care. Medical police was developed as a theory of health care delivery and a system for regulating all persons involved in that care (9). In varying ways, the national powers adopted codes and regulatory agencies that were designed to control epidemics, regulate apothecaries and pharmacists, supervise hospitals, develop health education programs for citizens, monitor medical education, and eliminate unqualified practitioners.

At least three kinds of police were included in this concept. In a more narrow sense, "medical" police referred to laws and regulations designed to monitor the activities of physicians and other health care providers, e.g., licensure laws. Another group of laws included those that would promote health and prevent disease, for example, regulations about sanitation. A third group included laws pertaining to occupations, often designated as industrial police. Because of their political traditions, governments of some continental countries enacted legal regulations which exemplified all three subdivisions of medical police or public health. These enactments continued throughout the nineteenth century—though not without vicissitudes (10).

The Anglo-American political tradition, buoyed with libertarian sentiments, resisted many of these notions of governmental regulation. This *laissez-faire* attitude, however, did not remove the acrid smoke and noxious vapors from the communities adjacent to British factories (11). How could the urge to wealth be reconciled with the quest for health? Presumed relationships between wealth and health, or poverty and disease, undergirded the evolution of medical care for the poor in England during the nineteenth century (Brand). As with licensure and anti-pollution legislation, care of the sick poor was characterized by a significant change in the role of the central government, a change that also led to a reform of licensing policies (12).

By distinguishing between qualified and unqualified practitioners, the Medical Act of 1858 thereby enabled numerous reforms for Poor Law Medical Officers. Although the 1858 act facilitated these reform efforts, the central authorities (the Poor Law Board) played essentially nominal roles until 1870 in the administrative consequences of the act. Afterwards, not a few medical officers must have been distressed at the ambivalences generated by the Local Government Board situated in London and the Boards of Guardians located in the parishes. The medical officers resented not only the lay inspectors sent by the Local Government Board, but also the counterproductive actions of the local guardians who, for example, would often rescind the physician's orders for dietary supplements.

That the British government was responsible for the care of the British poor was accepted grudgingly and gradually during the nineteenth century. When, in 1904, the Interdepartmental Committee on Physical Deterioration published its report about the physically degenerate condition of the British people, the effect was almost immediate (Gilbert). Physical weakness or deterioration meant social, economic, and military deterioration. No nation could maintain its political and economic power with an unhealthy citizenry. Within seven years, the British government accepted public responsibilities for feeding children in state schools, evaluating the health of school children, establishing old-age pensions, and creating compulsory national insurance. Echoes of mercantilist ideals were not faint.

American officials were equally slow in accepting governmental responsibility for certain public health needs. During epidemics boards of health would emerge in various cities, only to disappear after the epidemic had abated. It was in the form of sanitary police, though, that city and state governments began to identify their legal obligations to citizens desiring health. A singular example of post-Civil War legal reforms in sanitation was the passage of the Metropolitan Health Bill for New York City in 1866 (Brieger). As the first health legislation of its kind in the United States, this law served as a paradigm for other local and state laws adopted as efforts at sanitary police. After 1875, many state legislatures adopted statutes involving sanitation and environmental health, and most of these same governments adopted new licensure regulations which would, presumably, separate qualified from unqualified practitioners. The state governments were accepting a new set of responsibilities for securing and protecting the public's health (13).

The federal government became involved with medical care as early as 1798. As a form of compulsory health insurance, a marine hospital system was financed by monthly deductions from the wages of seamen aboard every American ship arriving from a foreign port (14). These seamen were treated by hospital surgeons whose position was not unlike that of the Poor Law Medical Officers in England. On the one hand, they were dependent upon the funds acquired by the clerks of the Revenue Marine Division of the Treasury Department, clerks who exercised no supervisory authority. On the other hand, they were subjected to the vagaries of the customs collectors in the various ports, vagaries that eventually included responsibilities for selecting and appointing the hospital surgeons. With passage of a new law in 1870, Congress began its policy of relatively constant attention to the needs and concerns of the Marine Hospital Service.

Throughout most of the nineteenth century, however, the federal government insisted, usually by inaction, that health care activities be entrusted to state and local governments (Roemer). These local and state authorities responded in a variety of ways: development of county health departments, construction of almshouses, insane asylums, and tuberculosis sanatoria, creation of city and state health boards, enactment of state medical practice acts, establishment of state-supported medical schools, and medical care of prisoners and other wards of the state.

Beginning around 1900, increased federalization has characterized much of the legislation pertaining to public health. In addition to the care of merchant seamen, the federal government has assumed responsibility for the medical care of Indians, employees of special governmental projects such as the Tennessee Valley Authority, migratory farm workers, members of the armed forces, and war veterans.

Public health legislation has reflected these changing patterns of federal/state/local government authority (Kagan). As its powers have been recognized and exercised by interpretations of constitutional law, the federal government has assumed many new roles in public health legislation. By the mid-twentieth century, the federal government was not necessarily trusted by American physicians and citizens any more than the original federal government had been trusted by Jeffersonian Democrats. Nevertheless, no other unit of American government had the power and resources to deal with the complex problems of health care for all American citizens.

Forensic Medicine

As the judicial systems of the modern national states expanded during the sixteenth and seventeenth centuries, the need for medical testimony became more explicit. Such physicians as Paré, Weyer, Augenius, Cardanus, Zacchias, and Fidelis responded to these circumstances by preparing treatises about forensic problems associated with wounds, insanity, pregnancy, and poisoning. These books were prepared primarily to help physicians who were called as expert witnesses during a variety of judicial proceedings.

One interesting example, involving the murder of Sarah Stout, occurred in England in 1699 (Rosenberg). Did Sarah Stout drown herself, or was she murdered? Was she pregnant at the time of her death? An autopsy was performed six weeks after the burial of her body. She was not pregnant. Was there evidence of murder; was there evidence of drowning? Answers to these questions were given by some of the most influential British physicians of the day: Hans Sloane, Samuel Garth, and William Cowper. The problem of determining the cause of sudden or accidental death was one of the most important problems of forensic medicine.

More than a century later, in 1821, the first definitive British monograph on forensic medicine was published by John Gordon Smith, an Edinburgh graduate who became the first professor of medical jurisprudence at London University (1829). Smith characterized forensic medicine as follows: (1) circumstances of death, especially if caused by violent means or occurring suddenly; (2) personal injuries; (3) circumstances disqualifying one for social and civil responsibilities; and (4) medical police, including whatever pertains to the preservation of public health. In the text itself, however, Smith did not discuss public health, and he omitted that category from later definitions of medical jurisprudence.

Smith's response was typical of a segregation that had occurred among the three major areas originally included in the concept of medical jurisprudence. By the turn of the nineteenth century, physicians were attending to the separate parts—medical ethics, forensic medicine, public health—but not the original whole. The most important American author of his day, Theodric Romeyn Beck, did not, in his text on medical jurisprudence issued in 1823, deal with medical ethics or public health. For Beck and many others, medical jurisprudence was synonymous with forensic medicine and involved the use of medical knowledge in court and judicial proceedings.

With the rise of psychiatry during the first half of the nineteenth century, legal problems associated with the care of the insane became very prominent. The trial of Daniel M'Naghten (1843) was one of the most important events in the history of Anglo-American jurisprudence of insanity during the nineteenth century (Quen). Were criminals mentally ill, either partially or completely? If so, could society punish them for their deeds? The medical problem was to determine if M'Naghten was insane. The legal problem was to determine if he could be punished for murdering Edward Drummond. The trial itself may not have been as important as the deliberations of the fifteen judges from the

Queen's Bench whose opinions have challenged lawyers and judges ever since they were uttered three months after M'Naghten's trial ended. Regardless, the events and aftermath of this trial established the jurisprudence of insanity as a major feature of Anglo-American forensic medicine.

A study of these essays will reveal a web of transactions between important legal and medical traditions in Western culture, especially as they pertain to Great Britain and the United States. The concluding essays (Ackerknecht, Spector, and Burns) suggest many possibilities for teachers and scholars who wish to explore the many uncharted territories of medico-legal history.

References and Notes

1. Chilperic Edwards, *The Hammurabi Code and the Sinaitic Legislation.* London: Watts, 1921.
2. Edward F. Hartung, "Medical Regulations of Frederick the Second of Hohenstaufen," *Med. Life,* 1934, *41*:587–601.
3. James Hitchcock, "A Sixteenth Century Midwife's License," *Bull. Hist. Med.,* 1967, *41*:75–76.
4. Leslie G. Matthews, "Licensed Mountebanks in Britain," *J. Hist. Med. All. Sci.,* 1964, *19*:30–45.
5. Joseph F. Kett, *The Formation of the American Medical Profession The Role of Institutions, 1780–1860.* New Haven: Yale University Press, 1968.
6. Richard H. Shryock, *Medical Licensing in America, 1650–1965.* Baltimore: The Johns Hopkins Press, 1967.
7. Charles J. Weigel, II, "Medical Malpractice in America's Middle Years," *Tex. Rep. Biol. Med.,* 1974, *32*:191–205.
8. See the forthcoming publication on the history of medical malpractice by Carleton B. Chapman.
9. George Rosen, *From Medical Police to Social Medicine Essays on the History of Health Care.* New York: Science History Publications, 1974.
10. Kirk Proskauer, "A Civil Ordinance of the Year 1846 to Combat Phosphorus Necrosis," *Bull. Hist. Med.,* 1942, *11*:561–569.
11. Ann Beck, "Some Aspects of the History of Anti-Pollution Legislation in England, 1819–1954" *J. Hist. Med. All. Sci.,* 1959, *14*:475–489.
12. For details of the period before 1870, see Ruth G. Hodgkinson, "Poor Law Medical Officers of England 1834–1871," *J. Hist. Med. All. Sci.,* 1956, *11*:299–338.
13. As examples of activities at the city and state level, see the following: John B. Blake, *Public Health in the Town of Boston, 1630–1822.* Cambridge: Harvard University Press, 1959; Philip D. Jordan, *The People's Health: A History of Public Health in Minnesota to 1948.* St. Paul: Minnesota Historical Society, 1953; Barbara G. Rosenkrantz, *Public Health and the State: Changing Views in Massachusetts, 1842–1936.* Cambridge: Harvard University Press, 1972; John Duffy, *A History of Public Health in New York City, 1625–1866.* New York: Russell Sage Foundation, 1968; John Duffy, *A History of Public Health in New York City, 1866–1966.* New York: Russell Sage Foundation, 1974.
14. Milton Terris, "An Early System of Compulsory Health Insurance in the United States, 1798–1894," *Bull. Hist. Med.,* 1944, *15*:433–444.

VISIGOTHIC MEDICAL LEGISLATION *

DARREL W. AMUNDSEN **

One hundred years before the fall of the Western Roman Empire, the Visigoths made their first inroad into Roman territory at the lower Danube and, extending slowly westward, by 476 controlled most of southern France and the Iberian Peninsula. Although the former area was soon lost, the latter was held under Visigothic sway until the Arab conquest of 711. The Visigoths brought with them their customary laws called *Belagines* into which some Christian principles had been introduced during the late fourth century.[1] It was during the reign of Euric, about 475, that there were promulgated the *Statuta Legum*, which were basically a codification drawn up according to Roman legislative principles, primarily Roman in form and content, into which were incorporated elements of Gothic custom.[2] Formulated by Euric's minister, Leon of Narbonne, this codification was the first of what were later to be collectively called the *Leges Visigothorum* and marks the initiation of a new epoch in legal history: the beginning of various legal systems and codices generally known as the *Leges Barbarorum*.

The then Arian Visigoths, who constituted a superstructure of power, were subject to the *Statuta Legum*. On the other hand, the Catholic Hispani, over whom the Visigoths ruled, had their own codes of personal law: the *Codex Gregorianus*, the *Codex Hermogenianus*, the *Codex Theodosianus*, the *Novella Constitutio* (*Novelles post-Theodosianae*) supplemented by various commentaries, such as those of Ulpian and Gaius, etc.[3] In 506, under the reign of Alaric, a compendium of these laws was promulgated for the Hispani, variously called the *Liber Legum*, the *Lex Romana Visigothorum* or the *Breviarum Alarici Regis*. This then existed side by side with the *Statuta Legum* until the former was superseded and the

* Read in abridged form at the 43rd annual meeting of the American Association for the History of Medicine, Birmingham, Ala., April 2, 1970.

** I wish to express my appreciation to Mr. Gary B. Ferngren, Department of History, Oregon State University, for his valuable advice and assistance.

[1] Marie R. Madden, *Political Theory and Law in Medieval Spain*, New York, 1930, p. 31.

[2] Ernst Levy, "Reflections on the first 'reception' of Roman law in Germanic states," *Am. Hist. Rev.*, 1942, *48*: 22.

[3] Madden, *op. cit.*, p. 32.

latter revised between 572 and 586 by order of Leovigild, thus making one code applicable to Visigoths and Hispani alike. Under the reign of Chindaswinth (642-653), the formulation of a new code of laws was begun which was completed and promulgated in 654 by his son Recceswinth. This became known as the *Liber Iudicum, Liber Iudicis, Liber Goticum, Liber Legum Gothorum, Liber Iudiciorum, Forum Iudicum* or most commonly, the *Lex Visigothorum*. Of the *Leges Visigothorum,* only the *Breviarum* of Alaric and the *Lex Visigothorum* of Recesswinth (with amendments of his successors) are extant in their entirety.[4] Over half of the laws contained in the *Lex Visigothorum* are labeled *Antiquae,* ancient laws, that is, from the codices of Euric or Leovigild.[5]

Of special interest to medical historians is Titulus I of Liber XI: *De medicis et egrotis* (concerning physicians and sick persons), which contains eight laws bearing the following titles:

I. Ne absentibus propinquis mulierem medicus flebotomare presumat. (A physician shall not presume to bleed a woman in the absence of her relatives.)

II. Ne medicus custodia retentos visitare presumat. (A physician shall not presume to visit those confined in prison.)

III. Si medicus pro egritudine ad placitum expetatur. (If a physician should be sought under contract on account of illness.)

IV. Si ad placitum susceptus moriatur infirmus. (If a sick person who has been treated under contract should die.)

V. Si de oculis medicus ipocemata tollat. (If a physician should remove cataracts from the eyes.)

VI. Si per flebotomum ingenuus vel servus mortem incurrat. (If a free man or a slave should die due to phlebotomy.)

VII. De mercede discipuli. (Concerning an apprentice's fee.)

VIII. Ne indiscussus medicus custodia deputetur. (A physician shall not be imprisoned without a hearing.)

These laws have been severely criticized by medical historians, particularly by Dr. Fielding H. Garrison and Dr. Max Neuburger: " Under the Visigoths in Spain, the activities of the medical profession were crushed by a Draconic code of laws." [6] " In Spain . . . the schools of the Imperial

---

[4] All are edited by Karl Zeumer in *Monumenta Germaniae Historica, Legum Sectio I, Tomus I,* Hanover and Leipzig, 1902.

[5] Levy, *op. cit.,* p. 21.

[6] F. H. Garrison, *An Introduction to the History of Medicine,* revised edition, Philadelphia, 1929, p. 146.

era degenerated . . . and with them also the medical status, the profession declining to the level of a trade. The small esteem in which it was held is shown by the legal enactments of the Visigoths. . . . Limitations of medical activity, such as are found amongst the Visigoths, are not known in the legal systems of other nations. . . . Such draconic enactments naturally hindered medical action, for none but itinerant quacks could escape the criminal dangers threatening treatment." [7]

It is my thesis that Drs. Garrison and Neuburger and many other medical historians have greatly exaggerated the severity of Visigothic medical legislation. I propose to show that, in the *Lex Visigothorum,* the *leges de medicis et egrotis* did provide certain safeguards both to the physician and the patient; were not, considering the absence of medical licensure regulations, unduly harsh; did not excessively hinder medical action; did not limit the medical profession to none but itinerant quacks; nor necessarily indicate that the medical profession was held in small esteem or that medical practice was at a low level.

Since the *Lex Visigothorum* is the product of a gradual blending of Roman law with Visigothic customary law, let us briefly consider the position of physicians and medical practice under Roman law. Beginning with Julius Caesar, physicians enjoyed a privileged position in Roman legal systems: in order to make physicians and teachers of the liberal arts more desirous of living in Rome and to induce others to move there, citizenship was conferred on all who practiced those professions.[8] Augustus, at a time of famine, expelled from Rome all foreigners except physicians and teachers.[9] After his personal physician, Musa, had restored Augustus to health, he gave, among other things, exemption from taxes both to him and to all members of his profession, as well as to future generations of physicians.[10] Additional privileges and exemptions were bestowed on members of the medical profession by the emperors Vespasian and Hadrian, the latter establishing rules defining the immunities which physicians could claim.[11] Thus there came into existence the *leges de medicis et professoribus* which bestowed many privileges on physicians and teachers, e. g. exemption from military and other public service and the duty of taking lodgers, freedom from the

[7] Max Neuburger, *History of Medicine,* translated by E. Playfair, Vol. II, Part I, Oxford, 1925, pp. 10 and 11.
[8] Suetonius, *De vita Caesarum,* " Divus Julius," 42, 1.
[9] *Ibid.,* " Divus Augustus," 42, 3.
[10] Dio Cassius, LIII, 30.
[11] *Digesta Justiniani,* L, 4, 18 and 30.

obligation of holding expensive and time-consuming offices, etc. There were no licensing requirements: virtually any free man could call himself *medicus* and enjoy these exemptions. It was during the reign of Antoninus Pius that the first restrictions were placed on the number of those who could qualify for these privileges, when he limited the number of eligible *medici* to five in villages, seven in middle-sized towns, and ten in larger cities. Appointed by the state magistracy, these *valde docti* could be deprived of their immunities if found guilty of culpable negligence.[12] This was not a condition of licensure: "there were still endless pseudo-physicians—but each city at least had a few doctors whose knowledge was guaranteed by the municipal authorities."[13] Nor was it the introduction of socialized medicine. In certain areas, particularly in Asia Minor, salaried public medical positions had existed since the Hellenistic era and earlier, and from the time of Antoninus Pius the number of communities supporting public physicians increased. It was under the reign of the co-emperors Valentinian I and Valens that the qualifications for holding the office of public medical officer were specified: examination and approval by a board consisting of the seven ranking public medical officers of the community.[14] Public medical officers henceforth were known as *archiatri populares*. The public physicians were, with certain restrictions, allowed to receive fees from individual patients but were apparently obligated to treat the poor without charge.[15] Additionally, there were

[12] *Ibid.*, XXVII, 1, 6 and 8.

[13] Henry E. Sigerist, "The history of medical licensure," *J. A. M. A.*, 1935, *104*: 1058.

[14] *Codex Theodosianus*, XIII, 3, 8 and 9.

[15] The view that the poor were treated gratuitously as a matter of policy, although generally accepted in the past, both in respect to the public physicians of the Greek city-states and the Roman public medical service, has been questioned by, among others, Edelstein (*Asclepius*, Baltimore, 1945, Vol. I, p. 175) regarding the former, and by Temkin (*Social Medicine: Its Derivations and Objectives*, ed. Galdston, New York, 1949, p. 11, n. 11) in respect to the latter. The most recent work dealing specifically with public physicians in the Greek city-states of the period prior to Roman domination is Cohn-Haft's *The Public Physicians of Ancient Greece* (Northampton, 1956). Cohn-Haft draws attention to the fact that there is virtually no reliable evidence to support the supposition that the Greek public physicians did, in fact, as a matter of policy offer free medical care to the poor.

The evidence normally cited in support of the policy of free medical care in fifth-century B. C. Athens is the comment of a scholiast on line 1030 of Aristophanes' *Acharnians*: οὐ δημοσιεύων τυγχάνω: οἱ δημοσίᾳ χειροτονούμενοι ἰατροὶ ὡς δημόσιοι προῖκα ἐθεράπευον. The Aristophanic scholia, from which this is quoted, according to W. G. Rutherford (*Scholia Aristophanica*, Vol. III: *A Chapter in the History of Annotation*, London, 1905, p. 368), date from after A. D. 400. This late date coupled with the general unreliability of the scholiast warrants the dismissal of this as evidence for conditions at Aristophanes' time by Cohn-Haft, who remarks: "The simplest answer—

military doctors, *medici* appointed for the circus and the gladiators, etc., and individuals could still practice medicine without being part of the public medical service.

Roman law had in it no restrictions regarding who could and who could not practice medicine. One can imagine the extent of ignorant malpractice that would prevail in any society where there is no system of medical licensure. This, of course, was alleviated to a great degree by the institution of Roman public medical service. There were almost

and perhaps the correct one—is that he [i. e. the scholiast] gave a patent interpretation to an unfamiliar word in order to make the word conform to something with which he and his contemporaries were familiar, in precisely the way that some of our contemporaries have dealt with the subject. . . . To offer such an answer, however, is to presume to read the scholiast's state of mind, a bootless undertaking with respect to an anonymous man who lived in an unknown place a millennium and a half ago" (p. 34, n. 9). Assuming a *terminus post quem* of A. D. 400, we could place the scholiast probably in the Eastern Empire. Since the *leges de medicis et professoribus* were adopted by the Justinian *Corpus Iuris Civilis*, if the scholiast does, in fact, reflect the practice of his own era, even if Byzantine, that would be consonant with the provisions of the *Codex Theodosianus*.

The passage from the latter (XIII, 3, 8) usually cited as evidence for the gratuitous treatment of the poor by members of the Roman public medical service is a law promulgated by Valentinian I and Valens in A.D. 368: "Qui [i. e. archiatri] scientes annonaria sibi commoda a populi commodis ministrari honeste obsequi tenuioribus malint quam turpiter servire divitibus." The force of the jussive subjunctive (malint) is that of a command, in this case for the *archiatri* "to accommodate themselves properly to the needs of the poor rather than to be basely subservient to the rich." For the *archiatri* to be commanded to accommodate themselves properly to the needs of the poor would not preclude the payment of an honorarium by those treated, be they rich or poor; however, the limitations on the conditions under which payment could be made is noteworthy: "Quos etiam ea patimur accipere, quae sani offerunt pro obsequiis, non ea, quae periclitantes pro salute promittunt." This, as I interpret it, stipulates that the *archiatri* could accept only what patients should offer them—patients who are *sani*, I assume, are those who had already been successfully treated—but could not accept payment offered in advance of treatment by those who are ill. Given the fact that the *archiatri* were ordered to accommodate themselves properly to the needs of the poor and the fact that they could accept only payment offered by those who had been restored to health, the onus would be on the patient to decide whether or not he desired, and could afford, to give the physician an honorarium. This in essence seems to amount to free medical care for the poor who could not afford to give an honorarium to the physician and free medical care as well for those who could afford, but would not elect, to bestow an honorarium. Should the provisions of this law have been enforced, the wealthy would not have been given special attention by the *archiatri* and often, if not usually, would have sought the services of private physicians.

The tone of this law indicates that it was not a new regulation promulgated by Valentinian I and Valens but rather an admonition for the *archiatri* to abide by the rules governing their responsibilities, by which rules they apparently had not been abiding. The quoted portions of this law were included in the *Codex Justinianus* (52, 9) which would have extended its provisions well into the Byzantine era.

no prohibitive stipulations of physicians' professional activities in Roman law, and generally cases of malpractice were not punished. Pliny the Elder's prejudice against the medical profession as a whole is well known, but perhaps his protestations were not totally unwarranted: " Besides this there is no law which would punish criminal ignorance, no manner of retribution. They learn from our perils and make experiments at the cost of our lives; only a physician can commit homicide with complete impunity." [16] However, according to Roman law, in the event of *imperitia* on the part of a physician, there was a distinction made between liability in tort and liability in contract. A physician, depending on the circumstances of the case, could be sued by a delictual action, *ex lege Aquilia*, or by a contractual one, *ex locato*. The former was originally limited strictly to instances involving injury to, or death of, a slave resulting from inexpert treatment. Later, delictual action could be taken against a physician for inexpert treatment of a free man.[17] In the event of the death of a free man owing to a physician's negligence or ignorance, the physician could be tried *ex lege Cornelia de sicariis et veneficis* for homicide. He could not, however, be punished on the basis of the act as such but only if intent were proved.[18] Facilities for redress for victims of malpractice were available under the Empire but at best were ill defined and did not afford the patient adequate protection, nor did they provide sufficient deterrent against the malpractice of the pseudophysician.

At what point public medicine, as provided by Roman law, had ceased to exist in Spain is impossible to determine with any accuracy.[19] Visigothic law, although it borrows much from Roman law, omits all the titles and laws of the *Codex Theodosianus* relative to physicians, professors, and education, and this omission includes the *leges de medicis et*

[16] Nulla praeterea lex quae puniat inscitiam capitalem, nullum exemplum vindictae. Discunt periculis nostris et experimenta per mortes agunt, medicoque tantum hominem occidisse inpunitas summa est. (*Historia naturalis*, XXIX, vii, 18).

[17] Adolf Berger, *Encyclopedic Dictionary of Roman Law*, Transactions of the American Philosophical Society, N. S., Vol. 43, Part 2, Philadelphia, 1953, p. 580.

[18] Paulus, *Sententiae*, V, 23, 3.

[19] Although public medical service died out throughout the western empire with the barbarian invasions, its reestablishment in Italy under Ostrogothic administration is attested by Cassiodorus, as praetorian prefect, under Theodoric (*Variae*, VI, xix, "Formula Comitis Archiatrorum," P. L., Vol. LXIX, 700 f.), who also adopted the *leges de medicis et professoribus* of the *Codex Theodosianus*. During the period of Byzantine rule in Central Italy (535-555), the practices were followed that had been in use in Theodoric's time (Justinian, *Nov.*, Ap. 7, 22), but, crushed by the Lombard invasion, Italy by 572 was forced to watch her social and intellectual standards decline to the Merovingian level.

professoribus. In lieu of these, the promulgators of the *Lex Visigothorum* instituted the *leges de medicis et egrotis,* drawing upon earlier Visigothic codes.

LEX III. ANTIQUA: " If a physician should be sought under contract on account of illness. If anyone should request that a physician treat him for a disease or cure his wound under contract, when the physician has seen the wound or diagnosed the illness, immediately he may undertake the treatment of the sick person under conditions agreed upon and set forth in writing." [20] This law provides for the physician-patient relationship to be contractual. It does not in any way specify content or form of contract, but leaves these up to the discretion of the individuals involved. This law is not inherently prejudicial either to physician or patient. If a physician should guarantee the results of an operation or treatment or sign any contract that he could not fulfill, if it were specified that the payment of his fee was contingent upon success, this would be the result of his own poor judgment, not the product of unfair legislation. Under Roman law a physician could not demand a fee for his services unless treatment were undertaken under contract. For services rendered without a contract a physician would not be compensated except by an honorarium, the amount being at the discretion of the patient. Although technically under American law a physician's liability in respect to his patient is in tort, any patient now who consults a physician assumes basically a contractual relationship that entitles him to sue the physician for damages resulting from incompetence or negligence. Likewise, the physician can sue the patient for the payment of fees. That in the eyes of the law in the United States there exists an unwritten contract between doctor and patient is evidenced by the risk taken by any physician who, unasked, treats an accident victim; in the absence of a " Good Samaritan " law this is true even if the lack of immediate medical attention might prove fatal.

LEX IV. ANTIQUA: " If a sick person who has been treated under contract should die. If any physician should undertake the care of a sick person under contract reduced to written obligation, let him restore the patient to health. Assuredly, if the patient should die, the physician shall definitely not require the fee specified in the contract; thereafter no malicious suit shall be brought against either party." [21] A physician, of

---

[20] Si medicus pro egritudine ad placitum expetatur. Si quis medicum ad placitum pro infirmo visitando aut vulnere curando poposcerit, cum viderit vulnus medicus aut dolores agnoverit, statim sub certo placito cautione emissa infirmum suscipiat.

[21] Si ad placitum susceptus moriatur infirmus. Si quis medicus infirmum ad placitum

course, is judged to a degree by the recovery or death of his patient, although the apparent results of treatment may be due to many causes other than the ability or incompetence of the physician. Obviously, a physician cannot be liable to criminal investigation for every instance in which a patient does not recover. Visigothic law alleviated the threat of malpractice suits to a great extent in the case of a patient's death by the promulgation of this law under which a doctor could not be charged with homicide after unfortunate termination of a case following his treatment. Of course, forfeiting a fee after one has conscientiously tried every possible means to help a patient is unfortunate, but immunity from criminal action brought by vindictive relatives of the deceased is some compensation. Unquestionably, members of the medical profession should be liable for prosecution in the event of willful, negligent, or ignorant malpractice, particularly in a society where there is no system of medical licensure. The formulation of legal procedures whereby a victim of malpractice or his relatives may seek redress presents a great problem: medical practice regulations should not be so unnecessarily repressive or restrictive as to hamper the proficiency and progress of medical science. The Code of Hammurabi, which stipulated that a physician whose patient should die in or following surgery should have his hand cut off, if enforced, would have stifled the practice of surgery. Likewise, quite recent codes of law have been unduly prejudicial to medical practice and advancement, e. g. in Romania, where, at about the turn of the century, merely the failure of a surgeon's or a physician's efforts sufficed to make him responsible, under law, for pecuniary damages.[22]

The only law in the *Lex Visigothorum* which deals specifically with the punishment for malpractice pertains to phlebotomy. In Recceswinth's code (654): LEX VI. ANTIQUA: "If a free man or a slave should die due to phlebotomy. If any physician, while he bleeds a patient, should debilitate a free man, let him be compelled to pay 150 solidi; if, however, the patient is a slave, let him replace the slave with one of equal value."[23] We often associate with medieval medicine the "barber surgeon" whose "surgical" panacea was phlebotomy. Discussing the popularity of this

susceperit, cautionis emisso vinculo, infirmum restituat sanitati. Certe si periculum contigerit mortis, mercedem placiti penitus non requirat; nec ulla exinde utrique parti calumnia moveatur.

[22] G. R. Fowler, "Surgical malpractice," in A. M. Hamilton and L. Godkin, *A System of Legal Medicine*, 2nd ed., New York, 1906, vol. 2, p. 574.

[23] Si per fleotomum ingenuus vel servus mortem incurrat. Si quis medicus, dum fleotomiam exercet, ingenuum debilitaverit, CL solidos coactus exolvat; si vero servum, huiusmodi servum restituat.

type of treatment in early medieval times, Professor MacKinney wrote: " Most prominent was the process of cupping or blood-letting. It was employed constantly for all sorts of ailments, especially fevers. Sometimes the results were admittedly precarious; early medieval literature contains references to the dangerous swellings that followed the operation. Many a person in medieval times must have been bled to death." [24]

The Visigoths, not borrowing this law from earlier known codes, indeed must have been cognizant of the possibly harmful results of this manner of treatment to have enacted legislation of this nature. Such a law, if enforced, ought to have discouraged the indiscriminate practice of phlebotomy; yet a need to enlarge its scope was apparently felt, as shown by the revision promulgated by Erwig (680-687): LEX VI. ANTIQUA: " If a free man or a slave should die due to phlebotomy. If any physician, while he bleeds a patient, should debilitate a free man, let him be compelled to pay 150 solidi. If, however, the patient should die, the physician must immediately be handed over to the relatives of the patient so that they would have the power to do with him whatever they wish. If, however, he should debilitate or kill a slave, let him replace the slave with one of equal value." [25] The provision for a physician being turned over for vengeance to the relatives of the patient whom he had bled to death seems to us to be extremely harsh. The degree of the harshness of a law can be evaluated in different terms. It can be compared to present standards of justice, in which case this law would seem most severe; it also can be analyzed in respect to its degree of severity in comparison with the concepts of justice inherent in the code in which the law is found. In the *Lex Visigothorum* punishments were relatively mild for the times and the extent of employment of the *lex talionis,* i. e., retribution in kind, was limited. There were certain crimes for which the principle of " an eye for an eye and a tooth for a tooth " was exacted and in some cases more severe punishment imposed so as to act as a deterrent: " The savage temerity of some persons must be legally punished by more severe penalties, so that, when anyone fears to suffer for what he has done, at least unwillingly he would abstain from the commission of crime." [26]

[24] L. C. MacKinney, *Early Medieval Medicine with Special Reference to France and Chartres,* Baltimore, 1937, p. 39.

[25] Si per flebotomum ingenuus vel servus mortem incurrat. Si quis medicus, dum flebotomiam exercet, ingenuum debilitaverit, CL solidos coactus exolvat. Si vero mortuus fuerit, propinquis continuo tradendus est, ut, quod de eo facere voluerint, habeant potestatem. Si vero servum debilitaverit aut occiderit, huiusmodi servum restituat.

[26] Quorumdam seva temeritas severioribus penis est legaliter ulciscenda, ut, dum metuit quisque pati quod fecerit, saltim ab inlicitis invitus abstineat. (*Lex Visigothorum,* XI, IV, III.)

The injured party could opt in certain cases for pecuniary compensation from his oppressor, in lieu of retribution in kind, with the amount at his discretion. In many instances, though, a fine was stipulated to be paid to the injured party, e. g. 50 solidi for the loss of a thumb, 100 solidi for the loss of a nose. The severity of the punishment of the physician who bleeds a free man to death is probably indicative of the extent of debilitations and deaths resulting from the indiscriminate practice of phlebotomy. After the enactment of Erwig's revision, it is likely that the practice of phlebotomy decreased to the mutual benefit of patients' health and physicians' reputations.

Another law dealing with phlebotomy is LEX I. ANTIQUA: "A physician shall not presume to bleed a woman in the absence of her relatives. No physician shall presume to perform a phlebotomy on a free woman without the presence of her father, mother, brother, son, or uncle or any other relative, *unless the exigency of the illness demands it. Now, when the above named persons are not present, then, in the presence of respectable neighbors or in the presence of suitable male and female slaves, let him apply what he knows according to the nature of the illness.* If he should presume *otherwise*, let him be compelled to pay ten solidi to her relatives or husband, because it is not very difficult, on such an occasion, for wantonness occasionally to occur." [27] Some medical historians wax exceedingly indignant about this law as if it were an insult to the integrity of the medical profession as a whole. Perhaps they do so justly; but let us consider the practical implications of this piece of legislation. I feel it reasonable to assume that the enactment of this law, unprecedented in other, earlier legal codes, was brought about by circumstances that made it at least seem to its enactor to be warranted. We cannot assume that the unlicensed *medici* of Visigothic Spain were one and all of extremely high moral fiber. Neither, on the basis of this law, can we relegate the Visigothic physicians as a whole to the unsavory category of wanton violators of debilitated women, nor can we interpret this as an indication that members of the medical profession were held in a position of deepest distrust by the Visigothic legislators. Even if there had not

[27] Ne absentibus propinquis mulierem medicus flebotomare presumat. Nullus medicus sine presentia patris, matris, fratris, filii aut avunculi vel cuiuscumque propinqui mulierem ingenuam flebotomare presumat, *excepto si necessitas emerserit egritudinis. Ubi etiam contingat supradictas personas minime adesse, tunc aut coram vicinis honestis aut coram servis et ancillabus idoneis secundum qualitatem egritudinis que novit inpendat.* Quod si *aliter* presumpserit, decem solidos propinquis aut marito coactus exolvat, quia difficillimum non est, ut sub tali occasione lubidrium interdum adcrescat. Sections in italics were added by Erwig's revision.

been one case in which a physician had actually abused a woman weakened by phlebotomy, it is not unlikely that there were some physicians accused of doing so. The debilitating and sometimes syncopic effect of phlebotomy could make it in some ways, although certainly not in all respects, analagous to anesthetization. Dr. George R. Fowler, in his essay entitled "Surgical Malpractice," stressed the importance of a physician not administering an anesthetic to a woman without a witness being present: "The necessity of always having witnesses at hand when anaesthetics are administered to female patients has been more than once insisted upon. Experience shows that young women often have voluptuous sensations while under the influence of an anaesthetic, during which time their clothing may become soiled with mucus. Upon awakening they will affirm, with the greatest positiveness, that they have been violated sexually during the anaesthesia. This may arise in part from the fact that women fear that the person administering the anaesthetic might take advantage of their helplessness. The impression may continue after awakening, the fear being changed into a belief of the impression as a reality. The importance of observations upon this point is apparent when the fact is borne in mind that more than a few persons thus accused have suffered punishment, although in the light of subsequent events it was deemed more than probable that they were innocent." [28] Even though the law under consideration was probably intended more for the protection of the patient than the physician, it undoubtedly served to benefit both.

Another prohibitive law is LEX II. ANTIQUA: [29] "A physician shall not presume to visit those confined in prison. No physician shall presume to enter where governors, tribunes, or deputies are held in custody, *without the keeper of the prison*, so that those through fear of their crime would not seek from him a means of death for themselves. For if anything deadly *should be furnished or administered* to these *by the physicians themselves*, the course of justice would be greatly obstructed. If any physician should presume to do this, let him receive judgement along with punishment." [30] We cannot assume the ethical standards of all who

---

[28] *Op. cit.*, p. 595. I assume that Dr. Fowler here is thinking specifically of the effect of ether. Such physiological effects would not necessarily occur in a woman rendered syncopic by phlebotomy, but nevertheless the psychological effects could be analagous.

[29] See note 27, above.

[30] Ne medicus custodia retentos visitare presumat. Nullus medicorum, ubi comites, tribuni aut vilici in custodia retruduntur, introire presumat *sine custode carceris*; ne illi per metum culpe sue mortem sibi ab eodem explorent. Nam si aliquid mortiferum his *ab ipsis medicis datum vel indultum fuerit,* [The earlier version of Recceswinth here reads: ". . . mortiferum his contigerit, . . ."] multum rationibus publicis deperit. Si quis hoc medicorum presumpserit, sententiam cum ultione percipiat.

would call themselves *medici* were as high as those imposed in the so-called Hippocratic Oath, and for the state to guard against activity of this nature and to punish those guilty of such action does not seem to be either unduly repressive or necessarily an adverse reflection on the ethical level of physicians of that period.

The only treatment for which a fee was fixed by law was that of cataract removal. LEX V. ANTIQUA: " If a physician should remove cataracts from the eyes. If any physician should remove a cataract from an eye and restore the patient to his former condition of health, let him receive five solidi for his services." [31] Under the Romans, ophthalmic surgery had reached a high level of development. Celsus [32] briefly discussed the couching of cataract and Paulus Aegineta (625-690) gave a very thorough description of the operation. [33] Some instruments used at that time for couching have survived. [34] There is no indication that in Visigothic Spain surgery had been relegated to the barber surgeons, generally a product of a somewhat later era; however, we cannot determine with any real certainty the level of proficiency employed in cataract removal at this period. Since the stipulation in this law concerns the fee for successful operation and since there is no mention of penalty for the physician if damage to the patient results, in light of the concern of Visigothic law for the welfare of the patient, it is probably reasonable to conclude that in this particular area of practice there were at least some physicians whose competence was relatively high.

Law VII establishes that there was continuation of the Graeco-Roman *medici-discipuli* educational system in Visigothic Spain: LEX VII. ANTIQUA: " Concerning an apprentice's fee. If any doctor should take an attendant into his instruction, let him receive twelve solidi for his services." [35] As in classical times, the level of medical education for physicians would depend in great part on the proficiency and philosophy of the individual instructor. In the education of Visigothic physicians we cannot ascertain the curricular ratio of precepts and oral instruction to that of observation and experience. Since the practice of medicine probably was for most Visigothic *medici* a craft, likely for the majority, as

[31] Si de oculis medicus ipocemata tollat. Si quis medicus hipocisim de oculis abstulerit et ad pristinam sanitatem infirmum revocaverit, V solidos pro suo beneficio consequatur.

[32] *De medicina*, VII, 7.

[33] *Epitome*, VI, 21.

[34] Some are pictured in J. S. Milne, *Surgical Instruments in Greek and Roman Times*, Oxford, 1907, pl. XVI.

[35] De mercede discipuli. Si quis medicus famulum in doctrinam susceperit, pro beneficio suo duodecim solidos consequatur.

was the case in Greece and Rome, the practical aspects of apprenticeship played the dominant if not the exclusive role.

The last law dealing with physicians is indeed favorable to members of the medical profession: LEX VIII. ANTIQUA: "A physician shall not be imprisoned without a hearing. No one shall confine a physician in prison without a hearing, except in the case of homicide. Nevertheless, when charged with debt, he must provide a surety."[36] This places the *medici* in an almost unique position in Visigothic law and raises the question of how legislators and judges determined who was and who was not a *medicus*. There is no evidence at all of any state-supported medical facilities; indeed, the evidence available is most conclusively indicative of their absence. Criteria used probably were somewhat arbitrary: those who had established practice in the community would likely qualify for this exemption whereas itinerants would not. It appears, then, that a physician charged with malpractice would be entitled to a formal hearing and would not be subject to retention pending trial in the event of an accusation having been filed against him. The clause excepting cases of homicide would not apply to cases of alleged malpractice resulting in the death of a patient since, as we have seen,[37] in the event of a patient's death, the physician was contractually protected against suit by virtue of the forfeiture of his fee, except, as noted, in the case of death resulting from phlebotomy.[38]

We can conclude from the above laws that in Visigothic Spain there was a distinct non-clerical, non-monastic, professional medical class, a non-licensed but legally recognized class whose conduct was regulated to a reasonable extent by laws that were neither unduly oppressive nor restrictive, neither excessively indulgent nor prejudicial. These laws were designed to regulate medical activity only to benefit patient and physician alike, to check abuses and encourage responsible practice: the peripatetic quack, charlatan, and general pseudophysician would have been hampered by these statutes, not the competent and ethical physician of that era. They certainly are not to be regarded as the veritable *leges optimae* of medical regulations, nor ought they to be condemned. Criticism, if deserved, should not be leveled against these laws as indiscriminately and vehemently as some medical historians have done.

[36] Ne indiscussus medicus custodia deputetur. Nullus medicum inauditum, excepto homicidii causam, in custodia retrudat. Pro debito tamen sub fideiussorem debet consistere.

[37] Above, p. 559 f.

[38] Above, p. 560 f. For Visigothic laws governing abortion, see below, pp. 566 ff.

Visigothic Laws Governing Abortion

In Roman law [39] a fetus was not held to be human [40] but a part of the maternal body; accordingly the destruction of the fetus *per se* was not a matter to which the law addressed itself since homicide was defined as the deliberate killing of a human being by weapon or drug. It was only when the rights of the father were violated by his wife's procuring an abortion without his consent that there was any penalty imposed for the commission of such an act.[41] Even after Christianity became the state religion, Roman legislators enacted no legislation punishing the practice of abortion if it was done with paternal consent, no injury was sustained by the mother, and no poisons were used.

Early Christians were, however, adamant in their condemnation of abortion [42] and ecclesiastical sanctions were imposed by church councils as early as *circa* A. D. 300 by a local Spanish council at Elvira.[43] Although the effect of action taken by church councils was negligible on Roman law in the area of abortion, in various codices of the *Leges Barbarorum,* particularly in Visigothic law, legislation began to be enacted in which the spirit of the law became consonant with church policy. Prior to the conversion of the Visigoths to Catholicism (587), under the reign of Recarred (586-601) there was promulgated in the *Statuta Legum* of Euric,[44] of which only fragments survive, a law which is extant only in part: " If any woman gives a potion to another in order to bring about an abortion, if she is a female slave, let her receive 200 lashes, and if she is a free woman, let her be deprived of liberty, being condemned to slavery to whom [we order]. If anyone causes a woman to abort by a blow to any place whatever, if the woman dies, let him be held as a murderer. If, however, only the fetus is destroyed ———." [45] There is here no stipulation made concerning penalty for voluntary abortion;

[39] See R. Hähnel, "Der künstliche Abortus im Altertum," *Sudhoffs Archiv für Geschichte der Medizin und der Naturwissenschaften,* 1936, *29*: 224-255, for a survey of sources illustrating the practice of abortion in classical antiquity.

[40] *Digesta Justiniani,* 25, 4, 1, 1; 35, 2, 9, 1.

[41] *Ibid.,* 47, 11, 4.

[42] E. g., *Didache,* II, 2; *Epistle of Barnabas,* 19, 5; Minucius Felix, *Octavius,* 30, 2; Tertullian, *Apologeticus,* IX, 8; Clement of Alexandria, *Paedagogus,* 2, 10, 96, 1; Augustine, *De nuptiis et concupiscentia,* II, 12; Jerome, *Epistles,* XXII, 13.

[43] See R. J. Huser, *The Crime of Abortion in Canon Law,* Washington, 1943.

[44] See above, p. 000.

[45] Si quae mulier alii potionem dederit, ut avorsum faceret, si ancilla est, CC flagella suscipiat, et si ingenua, careat libertatem, servitio deputanda cui [iusserimus]. Si quis mulier[em] ictu quolibet abor[tare] fecerit, si mulier mortua fuerit, tamquam homicida teneatur. Si autem tantum partus extinguitur ————. Zeumer, *op. cit.,* p. 29.

rather the law directs its attention toward the second party who voluntarily or involuntarily causes a woman to abort. The distinction is made much more elaborately in the *Lex Visigothorum* where, of the seven laws governing abortion,[46] six stipulate punishment for the second party, with one decreeing penalty for the woman who voluntarily causes herself to abort. Of the six laws addressed to the second party, one deals with those who intentionally cause a free woman to abort (Lex I), two with those who cause a free woman to abort where the abortion is merely the incidental result of other action (Leges II and III), and three with situations where intent has no bearing on the establishment of penalty (Leges IV, V and VI). Of these laws, all are *antiquae* with the exception of VII.

Lex I. Antiqua: " Concerning those who give a potion [47] to induce abortion. If anyone gives a potion to a pregnant woman to induce abortion or for the purpose of killing the unborn child, let him be put to death; and let the woman who seeks to prepare a potion for abortion, if she is a slave, receive 200 lashes; if she is a free woman, let her be deprived of the dignity of a *persona* [48] and be handed over as a slave to whom we order." [49]

Lex II. Antiqua: "If a free man causes a free woman to abort. If anyone strikes a pregnant woman by any blow whatever or through any circumstance causes a free woman to abort, and from this she dies, let him be punished for homicide.[50] If, however, only the fetus is destroyed, and the woman is in no way debilitated, and a free man is recognized as having inflicted this to a free woman, if he has destroyed a developed fetus, let him pay 150 solidi; if it is actually an undeveloped fetus, let him pay 100 solidi in restitution for the deed." [51]

---

[46] *Ibid.*, pp. 260-262, *Lex Visigothorum*, VI, III, I-VII.

[47] *Potio* may be translated a drink, draught, a potion, a magic potion, philter, a poisonous draught.

[48] *Persona* as a legal term means one having legal rights, as opposed to a slave.

[49] De his, qui potionem ad aborsum dederint. Si quis mulieri pregnanti potionem ad avorsum aut pro necando infante dederit, occidatur; et mulier, que potionem ad aborsum facere quesibit, si ancilla est, CC flagella suscipiat; si ingenua est, careat dignitate persone et cui iusserimus servitura tradatur.

[50] *Lex Visigothorum*, VI, V (Zeumer, *op. cit.*, pp. 269-285), contains 21 laws defining homicide. A free man who had killed another unintentionally was not held to be guilty of homicide when he, while intending to inflict a slight injury, had caused another's death.

[51] Si ingenuus ingenuam abortare fecerit. Si quis mulierem gravidam percusserit quocunique hictu aut per aliquam occasionem mulierem ingenuam abortare fecerit, et exinde mortua fuerit, pro homicidio puniatur. Si autem tantumodo partus excutiatur, et mulier in nullo debilitata fuerit, et ingenuus ingenue hoc intulisse cognoscitur, si formatum infantem extincxit, CL solidos reddat; si vero informem, C solidos pro facto restituat.

24

Lex III. Antiqua: " If a free woman compels a free woman to abort. If a free woman through any violence or circumstance destroys the fetus of a free woman or is known to have debilitated her by this, let her be punished by the penalty just as if for the injury of a superior free man." [52]

Lex IV. Antiqua: " If a free man causes a female slave to abort. If a free man causes a female slave to abort, let him be compelled to pay 20 solidi to the master of the female slave." [53]

Lex V. Antiqua: " If a slave destroys the fetus of a free woman. If a slave destroys the fetus of a free woman, let him be whipped with 200 lashes in public and handed over to the woman as a slave." [54]

Lex VI. Antiqua: " If a male slave causes a female slave to abort. If a male slave causes a female slave to abort, let the master of the male slave be compelled to pay ten solidi to the master of the female slave, and additionally, let the male slave himself receive 200 lashes." [55]

The one law that actually forbad the practice of abortion was also directed toward infanticide, following the provisions of Canon 17 of the Third Council of Toledo (A. D. 589): " Having been reported that in certain parts of Spain parents are killing their own children. . . . Accordingly so great a sin has been brought to the cognizance of our glorious master, King Reccared, whose honor has deigned to command the judges of these same areas to diligently seek out this horrible crime together with a priest and to forbid [it] by applied severity." [56]

Lex VII. " King Chindaswinth: Concerning those who kill their own children either already having been born or in utero. There is nothing worse than the depravity of those who, disregarding piety, become murderers of their own children. In as much as it is said that the crime of these has grown to such a degree throughout the provinces of our land that men as well as women are found to be the performers of this

[52] Si ingenua mulier ingenuam abortare conpulerit. Si mulier ingenua per aliquam violentiam aut occasionem ingenue partum excusserit aut eam ex hoc debilitasse cognoscitur, sicut et ingenui superioris damni pena multetur.

[53] Si ingenuus ancille partum effuderit. Si ingenuus ancille aborsum fecerit pati, XX solidos domino ancille cogatur inferre. One version adds: pro lesione autem legibus adicetur (let him be held liable under the laws for damage.)

[54] Si servus ingenue partum excusserit. Si servus ingenue partum excusserit, ducentenis flagellis publice verberetur et tradetur ingenue serviturus.

[55] Si servus ancille partitudinem leserit. Si ancillam servus abortare fecerit, X solidos dominus servi ancille domino dare cogatur, et ipse servus CC insuper flagella suscipiat.

[56] Nuntiatum, ut in quibusdam Hispaniae partibus filios suos parentes interimant. . . . Proinde tantum nefas ad cognitionem gl. d. n. Recaredi regis perlatum est, cuius gloria dignata est iudicibus earundem partium imperare, ut hoc horrendum facinus diligenter cum sacerdote perquirant et adhibita severitate prohibeant.

heinous action, we therefore, forbidding this dissoluteness, decree that, if a free woman or a female slave murders a son or a daughter which has been born, or, while having it still in utero, either takes a potion to induce abortion, or by any other means whatsoever presumes to destroy her own fetus, after the judge of the province or of the territory learns of such a deed, let him not only sentence the performer of this crime to public execution, or if he wishes to preserve her life, let him not hesitate to destroy the vision of her eyes, but also, if it is evident that the woman's husband ordered or permitted such things, let him not be reluctant to subject the same to a similar punishment." [57]

---

[57] Flavius Chindasvindus Rex: De his, qui filios suos aut natos aut in utero necant. Nihil est eorum pravitate deterius, qui, pietatis inmemores, filiorum suorum necatores existunt. Quorum quia vitium per provincias regni nostri sic inolevisse narratur, ut tam viri quam femine sceleris huius auctores esse repperiantur, ideo hanc licentiam proibentes decernimus, ut, seu libera seu ancilla natum filium filiamve necaverit, sive adhuc in utero habens, aut potionem ad avorsum acceperit, aut alio quocumque modo extinguere partum suum presumserit, mox provincie iudex aut territorii talem factum reppererit, non solum operatricem criminis huius publica morte condemnet, aut si vite reservare voluerit, omnem visionem oculorum eius non moretur extinguere, sed etiam si maritum eius talia iussisse vel permisisse patuerit, eundem etiam vindicte simili subdere non recuset.

The Court Mediciner and Medicine in the Laws of Wales

JOHN CULE*

NOT often has it been possible to define the social position of the physician with such accuracy as to know his exact precedence in a community, but in 10th century Wales he even appeared to know his place at table. Although we cannot be absolutely sure that he really did sit at the seat the Laws appointed for him, there does seem to have been what amounted to a table-plan for the officers of the royal court. And to the jurists of the Middle Ages there was a significance in its design.

A belief in the order of things, a natural scale of hierarchies, was of considerable importance in the emerging philosophy of the Middle Ages. Ultimately, the chain of being stretched from God to dust in which every object, animate and inanimate, had its appointed position. Tillyard says: "The idea began with Plato's *Timaeus,* was developed by Aristotle, was adopted by the Alexandrian Jews, . . . was spread by the Neo-Platonists, and from the Middle Ages till the eighteenth century was one of those accepted commonplaces, more often hinted at or taken for granted than set forth."

This order of the universe has found a most articulate expression in the scheme of Dante's *Commedia,* but centuries later perhaps its most beautiful form is to be read in William Shakespeare's concept of an ordered society.

> For so work the honey-bees,
> Creatures that by a rule in nature teach
> The act of order to a peopled kingdom.
> They have a king and officers of sorts;
> Where some, like magistrates, correct at home,
> Others, like merchants, venture trade abroad,
> Others, like soldiers, armèd in their stings,
> Make boot upon the summer's velvet buds;
> Which pillage they with merry march bring home
> To the tent-royal of their emperor:
> Who, busied in his majesty, surveys
> The singing masons building roofs of gold,
> The civil citizens kneading up the honey,
> The poor mechanic porters crowding in

* Camberley, Surrey, England.

> Their heavy burdens at his narrow gate,
> The sad-eyed justice, with his surly hum,
> Delivering o'er to executors pale
> The lazy yawning drone.

The value, and thus the order of persons and things, was attempted in 10th century Wales under the Laws of Hywel Dda, which set forth the privileges of his subjects and enumerated their worth as well. In the Wales of that time the people recognized the status differences due to office and acknowledged such class differences due to birth as existed between bond and free. There was thus in existence a social situation ready for ordering. Professor D. A. Binchy, writing of the Irish Laws, the texts of which were embodied in the 8th century, has noted there the emergence of a special caste—which he describes as "men of art"—between the Irish nobility and commoners. These were lawyers, leeches, wrights and jewellers, poets, historians and musicians. Later, when Christianity was accepted, the churchmen were fitted in—"not always very comfortably." In Wales a similar skilled class was forming.

Hywel ap Cadell, grandson of Rhodri Mawr, ruled in Wales for about forty years until his death in A.D. 950. He was at first king of the south (Seisyllwg, comprising Ceredigion and Ystrad Tywi), later by marriage acquiring the southwest (Dyfed) and then by conquest the northwest (Gwynedd) as well (Rees, W. 1959). During his reign there was an unwonted peace with the House of Alfred in the persons of Edward the Elder and his sons Athelstan, Edmund, and Edred, giving him time to earn the title granted by later generations of Hywel Dda, Howell the Good. It seemed to have been his policy to pay homage to the English Kings (Rhys) and in the golden age of the Anglo-Saxon Laws visited the court of Athelstan, in whose reign six series of laws were made (Sayles). This Hywel was the king to whom tradition, supported by a certain amount of evidence, gives the position of the great Welsh lawgiver.

This tradition was given its substance in the preambles to the various texts of the Laws in such words as the following, translated from Section 1 of Aled Rhys Wiliam's edition of *Llyfr Iorwerth*.

Hywel, the son of Cadell, prince of all Wales, summoned to him six men, from each *cantref* in Wales, to the White House on the Taf, and these of the most learned men in his dominion, four of them laics and two clerks. The clerks were summoned lest the laics should ordain anything contrary to the holy scripture. The time when they assembled together was Lent, and the reason they assembled in Lent was, because everyone should be pure at that holy time, and should do no wrong. And with mutual counsel and deliberation the wise men there assembled and examined the ancient laws; some of which they suffered to continue unaltered, some they amended, others they entirely abrogated; and they enacted some new laws.

The traditional site of the White House on the Taf is Whitland in Carmarthenshire, though this traditional association might have come about by the later influence of the 12th century Cistercian Abbey there. From the increasing and suspect detail with which later manuscript writers so often 'improve' earlier versions there emerged the claim that Blegywryd, Archdeacon of Llandaff, "the most learned scribe in Wales," was added to the selected twelve and then accompanied Hywel and his bishops on an apocryphal journey to Rome to seek the pope's blessing on their endeavours (Lloyd; also Edwards).

Of the ancient manuscript sources of the Laws of Hywel Dda some thirty-five were written before the 16th century, roughly between 1200 and 1500. About an equal number of late copies were made in the 16th, 17th, and 18th centuries. Sir John Lloyd, the eminent Welsh historian, has summarized the historical position of these documents succinctly.

It thus becomes clear that no MS in Welsh or Latin preserves for us the original code of Hywel. The Latin no less than the Welsh MSS speak of the time of the great legislator as a byegone age. The nearest approach to evidence of what was contained in the first law-book is the consensus of all codes and versions, and there is, in point of fact, so much in common between them as to make this criterion not unserviceable.

The most important 19th century study on the Laws of Wales was made by Aneurin Owen in *The Ancient Laws and Institutes of Wales* (2 vols., 8vo; 1 vol., folio. Record Commission. London, 1841). His method was to divide the Welsh MSS into three groups, being the later variants of the laws as they came to be applied in the three regions of Wales. Of these he made composite texts, the Venedotian Code referring to the northwest (Gwynedd), the Dimetian Code to the southwest of Wales (Dyfed), and the Gwentian Code to the south (Deheubarth), for, despite its name, it cannot refer to Gwent—roughly modern Monmouthshire—where Welsh rule came to an end before the MSS were written. These three codes are to be found in the first volume, some other Welsh legal MSS and three Latin versions, "Leges Wallicae," "Leges Howeli Boni," and "Statuta de Rothelan" in the second. There are some palaeographical and historical objections to Aneurin Owen's method, but it did make a classification into texts of common tradition and it did have an English translation. He based his Venedotian Code on the 13th century *Black Book of Chirk,* with interpolations from other Venedotian MSS, with the intention of making the whole a reconstruction of the presumed archetype. He used similar methods for the other two codes.

It is now recognized that the ancient legal MSS were essentially composed of individual treatises or tractates on particular aspects of the law gathered together as lawyers' textbooks. Aneurin Owen's nomenclature has been replaced by the not wholly satisfactory substitution of the names of Iorwerth, Blegywryd, and Cyfnerth and his composite texts of the Codes simplified. A characteristic of the Venedotian Code MSS was their reference to Iorwerth ap Madog as a jurist of repute, and in some it was stated that he compiled the 'Judges' Test Book' out of the best books that he found in Gwynedd, Deheubarth, and Powys. A discussion of the importance of Iorwerth is given in the introduction to *Llyfr Iorwerth* (The Book of Iorwerth), a critical text of the Venedotian Code, mainly derived from a single MS, BM Cotton Titus Dii, by its transcriber and editor Aled Rhys Wiliam. Professor Sir Goronwy Edwards has pointed out that, although this text consists of seven tractates dealing with specific subjects, it is only the last four of these that are attributed to Iorwerth in any Venedotian MS. Blegywryd, the Archdeacon of Llandaff, has in *Llyfr Blegywryd* (The Book of Blegywryd) his name doubtfully attached to a text of the Dimetian Code, and the name of Cyfnerth is now associated with a text of the Gwentian Code. It was, nevertheless, the individual tractates of particular jurists which formed the bases of the Laws, and the fact that the MSS between 1200 and 1500 were collections of these made with the intention of forming law books (only the later ones were antiquarian copies) gave to their contents a general mediaeval importance.

Llyfr Cyfnerth has been translated by Wade-Evans in *Welsh Medieval Law; Llyfr Blegywryd* has been translated by Melville Richards in the *Laws of Hywel Dda,* but at the time of writing there has been no published translation of *Llyfr Iorwerth.*

The preamble to Section 1 of *Llyfr Iorwerth* has already been translated above and Section 2 of this work enumerated the officers of the court. One source, B.M. Additional MS 14931, referred to them as servants of the court. It is here we get our first glimpse of the mediciner and his place amongst his fellows.

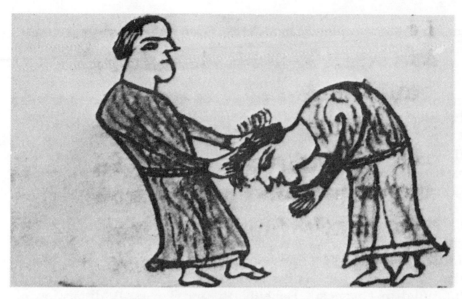

Fig. 1. The Peniarth MS figures. "Si quis mittat manum in capite alicuius per iram, reddat ei pro capillis duos denarios, et de pollice duos denarios, et unum de unoquoque digito, cum sua iniuria." Illustration from *De preciis humanorum membrorum* in the Latin *MS Peniarth 28* in The National Library of Wales. (By courtesy of The National Library of Wales.)

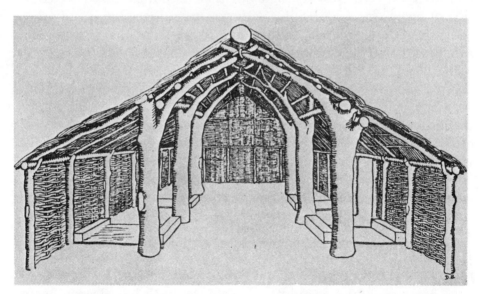

Fig. 2. Welsh Tribal House. The House of the Welsh Laws. (By courtesy of the Clarendon Press from Mary Salmon's *A Source Book of Welsh History*, Oxford University Press, 1927, p. 87.)

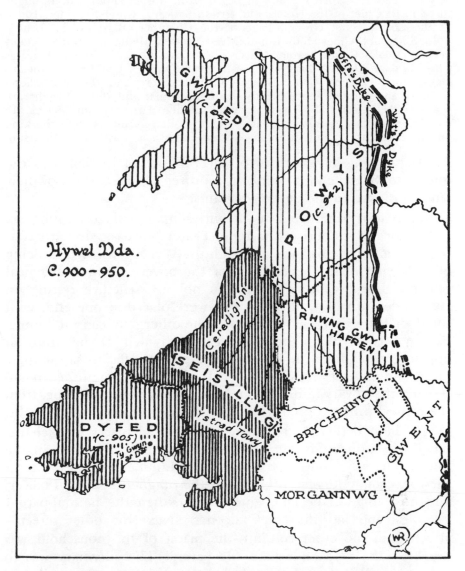

Fig. 3. Map of the Wales of Hywel Dda. (Reproduced by kind permission of Professor William Rees from pl. 23 of his book *An Historical Atlas of Wales*, London, Faber and Faber 1959.)

It was the court which he took to begin with. Twenty-Four officers ought to be in it: Chief of the Household, Priest, Steward, Chief Falconer, Judge of the Court, Chief Groom, Page of the Chamber, Bard of the Household, Silentiary, Chief Houndsman, Mead Brewer, Mediciner, Butler, Doorkeeper, Cook, Candlebearer, Queen's Steward, Queen's Priest, Queen's Chief Groom, Queen's Page of the Chamber, Queen's Handmaid, Queen's Doorkeeper, Queen's Cook, Queen's Candlebearer. And the first officers we have enumerated above are those of the court, and the last eight are those of the queen. Three times a year the above twenty-four officers are entitled to receive, according to law, their woollen garments from the king and their linen garments from the queen: Christmas, Easter and Whitsun.

As the king gave a third of the produce of his lands to the queen, so were the king's servants required to give a third of their land's produce to the queen's servants.[1]

The court conducted its activities in a hall containing six pillars for the support of the roof (Peate). In basic design it was reminiscent of the basilica, although the Welsh construction being of wood, not of stone, accounts for the poverty of archaeological remains. Lloyd describes it as "an oblong structure resting on six wooden uprights, of which two were placed at one end, with the door between them, and two at the other; the central couple, having between them the open hearth, divided the hall into an upper section where the king and the greater officials sat at their meat, and a lower section assigned to the less distinguished members of the royal train." Owen described screens running from the central pillars, on either side of the hearth, to the side walls.

In the hall there were fourteen appointed places with chairs, ten in the upper portion, "above the column", and four in the lower. The king himself sat next the column. Next the king sat the royal commote official known as the *canghellor,* a legal officer, and next to him the chief guest (*osb*), then the heir apparent (*edling*), and last the chief falconer.[2] Next the other screen—attached to the other column—the priest of the household was "to bless the food and chant the pater." The silentiary was to strike the pillar above his head, and this action prompted silence. Next to him sat the judge of the court, then the chaired bard, "the smith of the court on the end of the bench, before the two knees of the priest."[3] The footholder's function appeared to be to hold the king's feet in his lap during the arduous hours of revelry, "from the time he shall begin to sit at the banquet, until

---

[1] LI, s. 3, p. 2.
[2] *Canghellor* and *osb* are loanwords from the Latin *cancellārius* and *hospes,* whilst edling is a borrowing from the Anglo-Saxon *aedeling* (Binchy).
[3] LI, s. 5, p. 3.

he goes to sleep." During that time he was to rub the king, guarding him from every mischance, and eating from the same dish as the king, "with his back toward the fire."[4] His place was "on the side opposite the king's dish; and the mediciner *(meddyg)*[5] at the base of the pillar on the other side of the fire from him.[3] The mediciner's seat at table is confirmed in section 17 of *Llyfr Iorwerth* as being "at the base of the pillar attached to the screen near which the king sits." But there is a certain ambiguity (if not contradiction) in the description of the mediciner's exact place. There is a suggestion in Peniarth MS 164 that one of the duties of the mediciner was advising the king on what he should eat, and this would of course have required proximity.[6]

The chief of the household, who could either be a son or nephew of the king, presided in the lower end of the hall, "with his left hand to the end-door." Those of the household whom he chose sat with him and the rest on the other side of the door. The chief of the household was in effect the chief of the household troop, and thus his position between the king and the door had some defence significance. The other three places in the lower hall were given to the bard of the household, who sat on the one hand of the chief of the household, while the chief groom sat next the king but separated by the screen, and the chief houndsman next the priest of the household but separated by the screen.[3]

In the Dimetian Code as set out in *Llyfr Blegywryd* the mediciner appeared twenty-third[7] in order of precedence as compared with twenty-second[8] as set out in the Gwentian Code (or *Llyfr Cyfnerth*) and twelfth in *Llyfr Iorwerth*. *Llyfr Blegywryd* gave his usual place at table in the lower hall next to the chief of the household and at festival times accorded him no special place whatsoever, when amongst the court officers only the falconer was singled out for such distinction.[9]

Dr. H. D. Emanuel in a personal communication concerning the variants in court precedence of the various versions or redactions suggests that "the factual value of the whole of the Laws of the Court sections is problematic. The picture presented of the Court may be in the nature of a schematic or, to a certain extent,

[4] LI, s. 32, p. 18.
[5] Cotton Titus Dii gives mead-brewer *(medyd)* instead of mediciner *(medyc* or *meddyg)* in this position; but *The Black Book of Chirk* and BM Additional MS 14931 favour mediciner.
[6] AL, vol. 2, p. 587.
[7] LHD, p. 24.
[8] WML, p. 146.
[9] LHD, p. 26.

conventional picture." With this warning in mind, it is possible, using the BM Cotton Titus D ii of *Llyfr Iorwerth* as a guide, to make a table plan at which to sit the mediciner down.

To summarise the position of the mediciner in the court, Section 17 of *Llyfr Iorwerth* specifically dealing with the mediciner may be translated:

The mediciner is twelfth; he is entitled to have his land free and his horse kept in readiness and his woollen clothing from the king and his linen clothing from the queen. His place in the court in the hall [is] at the base of the pillar attached to the screen near which the king sits. His lodging is with the chief of the household. His protection over the safe conduct of an offender is from the time the king orders him to attend to a wounded man whether he be in the court or outside it until he returns from him.[10]

Each of the officers of the court had a privilege of protection, the power of granting temporary asylum, and in each case it was picturesquely associated with the office. The protection of the chief houndsman was so far as "where the sound of his horn can scarce be heard."[11]

There were, not unnaturally, conditions of service. The mediciner was to administer medicine gratuitously to all within the palace, and also particularly to the chief of the household, in whose house he lived. He was to accept nothing from them except their bloodstained clothes.[12] Only three types of injury were exempted from this rule and these were related to "the three mortal wounds," namely, "a stroke on the head unto the brain; a stroke on the body unto the bowels, and the breaking of one of the four limbs." These must have been perilous wounds with a very poor prognosis for a mediaeval victim! For each of these wounds, the mediciner was to be paid nine score pence and his

[10] *Llyfr Blegywryd* gave a similar account of the mediciner's protection: "The protection of the physician is from when he goes to his chamber at the king's command to visit the sick until he shall return to court." (LHD, p. 28.)

[11] LI, s. 15, p. 11.

[12] It has been suggested by Aled Rhys Wiliam in his notes on a later section of *Llyfr Iorwerth* (1. 1, s. 147) that *gwaet dyllat* should be translated as 'dressings or bandages' rather than its apparent meaning of 'blood-stained clothing.' This is an attractive idea, because if the passages in which these words occurred could be taken to mean that the mediciner was to receive nothing 'except *for* the bandages,' it would seem more reasonable for him and be comparable with the Irish system of *othrus* (*folog nothrusa*) in which the duty of meeting the costs of all the necessities of treatment and maintenance of the patient fell upon the assailant. Or if bandaging only was necessary then it was classed as *inindraig sē sēt*. (See also footnotes 14 & 53.)

However, although he quotes in his support a passage from his father's edition of *Llyfr Blegywryd*, (gwaetwisc), p. 8, lines 21-23—". . . *y waetwisc a geiff ef a'r tudedyn vchaf y'r brenhin, pan ymwelho gynntaf ac ef*"—this would seem to imply that he *did* also receive the bloodstained clothes on the first occasion, i.e., when they were taken off. Also on p. 26, lines 16 & 17, ". . . *kany cheif y gantunt namyn y dillat creulyt a torrer a heyrn*" does seem to make the mediciner the recipient of the bloodstained clothes torn with arms.

food, or a pound (240 pence) without his food and also the bloody clothes. The mediciner was further enjoined to make sure that he had an indemnification from the kindred of the wounded person, in case he should die from—or possibly just during the course of—treatment. And if he did not take it, he was to answer for the deed.[13] This could have had far-reaching consequences for the mediciner and his family, as may be seen in the sections of the laws relating to compensation.

John Pughe has translated the 13th century MS of the Myddfai physician Rhiwallon and his sons, a work unrelated to the Law MSS, where a similar fee was mentioned for a head wound with the addition of a few therapeutic tips.

As to a recent blow or fresh wound on the head, the sooner it is dressed the better, lest there should be extravasated blood upon the dura mater (*brain covering*) and that it should become concocted there. When the bone and the dura mater (*brain covering*) are exposed, take the violet and fresh butter, and pound together. If the violet cannot be gotten, take the white of eggs and linseed, pounding them together; or fresh butter and linseed, and apply thereto until (the pain) is assuaged. Then an ointment should be prepared of herbs, butter and tallow, and applied thereto until it is cured.

A pound is the mediciner's fee for this treatment as regards the deed of mercy simply, without victuals; or nine score (pence) with victuals.

There are some further itemized fees for treatments in the Laws given in *Llyfr Iorwerth*. The mediciner was to have twenty-four pence for applying a *goreth*, which may be translated by the late Middle English word tent, a sort of surgical drain made of soft material.[14] The fee for the treatment of a major blood vessel was twelve pence; a medicament of herbs for a swelling, eight pence; for blood-letting, four pence. The treatment of bleeding from a major blood vessel was evidently regarded as less difficult than the application of a *goreth*, for it merited only half its fee. Of course, if it included subsequent visits, then it might be expected that these could be protracted in treating a suppurating wound, requiring a drain. Immediate success or failure was likely to attend treatment of a major blood vessel.

13 LI, s. 17, p. 12-13.
14 The word tent (*goreth*) was used in late Middle English for "a roll or pledget, usually of soft absorbent material, often medicated, formerly much used to search or cleanse a wound, or to keep open or distend a wound, a sore or natural orifice." (*Shorter Oxford English Dictionary*, 1933.) There is an Irish word *inindraig*, 'that which requires a bandage (or tent),' from *indrach*. These 'bandage-wounds' formed a separate class in the tariff of injuries in many early systems (Binchy; see also fn. 12). If the wound only required bandaging and the patient was ambulant the question of *othrus* would presumably not arise, for it would not be necessary to provide for his complete maintenance.

The translation of the remainder of the full text of Section 17 of *Llyfr Iorwerth* reads:

He is to give free treatment to those in the court and to the household, and he is to have nothing from them but their bloodstained clothes, except for one of the three mortal wounds; these are namely, a blow on the head unto the brain; a blow on the body unto the bowels, and the breaking of one of the four limbs. For each of these three mortal wounds the mediciner should be given nine score (pence) and his food, or a pound without his food, also his bloody clothes. He is to have twenty-four (pence) for applying a tent. Treatment for a major blood-vessel, twelve pence; a medicament of herbs for a swelling eight pence; for blood-letting four pence. And his nightly food is worth one penny halfpenny; and his light is worth one penny. The worth of a medicament pan, one penny. He is entitled to take a guarantee from his kindred in respect of a wounded person if he die from the treatment he may give him, and if he does not take it let him answer for the deed. He is to go to the hostings. He is not to leave the court except by the king's permission. His *sarhad* is six kine and six score of silver; his worth is six kine and six score (more) with the augmentation.

Llyfr Blegywryd agrees with *Llyfr Iorwerth* on the three mortal wounds.

If a person be struck upon his head so that the brain be seen; or if he be stabbed in his middle so that the bowels come out; or if the thigh bone or the arm bone of a person be broken, for each of them three pounds are to be paid to him, for he is in danger of his life by every one of them.[15]

The Lawbooks also recorded the value of the mediciner's equipment. The medicament pan, which was stated to be worth one penny in *Llyfr Iorwerth,* was valued at four times that amount in *Llyfr Blegywryd.* Medical costs were awarded automatically. If it were necessary for the wounded person to have medical aid, there was besides his *sarhad* or honour price, a specific allowance made in *Llyfr Blegywryd* of "four pence for a pan to prepare medicaments for him; four pence for tallow: a penny for his light nightly; a penny for the food of the physician nightly; and a penny for the food of the wounded person daily."[15]

Although the Welsh custom at that time appeared to consist in having two meals a day, (*borefwyd* and *cwynos*) morning and evening, it is probable that 'nightly' merely recorded the passage of time as in the modern word fortnight. In comparison with the messing allowance the tariff for specific treatments seemed generous. It is possible that the monetary allowances were for permitted private practice outside the court and household, and the origin was most likely to have been that, as in the earliest texts of the

15 LHD, p. 64.

old Irish Law, the injurer instead of paying the leech fee (the *laecefeoh* of the Anglo-Saxons) had to undertake the duty of nursing his victim back to health and providing him with medical attendance (Binchy). This was frequently referred to in Irish as *folog nothrusa* or 'maintenance of sickness,' and in time this primitive obligation was commuted for a fixed payment. The statement made in Section 17 of *Llyfr Iorwerth* that "the mediciner should be given nine score (pence) and his food, or a pound without his food" is amplified in Section 147 translated below as being payable "by the person who has wounded him." The Welsh Laws may therefore represent a transitional stage between the *folog nothrusa* and the *laecefeoh*. It would also seem that the expected duration of medical attendance for one of the "mortal wounds" was forty days if the assessment in *Llyfr Iorwerth* of a commutation of sixty pence for the food at a rate of one penny halfpenny a day was reasonably accurate.

Gifts from patients were also customary and *Llyfr Blegywryd* made special mention of them, drawing attention to their protection from any later claims of wrongful title: "Three chattels for which no surety is necessary, chattels given by a lord to his man, and a bequest received by a priest from the dead, and chattels received by a physician from the person whom he attends."[16]

Llyfr Blegywryd also recorded the value of needles: "There are three legal needles: the needle of a queen's serving maid: and the physician's needle to sew up wounds; and the chief huntsman's needle to sew up torn dogs. The worth of each of those, four legal pence."[17]

None of the apparatus of the mediciner seems to have survived and this is probably because of its construction. Trease, writing of the Anglo-Saxon mediaeval apothecary, comments that archaeologists have discovered little pottery which can definitely be called pharmaceutical.

The explanation for this would seem to be firstly that wooden boxes and similar perishable containers were more convenient for carrying to fairs or, in the case of a court apothecary, for following an army or itinerant court; and, secondly, that where pots, bowls and pans were used by apothecaries they were of types already used for domestic and other purposes and therefore cannot be recognized unless they contain the remains of drugs.

It was expensive to apply herbs to a swelling for the fee was eight pence. Herbs were specially cultivated, and the stealer of them

16 LHD, p. 108.   17 LHD, p. 107.

38

when they grew in the ground was subject to the special fine of *camlwrw*.[18] *Camlwrw* appeared to be fine of three cows, sometimes doubled, and paid directly to the king (Lloyd). It was thus an offense against the state in the person of the king.[19]

Herbs and medicaments were mentioned only in the context of trauma, as perhaps might have been expected in a lawbook. No prescriptions were given, but a type of remedy used in 13th century Wales, again taken from Pughe's translation of the MS of Rhiwallon, indeed might have been the remedy used for swelling after an injury referred to in the Laws. "Take the juice of the yellow bedstraw, the juice of the plaintain, rye meal, honey and the white of eggs. Make into a plaster, and apply thereto."

The fees of the mediciner thus varied from the pound permitted for the treatment of one of "the three mortal wounds" to four pence for blood-letting. These may be considered in relation to those of the judge of the court, who received twenty-four pence for each judge he examined.[20] By the Law of Hywel, for theft to the value of four pence a thief was saleable; and for a greater amount he forfeited his life. "Seven pounds is the worth of a thief who is to be sold."[21] The Laws deal extensively with values, giving us the opportunity of comparing them with the mediciner's scale.[22] A palfrey was worth six score pence and a

18 LHD, p. 112. cf. "Every invalid in Irish Law is to be fed according to the direction of a leech. No person on sick maintenance is entitled in Irish Law to any condiment except garden herbs; for it is for this purpose that gardens have been made, viz. for care of the sick." (*Ériu*, 1934, vol. 12, p. 23.)

19 There were two kinds of fine: *dirwy*, for major offences, of twelve cows or three pounds; and *camlwrw*, for lesser offences, of three cows or nine score pence.

20 LI, s. 10, p. 8.

21 LI, s. 115, p. 79.

22 *Ceiniog*. The penny was the unit of money. In his glossary Aneurin Owen defines *Ceiniog*: "The common or curt penny is meant generally when penny is mentioned; the legal penny was one third higher in value; the halfpenny or *dimai* was half the curt, one third of the legal penny. It is possible that this enumeration of two descriptions of pennies might have had its origin from the existence and use of the two species of denarii common during the Lower Empire, of the same relative proportions. The number of pence in the pound was 240."

In his notes to *Llyfr Iorwerth*, Aled Rhys Wiliam comments that two thirds of eightpence was apparently a payable sum, for the legal penny was worth three halfpennies, and the *ceiniog gota* (curt penny) was worth two halfpennies. The halfpenny was also divisible in thirds, thus two thirds of a legal penny was equal to a curt penny and two thirds of a halfpenny was equal to a third of a curt penny. An appreciation of these numismatic oddities will help in understanding of the computation of the worth of life and limb of Hywel's subjects and helps the pattern of the order of his society to emerge.

Dolley states: ". . . a coin deserves mention which is known to us from one specimen only, now in the British Museum. It is of the common English type of this period but bears the title 'Howael Rex' and the name of the moneyer Gillys. The date of the coin, tempore Edmund, assigns it without doubt to Howel Dda. . . . The coin was struck by a Chester moneyer, and is the only piece known that can be attributed to a Welsh Prince."

working horse three score pence.[23] A calf was worth four pence, a cow in calf, two score pence, and a cow of full worth, three score pence.[24] A lamb was worth one penny and a sheep, four pence;[25] a kitten before it opened its eyes and a mouse-killing cat ranked equally with a newborn lamb and a sheep.[26] The plaid of an *uchelwr*[27] was worth sixty pence, a yew pail, four pence, a bill-hook, one penny, a wooden shovel, a fork and a rake were worth a farthing each. A salmon net was valued at twenty-four pence but the lordly salmon itself at only two pence.[28]

There is an interesting wage differential given in Min. Acc 1221/16 Crown Lands (9R.II) Rees, 1924).

Wages of Welshmen of Builth for York.—Paid David ap Ieuan, leader of 213 Welshmen, *centeners, vinteners,* and archers, going from Builth to York, 10 days beginning July 5th 9R.II, viz, Wages of David 2s a day, 2 *centeners* 1s each a day, chaplain 4d, one man carrying the standard 6d, one Ringild called Ringild Du 6d a day, 13 *vinteners* each 4d, 1 doctor 4d, 255 archers on foot each 2d a day.

The mediciner lodged with the chief of the household in the largest and most central house in the town, together with the bard of the household. The rest of those who lived with the chief of the household were chosen by him, as were others "around his lodging, so as to be near at hand to administer to his service."[29] The steward apportioned the lodgings and he himself, the silentiary who superintended the meat and drink on his behalf, together with his other servants lodged in the one nearest the court.[30] The priest and the clerks lived in the bellman's house.[31] The chief falconer lived in the king's barn "lest the smoke should affect his birds,"[32] the chief groom in the house nearest the barn "as his duty is to distribute the provender,"[33] and the chief hounds-man in the kiln.[34] The judge and the page of the chamber slept in the king's apartment.[35]

23 LI, s. 121, p. 82.
24 LI, s. 127, p. 85.
25 LI, s. 130, p. 87.
26 LI, s. 131, p. 87.
27 *Uchelwr.* T. Gwynn Jones distinguishes three free Welsh classes: (1) Royal. (2) *Uchelwyr* or nobles with bloodfines of 126 cows. (3) *Boneddigyon* with bloodfines of 63 cows. The son of an *uchelwr* became a *bonheddig* at fourteen, "as he ascends not to the privilege of his father until his father's death." (*Aberystwyth Studies*, 1928, vol. 10, p. 104.)
28 LI, s. 140, pp. 92, 93.
29 LI, s. 6, p. 4.
30 LI, s. 8, p. 6.
31 LI, s. 7, p. 5.
32 LI, s. 9, p. 7.
33 LI, s. 11, p. 9.
34 LI, s. 15, p. 11.
35 LI, ss. 10 & 12, pp. 8 & 9.

The mediciner thus lived and was treated as one of the royal officers or servants. The so-called tribal system then extant in Wales was founded on the kindred or family in its broadest sense (*cenedl*), the village community (*tref*), the region or hundred (*cantref*) , and the king (*brenin*). The *brenin,* who was head of the tribe, was also sometimes known as *arglwydd* or *tywysog,* and his dominion might be over one or many *cantrefi.* The peoples were divided into free and unfree. The unfree were further divided into three classes. The Welsh and unfree man, called an *aillt* or *taeog,* might have been a survivor of an earlier invasion. A foreign and unfree man was known as an *alltud,* and the actual slave or bondman, a *caeth* (Ellis). The freemen were originally an aristocratic minority, related to the local chieftains and performing the obligations of kindred amongst themselves, but from 1100 onward they gradually became the majority. In the 13th century the bond population was only a third of the total, and by this time Wales could be regarded as a land of settled hamlet dwellers. It was to the groups of bond hamlets that social organization was first applied. Under certain circumstances a bondman might become free, for instance rather romantically if he became a poet, but then logically it was for his life tenure only (Jones).

Civilisation and survival depended on overcoming the greatest disability of the powerful family feeling described by Giraldus Cambrensis in the 12th century.

> Being particularly attached to family descent, they revenge with vehemence the injuries which may tend to the disgrace of their blood; and being naturally of a vindictive and passionate disposition, they are ever ready to avenge not only recent but ancient affronts. (Hoare.)

The blood feud with its destructive terror had to be mitigated by a method of financial compensation. Revenge was meticulously controlled by setting out in detail the payment for insult to honor (*sarhad*) and for homicide (*galanas*) whether the killing was intentional or unintentional. The word *sarhad* was used both for the honor-price and the act of insult. Similarly, the word *galanas* was used to mean the compensation for killing a person and for the act of killing (Ellis). These sums varied with the rank of the victim and were paid by the family of the offender within specified relationships on both the male and female sides. Failure to meet the compensation by the last penny "set vengeance free." Aneurin Owen translating from the NLW MS Wynnstay 36 in the "Judges' Test Book" puts the question, "Is there a single penny for which a person's life is forfeited? There is: a penny wanting of *galanus*." This attention to a man's physical worth and that of his honor was but one aspect of this great collection of laws which Sir Paul Vinogradoff once described as elucidating "the working of the tribal system more completely than any other document in European history."

Blood feuds were, of course, not uncommon in England. Alfred's Laws state that "a man may fight on behalf of his lord if his lord is attacked, without becoming liable to a blood feud." The Laws of Edmund and Canute show that the blood feud was still a custom even in their days, and as early as the 5th century there had been attempts by offering 'wergild' compensation to stop the blood feud of family against family (Trevelyan). The law of the blood fine was in no way particular to Wales and can be seen to have formed part of the 'Jus Gentium' of Western Europe.

In Wales *galanas* and *sarhad* were determined by status and this gave the opportunity of determining the values of the officers, alive, dead, or in pieces.

The *sarhad* of most of these officers was six kine and six score of silver, except for the chief of the household troop, whose rank entitled him to a third of the *sarhad* of a king—without the gold—while the priest's *sarhad* could only be determined by a decision of the synod: the steward rated nine score of silver and nine kine. The worth of the officers for *galanas* was usually augmented to three times that of the *sarhad,* though in the case of the silentiary once only is specified.[36] The *sarhad* and *galanas* for the male officers shows the equality characteristic of this society and demonstrates a high regard for human worth and dignity in that turbulent age. Only the apparitor (*rhingyll* or court summoner), "who watched lest the house be burned whilst the king was at meat," ranked below at three kine and three score of silver. And even this should "according to some be equal to the *sarhad* payable to the person on whose land he was insulted."[37]*Llyfr Blegywryd* gave a *sarhad* of nine cows and nine score of silver for the steward, chief groom, court judge, falconer, chamberlain, and maid of the chamber, while the mediciner ranked with the rest at six cows and six score of silver.[38]

It is probable that the social status of the mediciner was at least equivalent to that of the bard for his daughter was granted

36 LI, ss. 6-25, pp. 4-16.
37 LI, s. 34, p. 19.
38 LHD, p. 29.

the same privileges according to *Llyfr Blegywryd*,[39] which in other ways perhaps tended to give the mediciner a more lowly status than that of *Llyfr Iorwerth*. Bardism ranked with clerkship and smithcraft as one of the three vocations which a villein might not follow, for this would mean the loss of his services to his lord.

Three arts which a bondman cannot teach his son without the consent of his lord: clerkship and smithcraft, and bardism; for if the lord be passive until the clerk be tonsured, or until the smith enter his smithy, or until a bard graduate, he can never enslave them after that.[40]

Thus, under certain circumstances a slave could become a bard, achieving freedom for his life tenure. There were no specific restrictions on the study of medicine.

The exact order of the officers given in the court sections of the laws was probably somewhat arbitrary, although the general position of the mediciner toward the bottom of the list must have been indicative of his status. Of the three professions, the Church, Law, and Medicine, there seems no doubt that Medicine was least regarded. In the Triads of *Llyfr Blegywryd,* however, the three are ranked with equal responsibility.

Three kinds of *sarhad* not to be compensated if received when intoxicated: *sarhad* done to the priest of the household, and to the judge of the court, and to the physician of the court, for it is not right that any of those three should ever be drunk, as they know not at what time the king may have need of them.[41]

They are grouped together again in the matter of privileged communication. "Three private conversations which the king is entitled to have without his judge: with his wife, with his priest, and with his physician."[17]

The judge, the priest and the mediciner were also free to communicate with the king when they wished.[42] They were also exempt from pledge.[43]

The mediciner was also granted a safe conduct when visiting the sick.

There are three persons who are free to travel the road, and out of the road: a priest, to visit the sick, along with his messenger; the second is, an apparitor, upon his lord's commission; the third is, a mediciner, along with the messenger of the sick.[44]

39 LHD, p. 41.
40 LHD, p. 102.
41 LHD, pp. 103-104.
42 AL, vol. 2, p. 605.
43 AL, vol. 2, p. 641.
44 AL, vol. 1, p. 781.

A messenger for the sick appeared to have the further liberty of commandeering a horse to summon either a priest or a mediciner for a patient in danger of his life.[45]

There is no evidence in the Laws of a professional standard required of the mediciner, rather the little evidence that exists refers to the apparently timeless problems of his ethical behaviour and his fees. The law officers did have a professional standard, for the judges were appointed after examination by the court judge,[20] and the priests were subject to the discipline of the Church. There is evidence, too, of bardic organisation. Bards were admitted to the order by the *pencerdd* after careful instruction and payment of a fee of twenty-four pence.[46] The *pencerdd,* the 'chief poet'—sometimes styled the 'chaired bard'—although senior to the *bardd teulu* or court bard, was not himself strictly an officer of the court.[39] That is, he did not rank amongst the twenty-four, but he was an officer of the court "by custom and usage."[47] Nor is there any evidence of an organisation into medical guilds if we ignore the ambiguous statement in the spurious "Triads of Dyvnwal Moelmud" translated by Aneurin Owen. Indeed, from the Laws the court mediciner emerged as rather a solitary figure, pre-occupied with casualty surgery and in common with casualty officers of a later age beset with a threat of litigation for his omissions in times of stress. Nevertheless he was regarded as a responsible officer in his grouping with the judge and the priest, and in a more homely light as the social equivalent of the bard. His duties extended beyond the personal attendance on the officers of the court to the care of the household, and the specific mention of the provision of free treatment for these would suggest that he was able to offer his services to the rest of the community for a fee. There is no mention of any assistants.[48]

The Laws relating to compensation for injury again indicated the striving of this society toward a belief in the basic equality of human beings. The pieces of the mediciner were worth the same as anyone else's, for the worth of the limbs of all persons

45 AL, vol. 2, p. 583.
46 LI, s. 40, p. 21.
47 LI, s. 30, p. 17.
48 Trease states that in the English royal court of the 13th century the spicer or apothecary had a multiplicity of duties and was as frequently referred to as the king's clerk, king's serjeant or under-usher as by his medical title. This officer was not strictly comparable with the Welsh royal mediciner and Trease doubts if the English office existed before the 13th century. I can find no evidence of a man with similar duties in the Welsh Laws.

There is a reference to the criminal use of poison—which was regarded as particularly heinous—and to "the making of poisons to destroy others" in *The Black Book of Chirk* (AL, vol. 2, p. 23).

was equal, whereas the worth of the whole person varied according to status. This implied recognition both of the equality of the physical worths of human beings, giving man a logical place in the natural scale, and of the variations that individuals were able to achieve by the attainment of office. The total value of all the fourteen members of the human body came to £88 or 264 kine and 5,280 pence. This was a higher price than that set on any one's life except that of a royal personage and, as Ellis also pointed out, it meant that a bondman's hand was worth more than his life. In these matters the Anglo-Saxon and the Germanic laws differed from those of the Welsh in varying the worth of a man's limbs with his status. Ellis conjectured that the Welsh attitude was possibly influenced by the Celtic Church.

Llyfr Iorwerth, Section 146, deals with the worth of limbs.

This relates to the nine co-ordinate members. Namely they are, the two hands and the two eyes and the two lips and the two feet and the nose. The worth of each of these separately is six kine and six score of silver. The worth of the ear, if cut off, two kine and two score of silver; if it closes so as to prevent hearing, six kine and six score of silver. The worth of the two testicles is equal in worth to the nine co-ordinate members. The worth of the tongue is equal to the worth of all these, because the tongue is their defence. The worth of a toe, a cow and one score of silver. The worth of a great toe, two kine and two score of silver. The worth of a finger, one cow and one score of silver. The worth of the thumb, two kine and two score of silver. The worth of the nail 30 (pence). The worth of the top joint of the finger, twenty-six (pence) and a halfpenny and a third of a halfpenny. The worth of the middle joint, thirty-three (pence) and two parts of a halfpenny. The worth of the lowest joint, four score (pence): and this is the worth of the finger. The worth of each of the teeth, one cow and one score of silver. The worth of each of the fang teeth, two kine and two score of silver, because they are the shepherd of the teeth. Equal to all these is the worth of the trunk itself. The trunk being namely, the head and the body and the penis, because the vital force can be in these: on that account that is equivalent to all these.

Perhaps the most surprising of the above values was the poor price of a thumb. Its value as a prehensile digit is certainly greater than that of two fingers and scarcely comparable with the value of a great toe. Professor H. A. Harris used to remark that the prehensile thumb was the feature which most distinguished man from the ape. A late 15th century MS (BM add. MS 22.356: BM Welsh MS 9) improved this somewhat "Whoever shall cut off the thumb by the hand, let there be paid half the worth of the hand."[49] That would make its worth three cows and three score of silver, i.e. two hundred and forty pence instead of the one hundred and sixty

49 AL, vol. 2, p. 425.

The Values of Limbs

Part of body lost	Value in *Book of Iorwerth*	Value in Ministry of Pensions and National Insurance Scale as proposed for 1965 *Officers Other ranks* *Below 20%*	
Fingers			
Index, whole	One cow & one score of silver, or 80 pence	£389 (14%)	£359
2 phalanges	60 pence	£310 (11%)	£285
1 phalanx	26⅔ pence	£259 (9%)	£239
Middle, whole		£339 (12%)	£314
2 phalanges		£259 (9%)	£239
1 phalanx	as for index finger	£209 (7%)	£194
Ring or little, whole		£209 (7%)	£194
2 phalanges		£181 (6%)	£166
1 phalanx		£161 (5%)	£151
Toes			
Great, whole	Two cows & two score of silver, or 160 pence	£389 (14%)	£359
One other toe	80 pence	£111 (3%)	£106
Two toes	160 pence	£161 (5%)	£151
Three toes	240 pence	£181 (6%)	£166
Four toes	320 pence	£259 (9%)	£239
Thumb	160 pence	*Above 20%*	
including 2 phalanges		30%	
including metacarpal		40%	
Hand	480 pence	60%	
Foot	480 pence	30%	
Lip or nose	480 pence		
Severe facial disfigurement		100%	
Total deafness	480 pence x 2	100%	
Ear (loss of)	160 pence	7%	
Eye	480 pence	40%	

Note: The figures from the *Book of Iorwerth* do not include *sarhad* or "honour price," which was always paid in addition to any specific worth of an injury and varied with the rank of the injured. If a limb was severed the price of the blood shed was also added.

The modern scale appears to perpetuate the old Anglo-Saxon law in varying the worth of a man's limbs directly with his status.

pence of the earlier MS. Sight and hearing were equally valued with locomotion. Although the loss of an ear and the loss of hearing were distinguished, no such comparison was made with the nose and smell.

Aled Rhys Wiliam has worked out the cost of a finger and demonstrated the inescapable logic of the lawmaker that the loss of the lowest joint meant the loss of the whole finger. The middle part was thus worth sixty pence being $33\frac{1}{3} + 26\frac{2}{3}$, that is, plus the worth of the fingertip. On the basis of units of $6\frac{2}{3}$d. the relative values of the three parts are in the ratio $4:5:12$.[50]

Llyfr Cyfnerth gives the worth of the middle joint of a finger as "fifty & a halfpenny & two parts of a halfpenny."[51]

Section 147 of *Llyfr Iorwerth* continues with the worth of injury and compensation.

Three losses of blood which cannot be made good; blood from the teeth, blood from the nose and blood from a scab. It is to the lord that *dirwy* is paid for them, and nothing is payable to whom they belong for it is lost blood;[52] nevertheless *sarhad* is to be paid to him. Three mortal wounds for a man: a blow on the head unto the brain, a blow on the body unto the bowels, and the breaking of one of the four limbs. For each of these three pounds is to be awarded to the person wounded by the person who wounds him. This is the amount of the payment for the treatment by the person who has wounded him, a pound without food or nine score (pence) with food and his bloody clothes.[53] A tent, twenty-four (pence). Treatment for a major blood vessel, 12 pence. Medicament of herbs, four pence. One penny to be paid for the food of the mediciner each night: one penny to be paid for his light nightly. There are three conspicuous scars: one on the face and the other on the hand and the third on the foot; 30 (pence) on the foot; 60 (pence) on the hand; 120 (pence) on the face. Every hidden scar 4 (pence). Cranium, four pence. Each broken bone, twenty (pence) unless there be a dispute about its smallness; and if there be a dispute, let the mediciner take a brass basin, place his elbow on the ground and his hand above the basin, and if its sound be heard, 4 pence; and if it not be heard nothing is to be paid.[54] The worth of hair plucked from the root, one penny for each finger used in the plucking and two for the thumb.

50 LI, p. 131.

51 WML, p. 190.

52 Aled Rhys Wiliam suggests that *guaet ellygedyc* should be translated 'blood liable to be lost' thus making the line in the second sentence "and nothing is payable to whom they belong for it is blood liable to be lost."

53 In Welsh Law if the mediciner was supplied with food, his fee was correspondingly diminished. In Irish Law if the patient was treated in his own home instead of being maintained and treated elsewhere at the expense of the injurer, he was supplied with "food and leech." This latter development of *othrus* was known as *tincisin*. (Binchy).

54 The somewhat obscure reference to a basin is clarified in *Llyfr Blegywryd.* "Four curt pennies are to be paid to a person for every bone taken from the upper part of the cranium which shall sound on falling into a copper basin. For every bone from the lower cranium he is to have four legal pence." (LHD, p. 64.)

The worth of blood from a freeman, twenty-four (pence). The worth of blood from a bondman, 6 (pence). The *sarhad* of each man is to be paid according to his privilege.

This passage indicated that the mediciner was required to help in the assessment of the severity of an injury such as a comminuted fracture of the skull, although his method of obtaining the fragment was not given. Another 15th century MS suggested that he was also required to give 'sick certificates' to excuse attendance at a court of law.

There are three persons, against whom, according to law, no one is to be received, or heard, preferring any plaints in an established session of law, as the pleas of the king; and the law as to contempt is not to affect them, in any matter or cause, on the day when they may be called. . . . The third is, one who is bed-ridden from any natural disorder, or a blow, or a bruise, or a wound: the testimony of a mediciner, or a confessor, is to be credited, in that case, swearing, that the sick person could not without peril come to abide the law.[55]

The assailant causing a nose-bleed did not escape scot free. He had to pay a fine to the lord and a *sarhad* for insult to the victim. The *sarhad* was always paid in addition to any specific worth of an injury. Even a hair had its value. *Llyfr Blegywryd* enlarges on blood losses. "Three bloods not amenable to the law are: blood from the head of a scab, and blood from the teeth, and blood from a nose, unless shed through anger."[56] In the Triads, bleeding is still further classified, depending on its extent. The first was from head to breast, the second from breast to girdle, and the third from girdle to ground; but if from head to ground it was known as "complete blood."[57] If a limb was severed, the price of the blood shed was also added (Ellis).

The value of limbs compares closely in the various redactions, and *Llyfr Blegywryd* explains the reason for the assessment of the cost of blood.

Twenty-four pence is the worth of the blood of every kind of person. Thirty pence was the worth of the blood of Christ, and it was seen to be unworthy that the blood of God and the blood of man be of equal value, and therefore the blood of man is of less worth.[58]

However, the worth of the blood of a foetus was more, according to *Llyfr Cyfnerth*. "The first is, blood before formation, if it perish through cruelty, of the value of forty-eight (pence)." This was presumably for a miscarriage before the twelfth week.

55 AL, vol. 2, p. 385.
56 LHD, p. 106.
57 LHD, pp. 109, 110.
58 LHD, pp. 63, 64.

"The second is, before life (*eneit*) enters into it, if it perish through cruelty, the third of its *galanas* is to be paid for it"— perhaps up to eighteen weeks of gestation, the time of foetal movements. "The third is after that life has entered into it" when the whole of its *galanas* was to be paid. But this last, of course, was entering the law relating to killing.[59]

After dealing with the worth of blood loss, *Llyfr Blegywryd* continues with the worth of teeth and scars.

The worth of a man's fore tooth is twenty-four pence, with three augmentations.[60] The worth of a person's back tooth is thirty pence. When the front tooth of a person is to be paid for, the worth of a conspicuous scar is to be paid with it. The worth of a conspicuous scar upon a person's face is six score pence; if it be upon his hand, three score pence. It is worth thirty pence, if it be upon the foot. The *sarhad* of a person, when a conspicuous scar is left upon his foot, is to be paid with one augmentation; if it be upon his hand, with two augmentations; if it be upon his face with three augmentations."[16]

Llyfr Cyfnerth gives the worth of a back tooth as fifty pence, and the worth of an eyelid "as long as the hair is on it," as one legal penny for every hair. "If a part be cut away from it, then the worth of a conspicuous scar is paid."[61] Conspicuous scars were obviously regarded as a disfigurement more than as a trophy even in those violent days, although many must have possessed them. The payment of thirty pence for a conspicuous scar on the foot suggests that the feet were uncovered and this is confirmed by Giraldus (Hoare). A hidden scar was worth only four pence.

There is a passage in Aneurin Owen's Dimetian Code which leaves one a little breathless.

The worth of a man's fore tooth is twenty-four pence, with three augmentations; and it is thus augmented; the first augmentation is eight pence; the second augmentation is ten pence halfpenny and the third of a halfpenny; the third is fourteen pence halfpenny and the third of a halfpenny and the ninth part of a halfpenny; which, when all reckoned together is fifty-six pence and a halfpenny and two parts of a halfpenny and the ninth part of a halfpenny.[62]

The severity of bruising was measured by its duration.[63]

59 WML, p. 272. Owen translates a section of Peniarth MS 32: "If the foetus of a pregnant woman be injured: while white, three score pence; when quick, let there be paid half the *galanas* of a male; if before quickening the third of the *galanas*." AL, vol. 2, p. 201.

60 The augmentations of *sarhad* were generally calculated in thirds. Thus a first augmentation was by the addition of a third to the basic figure, the second augmentation a third of the new total added to itself, and for the third augmentation a third of the last figure was added to itself. Thus a basic figure of 90 would become 120, then 160 and then 213⅓ (Ellis).

61 WML, p. 191.

62 AL, vol. 1, p. 505.

63 AL, vol. 1, p. 701. Also WML, pp. 62-3.

Unintentional wounding was excluded from a legal right to *sarhad*, but it was considered the right and proper thing to do "to compensate the blood, the wound and the conspicuous scar if there be such."[64]

Hairpulling was evidently sufficiently in vogue to justify again dealing with its consequences in *Llyfr Blegywryd*. Apart from the *sarhad* that the attack itself justified, there was to be paid "a penny for every finger that touches his head, and two pence for the thumb, and a penny for every hair pulled by the root from his head, and twenty-four pence for the hair cut at the ends."[16] *Llyfr Cyfnerth* also deals with it succinctly.

Whoever shall strike a person, let him pay his *sarhad* first, because attack and onset constitute a *sarhad* to every person; and a penny for every hair pulled out from his head by the root; and a penny for every finger which shall touch the head; and twenty-four pence for the front hair. Let every one choose his status, whether by the status of his chief of kindred or by the status of his father or by the status of his office.[65]

This must have given great possibilities for legal dispute, and as if to drive the matter home there is an illustration in the Latin MS Peniarth 28 of this somewhat feminine habit. It is in the section *De preciis humanorum membrorum* and it is reproduced and wrongly captioned "A twelfth century leech at work" in T. Lewis's *A Welsh Leech Book*. The text of the MS makes the action of the drawing clear. There are many illustrations of the court officers in Peniarth 28, but unfortunately none of the mediciner.

The importance of the Welsh Laws in a study of Mediaeval Wales is that it is reasonable to suppose—granting their origin in the 10th century—that their later compilation as lawyers' textbooks implied a continued application in later centuries. In support of this Sir John Lloyd has written:

It is no doubt the case that the Welsh Laws, as preserved for us in the MSS of the thirteenth and fourteenth centuries, can be profitably studied as a body of mediaeval usage, quite independently of their supposed origin in the tenth century, and without reference to the particular ruler whose name they bear.

About one hundred years after the Norman Conquest, in the second half of the 12th century, the old Anglo-Saxon Laws disappeared, as Maitland said, with "marvellous suddeness." The

---

[64] WML, p. 255. Unintentional killing did permit of a legal right to *galanas*. (AL, vol. 2, p. 383.)
[65] WML, pp. 193-4.

old Welsh Law continued in Welsh Wales and in the March in varying degree until the middle of the 16th century when it was finally displaced by English Law. And although the picture of the court that has been left may indeed be often no more than a conventional one, like Shakespeare's honey-bees, it showed that in the Wales of the Middle Ages there existed in the order of things, a mediciner of non-academic status who was partly paid by the state as embodied in the king and the royal court; partly paid by the patient, or his assailant, as shown in the permitted fees; giving medico-legal certificates and allowed certain privileges related to his office. It was a step of significance in the social history of medicine that there were legal arrangements to relieve the patient under certain circumstances of medical costs, and from this custom it is reasonable to suppose that there developed the system of direct financial reward for the mediciner's services. The Laws of Hywel Dda gave the patient a right to medical treatment and gave the mediciner the right to collect fees for it.

ACKNOWLEDGMENTS

I should like to express my indebtedness to Mr. R. J. Thomas of the National Library of Wales and his colleagues for their advice on etymology and to Professor Idris Foster of Jesus College, Oxford not only for his invaluable help in the translation of the passages from *Llyfr Iorwerth* but for his constructive advice after very kindly reading the original manuscript of this paper. Dr. H. D. Emanuel made valuable suggestions on the significance of the Court Sections of the Laws, and I should also like to thank Dr. E. G. Dryburgh for so courteously answering my questions on modern pension practice.

In the libraries, Mr. B. G. Owens, Keeper of MSS and Records, and Mr. David Jenkins, Keeper of the Printed Books, and their staffs at the National Library of Wales, Mr. A. L. Bamber with the resources of the Surrey County Library Service and Miss Sue Goldie of the Wellcome Historical Medical Library gave their unfailing support.

This paper was read at a meeting of the History of Medicine Section of the Royal Society of Medicine on 7 April 1965, and is published here by courtesy of the Honorary Editors of the *Proceedings of the Royal Society of Medicine*.

REFERENCES

Binchy, D. A. "Secular Institutions" in Dillon, Myles, Ed., *Early Irish Society*, Dublin, 1954, pp. 52-65; "Bretha Crólige" in *Ériu*, 1934, *12*, 1-77; "Sick-maintenance in Irish Law," *ibid.*, pp. 78-134; "Some Celtic Legal Terms" in *Celtica*, 1956, *3*, 221-231.

Dolley, R. H. "Coinage" in Poole, A. L., Ed. *Mediaeval England*, 2 vols., Oxford, 1958, vol. 1, p. 276 and plate 30, i, facing p. 271.

Edwards, G. "Studies in the Welsh Laws since 1928," in *The Welsh History Review*, 1963, Special Number The Welsh Laws, pp. 1-17.

Edwards, J. G. "The Laws of Hywel Dda" in Roderick, A. J., Ed., *Wales through the Ages*, 2 vols., Llandybie, Christopher Davies, 1959, pp. 68-71.

Ellis, T. P. *Welsh Tribal Law and Custom in the Middle Ages*, 2 vols., Oxford, 1926, vol. 1, pp. 158-173 & 355-372.

Hoare, R. C., Ed. & Tr. *The Itinerary of Archbishop Baldwin through Wales, 1688 by Giraldus de Barri*, 2 vols., London, 1806. Vol. 2, Description of Wales, book 1, chap. XVII, pp. 290 and 331-2.

Jones, G. R. J. "The tribal system in Wales; a re-assessment in the light of settlement studies." *Welsh History Review*, 1961, *1*, 111-132.

Lewis, T. *A Welsh Leech Book*, Liverpool, 1914. Plate I, opp. p. xvi.

Lloyd, J. E. *A History of Wales*, 2 vols., 3d ed., London, Longmans, 1939, pp. 285-6, 309-11, p. 314, fn. 55 on p. 335, p. 340, p. 356; *Aberystwyth Studies*, 1928, *10*, 1.

Owen, A. *The Ancient Laws and Institutes of Wales*, 2 vols., Record Commission, London, 1841. (Referred to as AL in footnotes.) Vol. 1, fn. b on p. 11.

Peate, I. *The Welsh House*, Liverpool, Brython Press, 1946, pp. 112-33.

Pughe, J., Tr. & Williams ab Ithel, J., Ed. *The Physicians of Myddvai*, Llandovery, 1861, s. 7, p. 2, & s. 162, p. 28.

Rees W. *An Historical Atlas of Wales*, Cardiff, Faber & Faber, 1959, p. 20.

Rees, W. *South Wales and the March 1284-1415. A Social and Agrarian Study*, Oxford, 1924, fn. 2 on p. 264.

Rhys. J. & Brynmor-Jones, D. *The Welsh People*, London, 1900, p. 149.

Richards, M. *The Laws of Hywel Dda* (The Book of Blegywryd), Liverpool, University Press, 1954. (Referred to in footnotes as LHD.)

Sayles, G. O. *The Mediaeval Foundations of England*, 2d ed., London, 1950, p. 177.

Shakespeare, W. *Henry V*, 1, ii, 187.

Tillyard, E. M. W. *The Elizabethan World Picture*, London, Peregrine Book, 1963, p. 38.

Trease, G. E. "The Spicers & Apothecaries of the Royal Household in the Reigns of Henry III, Edward I and Edward II." *Nottingham Mediaeval Studies*, 1959, *3*, 21-23.

Trevelyan, G. M. *History of England*, 1st ed., London, Longmans, 1928, fn. 1 on p. 83.

Wade-Evans, A. W. *Welsh Mediaeval Law*, Oxford, 1909. (Referred to in footnotes as WML.)

Wiliam, A. R., Ed., *Llyfr Iorwerth*, Cardiff, University of Wales Press, 1960. (Referred to in footnotes as LI.)

Williams, S. J. & Powell, J. E. *Llyfr Blegywryd*, Cardiff, Gwasg Prifysgol Cymru, 1942.

ABBREVIATIONS

LI; *Llyfr Iorwerth*, (Wiliam, A. R.)

WML; *Welsh Mediaeval Law*, (Wade-Evans, A. W.)

LHD; *Laws of Hywel Dda*, (Richards, M.)

AL; *Ancient Laws & Institutes of Wales*, (Owen, A.)

THE FACULTY OF MEDICINE AT PARIS, CHARLATANISM, AND UNLICENSED MEDICAL PRACTICES IN THE LATER MIDDLE AGES

PEARL KIBRE

The rôle of the medical faculty of the university of Paris [1] in matters affecting the health of residents of the city of Paris was an active and important one. Not only did the faculty respond to the requests for aid in the periodic outbreaks of pestilence and plague from 1348 onward, [2]

---

[1] Material for the present article, read in part before the New York Society for Medical History, and constituting part of a larger study now in progress on " The Rights, Privileges, and Immunities of Mediaeval Universities and University Scholars," was gathered during a year abroad under a Fellowship Grant from the John Simon Guggenheim Memorial Foundation for 1950-1951.

A list of the extended titles for those works frequently cited in abbreviated form in the notes will be found at the close of the article.

[2] In 1348 King Philip IV asked for aid from the university faculty of medicine: *Chart. univ. Paris.*, II, no. 1159, p. 623; A. M. Campbell, *The Black Death and Men of Learning*, New York, 1931, pp. 14-17; and cf. *ibid.*, p. 97. In the fifteenth century so many masters, because of the great multitude of the sick, were occupied with practice that they were unable to carry on their teaching: *Chart. univ. Paris.*, IV, pp. 351-352. See also *ibid.*, III, p. 107, no. 1284. In the year 1500 when the provost of the city of Paris asked the faculty's aid in combating the plague, the faculty requested in return the provost's assistance in combating illegal medical practice by charlatans and empirics: Wickersheimer, *Commentaires*, Paris, 1915, introduction, particularly, pp. lxxxviii-xci; also pp. 425 (1499-1500), and 448 (1500-1501).

but on its own initiative it undertook the less spectacular task of attempting to stamp out charlatanism and medical practice by empirics. It also endeavored, " in the public interest," to establish an effective surveillance over apothecaries, herbalists, and surgeons. To realize these aims, the faculty relied not only on the issuance of regulations and statutes but even more particularly upon the active prosecution, with the aid of the bishop's court, of those who engaged in illicit practices. The regulations and the records of the court proceedings in specific instances, in the fourteenth and fifteenth centuries, which have been utilized in the present study, reveal the steps taken to punish charlatans and empirics and the difficulties of enforcing the university regulations.[8]

The university's right to prosecute unlicensed persons who were practicing medicine was based, it asserted, upon a regulation issued at some earlier date by the bishop's court at Paris. The intent of this regulation which, in 1311 and 1322, was said to have been made some two hundred years before, was to prohibit from engaging in medical practice in Paris anyone who had not been examined and approved by the faculty. Both the authenticity and dating of such a statute appear doubtful since so far no text of such a pronouncement seems to have been found. There is also no apparent evidence that an organized faculty of medicine was functioning in Paris before 1200.[4] It is of course possible that the term " two hundred years " was a mere figure of speech to establish the hoary antiquity of the faculty's jurisdiction.

There were some precedents outside of Paris for the principles of examination and licensing of practicing physicians but no records of such regulations appear to be extant before the first quarter of the twelfth century. Such regulations would appear therefore to be a distinctly medieval phenomenon. No legal restrictions on practicing physicians prevailed in antiquity, despite the emphasis of the Hippocratic school of physicians upon adherence to a strict code of professional ethics. And although this code of ethics, preserved in the Hippocratic Oath, persisted into the middle

[8] The most interesting collection of materials for this purpose is that contained in the seventeenth century manuscript in the Paris Archives nationales: MM 226: " Extrait sommaire des divers procès de contestatione de la faculté de medecine depuis contra divers particulaires exercant illicitime la medicine. Pour l'utilité publique et d'histoire . . . ab anno 1311 ad annum 1395." Most of the materials in this collection have already been published in the *Chart. univ. Paris.*, which at II, xxi, reports on it.

[4] Medicine along with Civil Law was being taught at Paris between 1175 and 1190 and very probably earlier, but it is doubtful that the medical faculty was organized at that early period: *Chart. univ. Paris.*, I, pp. 55-56, no. 54.

54

ages,[5] there were no laws against medical practice by ignorant and untrained persons who might never have heard of the Hippocratic oath. Thus Pliny the Elder caustically remarked that there " is no law which punishes ignorance, no example of redress for this capital crime, that they (the physicians) learn by endangering our lives and carry on experiments by causing deaths, to such an extent that the greatest impunity is given to a physician for having killed a man." [6] Only in the fourth century of the Roman Empire do we encounter any legislation in this regard. But the laws made under Valentinian I and Valens providing for the examination of those preparing to practice medicine pertained only to the chief physicians, the *archiatri* or the physicians associated with the royal or imperial person. The Theodosian Code further added that after the prospective *archiatri* had submitted to an examination by a college or royal council of the chief physicians, they must have the emperor's consent before they could practice in the palace.[7] It was apparently to this royal council of chief physicians that Cassiodorus addressed his *Formula comitis archiatrorum,* in the early sixth century.[8]

But even such scanty legislation became a dead letter with the breakdown of Roman imperial authority in western Europe. From the sixth century onward, medical learning and skill, transmitted from antiquity together with the code of medical ethics embodied in the Hippocratic oath, were obliged with other classical learning to take refuge in monastic centers. There under ecclesiastical supervision medical study and practice were at first encouraged and cultivated probably for purely practical reasons and in accordance with the clear admonitions of the " Book of Ecclesiasticus " [9] that the physician and medicine are to be honored because they are created by God. Cassiodorus in his monastic retreat at Vivarium urged the monks to become acquainted with the medical works that he had collected for their use; [10] and Rabanus Maurus two centuries later, in both

---

[5] In this regard see especially L. C. MacKinney, " Medical Ethics and Etiquette in the Early Middle Ages: the persistence of Hippocratic Ideals," *Bulletin of the History of Medicine,* 1952, vol. 26, 1 *et seq.,* and the references there cited.

[6] Pliny, Nat. Hist., lib. XXIX, cap. 8 (*Bibl. classica latina,* 1829, vol. 79: viii, p. 198).

[7] See H. Conring, *De antiquit.,* pp. 57-59, 259-261, citing " Const. Valentiniani et Valentis "; and *The Theodosian Code and Novels and the Sirmondian Constitutions, a translation with Commentary, Glossary, and Bibliography,* by C. Pharr, Princeton University Press, 1952, p. 388.

[8] Variarum, liber VI, paragraph xix (Migne, vol. 69, cols. 700-701).

[9] Liber Ecclesiasticus, 38, 1-11 (*Biblia Sacra Vulgatae Editionis Sixti V Pont. Max.,* 1922, p. 655) : " Honora medicum propter necessitatem: etenim illum creavit Altissimus . . . Altissimus creavit de terra medicamenta. et vir prudens non abhorrebit illa."

[10] De inst. divin. lett., cap. 31 (Migne, vol. 70, cols. 1146-47).

his encyclopedic " De universo " and in his " Commentary on the Book of Ecclesiasticus," urged that out of necessity medicine should be cultivated and honored rather than spurned.[11]

By the twelfth century, however, the increasing tendency of members of monastic orders to engage· in medical practice to the neglect of their religious duties was cause for alarm and regulation by the ecclesiastical authorities. Prohibitions of such practice, at first directed only to monks who practiced medicine for gain, were later extended to any or all medical practice or study outside the monasteries by members of the orders.[12] In the thirteenth century Pope Honorius III renewed the prohibitions and extended them to all clerics regular or secular.[13] But by the middle of the fourteenth century such restrictions were being set aside by papal dispensations, and clerics, regular or secular, were given permission to study, to lecture, and to practice medicine at Paris or elsewhere in accordance with the university regulations.[14]

Direct regulation of those who wished to teach medicine and to practice among the populace first appeared in southern Italy where the school of Salerno was already a flourishing medical school in the eleventh century. Legislation relating to the examining and licensing of prospective physicians is extant, however, only from the twelfth century.[15] On the other

[11] De universo, liber XVIII, cap. 5 (Migne, vol. 111, col. 501) : " Medicinae curatio spernanda non est quia et sanctos viros ea uti legimus . . . Eccl. Honora medicina propter necessitatem." Comm. in Ecclesiasticum, liber VIII, cap. 13, De medico honorando (Migne, vol. 109, col. 1030).

[12] This was done at the councils of Reims in 1131 and at the Lateran council in 1139: E. Lesne, *Histoire*, pp. 679, 688. For the prohibitions of 1163 and 1179 (1180), see *Chart. univ. Paris.*, I, pp. 3 (no. 1) ; 78, note.

[13] For the prohibitions of Pope Honorius III in 1213 and 1219, see *Chart. univ. Paris.*, I, pp. 77-78; 90-93; and for those of 1227-1268, see *ibid.*, I, pp. 478-479.

[14] On January 9, 1364, clerics were permitted to enter the faculty of medicine and to be given a license; and on November 1, 1380, pope Clement VII granted to Guibertus de Celceto, a canon of the church of S. Germain and master of medicine, the right to lecture on and to practice medicine at Paris. A similar dispensation was given to Guibertus de " Saliceto," physician of Charles V, on September 25, 1377, by Gregory XI : *Chart. univ. Paris.*, III, pp. 109-110; 292, no. 1452; 331, 339, no. 1501; Arch. Nat. MM 266, p. 166. See also *Chart. univ. Paris.*, IV, pp. 55, 138, 197, 209, 578, 604, for such dispensations in the fifteenth century; Wickersheimer, *Commentaires*, introduction, pp. xlv-xlvii.

[15] For Salerno and Naples, see H. Conring, *De antiquit.*, pp. 60-61, 104, 106-107; H. Rashdall, *The Universities of Europe in the Middle Ages* (new ed. by F. M. Powicke and A. B. Emden, 3 vols.), Oxford, 1936, I, 76 *et seq.*; 83-85; also F. R. Packard, *History of the School of Salernum*, New York, 1920, pp. 34-36. The English translation of the ordinances was published by E. F. Hartung, " Medical Regulations of Frederick the Second of Hohenstaufen," in *Medical Life*, 1934, vol. 41, pp. 587-601.

hand ecclesiastical supervision of those who wished to teach medicine in the university is revealed at Montpellier in 1220, when Cardinal Conrad, the papal legate, made a ruling in this regard. He stated that although the science of medicine had flourished for a long time at Montpellier, henceforth no one ought to be free to teach medicine publicly there unless he received the license to teach (licentia docendi) from the bishop of Maguelone after he had been examined and recognized as qualified.[16] Earlier, in January, 1181, Guilhem VII, lord of Montpellier, had declared that the teaching of medicine in the schools of Montpellier should be free from outside interference.[17]

Although many of the provisions enacted by the medical faculty at Paris, for the examination and licensing of prospective physicians, resembled the imperial legislation at Salerno and Naples, the action of the faculty of the northern university provides a distinct contrast to the other centers. For unlike either Salerno or Montpellier, the initiative for the active prosecution of those practicing without a license came not from the imperial, ecclesiastical, or royal authorities but from the university medical faculty itself. In 1271 and 1272, the faculty at Paris took occasion to define more clearly the requirements for obtaining the license which was conferred by the chancellor of the Cathedral of Notre Dame.[18] At the same time the faculty proceeded to legislate against persons who were practicing illegally without a license and without the approval of the faculty, or more explicitly against those who " by shameful and brazen usurpation," assumed the office of medical practitioner at Paris. The members of the faculty denounced those empirics, who, without the approval and counsel of the more learned members of the profession, were administering to all comers medicines which they had concocted out of their own heads. They were declared by their treatment of the sick, based only on the whims of chance and fortune, to be guilty of criminally handing over many to suffering and even to death. The faculty pointed out that by practicing without authorization such persons were imperilling the safety of their own souls and were daily incurring the penalty of the ban of excommunication which would be launched by the official of the bishop of

[16] *Cartulaire de l'université de Montpellier* (2 vols.), *Montpellier*, 1890, I, pp. 180-183.
[17] *Ibid.*, pp. 179-180. See also E. Nicaise, introduction to his edition of *La Grande Chirurgie de Guy de Chauliac*, Paris, 1890, pp. li *et seq*.
[18] *Chart. univ. Paris.*, I, p. 517, no. 453; English translation by L. Thorndike, *University Records*, pp. 81-82. For other documents on license requirements, see *Chart. univ. Paris.*, I, nos. 444, 451-456; II, nos. 921, 996; IV, no. 2659. See also Wickersheimer, *Commentaires*, introduction, pp. xi-xvii, xviii *et seq*.

Paris against them. By their practices these empirics were said to constitute a distinct threat to the welfare of the residents of Paris as well as a serious discredit to the good name and repute of the more learned members of the medical profession. The faculty went on further to assert that it had been urged to take action to correct the existing critical situation by clergy and laymen alike. To prevent the continuation or perpetuation of such errors, perils, and resulting scandals, the faculty drew up, therefore, the regulations which were, it insisted, in confirmation of a statute made long ago, a statute which was said to be supported by letters of the official of the bishop of Paris, by royal authority, and the oaths taken by the individual members of the faculty of medicine.[19]

The regulations of 1271 were directed particularly against " certain manual operators," who made or possessed various medicaments which they administered without knowing the relation which these medicines had to diseases. Under every penalty allowed by civil and canon law for noncompliance with the law it was provided that no surgeon, male or female, no apothecary nor herbalist, was to exceed or overstep the limits or bounds of his craft, either secretly or publicly. The surgeon was to engage only in manual practice, the apothecary and herbalist were only to mix drugs which were to be administered exclusively by masters in medicine or under their express license. No one of the aforementioned was to visit any sick person nor " to administer to him any alterative medicine or laxative or anything else " that pertained to a physician, nor was he to advise that it be administered except by a master in medicine. Surgeons, apothecaries, and herbalists, were to be bound by oath to obey these provisions. Furthermore, bachelors in medicine,[20] that is those who had been permitted to lecture but were not yet licensed as masters in the medical faculty, under penalty of having their promotions withheld, were strictly forbidden to visit patients or to administer to them any drugs unless they were accompanied by or were in the presence of a master of the medical faculty. Information regarding anyone acting contrary to this statute was to be revealed secretly and under oath to the dean or to some teaching master in the medical faculty. The one to whom such information was given was to be obliged to shield the informer.[21]

[19] *Chart. univ. Paris.*, I, p. 488-490, no. 434. The document is translated into English by L. Thorndike, *University Records*, pp. 83-85.

[20] For the use of the term " baccalarius," or " bachelarius," in medicine, see Wickersheimer, *Commentaires*, introduction, p. xviii and note.

[21] *Chart. univ. Paris.*, I, pp. 489-490; Thorndike, *op. cit.*, pp. 84-85; Wickersheimer, *op. cit.*, introduction, pp. lxxii *et seq.*

Thus armed with laws of its own making, the faculty through its dean undertook the more difficult task of securing their enforcement. In 1311, a charlatan or empiric against whom the dean of the faculty brought charges of illegal practice demanded to know by what right the faculty dared to trouble him in his medical practice. To this demand the faculty made the reply noted above that their authority dated back to a statute of the official of the bishop of Paris made two hundred years earlier. By this statute, it was asserted, the right to practice medicine in Paris was denied to anyone who was not a master or who had not been licensed in the faculty of medicine.[22] The case, in 1312, of Clarice de Rothomago, wife of a certain Peter Faverel, revealed the steps taken against unlicensed persons. In this case, which ran from January 17 to June 15, 1312, Clarice was accused of practicing medicine illegally in Paris and was arrested at the instance of the dean of the faculty of medicine. She was then put under ban of excommunication by the official of the bishop's court at Paris. From this penalty she appealed to the official of the bishop of Senlis, the so-called conservator of the apostolic privileges of the university.[23] Her appeal was, however, of no avail since the dean of the medical faculty was able to obtain from the bishop of Senlis a reaffirmation of the sentence of excommunication against Clarice and against her husband as well. They were both to be denounced in all the churches and anyone who associated with them was to be subject to the same penalty.[24]

The effectiveness of this ban of excommunication and oral denunciation, applied against Clarice and her husband, as a means of frightening off other unlicensed persons from medical practice, appears to have been slight. Numerous cases of illegal practice continued to come to the

[22] Pajon de Moncets, *De l'origine des appariteurs des universités et de leurs masses*, Paris, 1782, pp. 122-123. Wickersheimer, *op. cit.*, pp. lxxii-lxxiii, indicates that it was probably toward 1220 that the faculty of medicine obtained from the diocesan official a sentence reserving the right to practice medicine at Paris and in the faubourgs to those who had obtained the master's degree in medicine with the approval of the chancellor of the university.

[23] The conservator of apostolic privileges of the university had the general power of protecting the university in its enjoyment of the privileges granted to it, and to secure respect for these privileges by punishing those who infringed upon them by ecclesiastical censure: Rashdall, *The Universities of Europe in the Middle Ages*, 1936. I, 342-343; 417-419.

[24] Paris, Arch. Nat. MM 266, pp. 3-13; *Chart. univ. Paris.*, II, pp. 149-153, nos. 693, 693a-c. The husband of Clarice, Petrus Faverel, was excommunicated as "empeiricus" on June 13; *ibid.*, pp. 150-151. He had sent no witnesses and had failed to appear himself after the appeal. He was therefore judged contumacious and the costs of the case were adjudged against him. The sentence against Clarice was issued on June 14, 1312; *ibid.*, pp. 151-152.

attention of the faculty. One of the most interesting of these was the case of Jacqueline Félicie de Almania. Her involvement began with her citation on August 11, 1322, for illegal practice, before the official of the bishop of Paris by the proctor of the dean of the medical faculty. She was duly excommunicated and, like Clarice, appealed against this sentence.[25] In the course of her trial, the proceedings of which continued for several months, a great many witnesses were called to testify on each side. Among the witnesses for the prosecution, on the side of the faculty, was the military knight and surgeon, John of Padua, who had been, as early as 1301, surgeon to the king of France, Philip IV.[26] John asserted that the penalities of prohibition and excommunication had been in operation for more than sixty years against ignorant and illicit empirics practicing in Paris and its environs. These penalties had been applied with the full approval of the venerable official of the bishop's court at Paris as well as with that of the illustrious kings of France. Yet contrary to these well known facts the defendant in question had persisted in acting as a physician although she was totally ignorant of the art of medicine. She was not lettered, nor had she been approved as competent in those things which she presumed to treat.

Furthermore, John pointed out, as it was forbidden by law that a woman practice law or be a witness in a criminal case,[27] so it was of far greater moment that she be likewise barred from the practice of medicine. Such practice required her to prescribe for patients foods and drinks for internal consumption and to apply clysters when in truth she knew neither the causes of the diseases from which they were suffering nor understood the letter or art of medicine. How much more serious therefore, John argued, was the danger that she might thus kill a man by these potions and clysters than that she might lose a civil suit through ignorance of the law. For through lack of knowledge in the former she might commit murder, and such a death would be a mortal sin over which the church would have jurisdiction. Hence in John of Padua's opinion the admonition

[25] *Chart. univ. Paris.*, II, pp. 255-256, no. 811; Arch. Nat., MM 266, pp. 13, 22, 23. Of this case Wickersheimer, *Commentaires*, introduction, p. lxxv, states: " C'est dans les pièces du procès intenté en 1322 à Jacqueline Félicie que nous trouvons les détails les plus intéressants pour l'histoire du charlatanisme à Paris au moyen âge."

[26] For John of Padua, see *Chart. univ. Paris.*, II, p. 256, note 1; also *ibid.*, II, no. 812, note; and Wickersheimer, *Dictionnaire*, II, 459.

[27] For the prohibition against the admission of women to the corporation of barristers or lawyers, see Paul Fournier, *Les Officialités, au moyen âge. Etude sur l'organisation, la compétence et la procédure des tribunaux ecclésiastiques ordinaires en France, de 1180 à 1328*, Paris, 1880, pp. 32-33; and for the prohibition against their appearing in civil courts as accusers, *ibid.*, p. 238.

and decree of excommunication launched by the official of the episcopal court at Paris should be binding.[28]

Equally emphatic were the arguments put forth by the defending counsel. He pointed out that Jacqueline Félicie had treated and cured many sick persons; that she had brought them comfort when other physicians had failed to do so; and that she had visited and cared for her patients assiduously until they were cured. This was corroborated by several witnesses who were brought to give testimony in Jacqueline's behalf. To each of these witnesses in turn the court put the questions of how they had learned about Jacqueline; whether she had acted as if she were a qualified physician; whether she had attempted to extort money from them; and finally, whether they knew that she had not been approved in any *studium generale*,[29] at Paris or elsewhere, or if they had seen her at Montpellier. In each instance the replies were similar. They had learned of her through a friend; she had proceeded as did most physicians in examining a patient; she had consistently refused to take any money until the patient had been cured; and they had not inquired into the matter of her qualifications. Among the witnesses for the defense was John of St. Omer. He testified that he had been cured of an illness by Jacqueline who had visited him several times and had done more for him than had any of the other physicians who were called in during his illness. She had given him a drink of some kind of clear liquid, which she or some one else had first sampled. Matilda, the wife of John of St. Omer, also attested the cure and added further that Jacqueline had applied poultices to John's chest.[30] Another witness, John Faber, asserted that Jacqueline had cured him by administering certain potions, one of them green in color, the other clear and colorless, but of what they were made, he did not know.[31]

An even more telling witness was a woman named Yvo Tueleu, a servant at the bishop's court in Paris. She related that she had been ill of a fever for which she had been visited by several physicians, none of whom had been able to cure her. Then at her request Jacqueline had come to her bedside, had given her a glass of the very clear liquid which had acted as a purge, and had successfully cured her of the fever.[32] Various other

[28] *Chart. univ. Paris.*, II, p. 256, no. 812; Arch. Nat. MM 266, p. 14.
[29] The usual term for the place in which the university associations were established; for its use see especially, Rashdall, *The Medieval Universities*, 1936, I, pp. 6-8.
[30] *Chart. univ. Paris.*, II, pp. 257-262; 261-262; Arch. Nat. MM 266, pp. 17-21.
[31] *Chart. univ. Paris.*, II, p. 259.
[32] *Ibid.*, II, p. 262.

persons who had been treated by the defendant testified to her ability and skill. One of them, Dominus Odo de Cornessiaco, a friar of the Hotel Dieu at Paris, stated that he too in his illness had been visited by several prominent physicians including John de Turre,[33] and the physicians Martin, Herman, and others. But none of them had been able to cure him. Then Jacqueline had come and had brought him back to health. Her course of treatments had included steam baths, massages with oil, and applications of herbs including leaves of camomile, melilot, and others. He stated that she had worked incessantly until he was entirely cured. Another former and grateful patient, Johanna, the wife of a certain Dionysius, stated that she too had been ill of a fever for which she had been visited by several physicians, including a certain Friar de Cordelis, the masters Herman, Manfred, and several others. All of them had given her up for certain death. Then Jacqueline had come and saved her. And still a further former patient, Johanna de Monciaco, a storekeeper or haberdasher, testified that she had been ill of an affliction of the kidneys, and that she had been for eleven days at St. Sulpice where she too was visited by the physicians, Guilbert, Herman, Manfred, and Thomas, none of whom had been able to help her. Then Jacqueline had succeeded in doing so by administering a glass of the clear liquid mentioned earlier.[34]

Also pointed out, in Jacqueline's defense, was the fact that there were many persons, practicing daily in Paris, who had not been approved in any university either at Paris or elsewhere and these persons similarly were without licenses either from the chancellor, the bishop of Paris, or from the said dean and masters of the medical faculty.[35] The defense then went on to attack the legality of the university statute.[36] This law, it was claimed, which had been invoked by the medical faculty had no legal validity, since it had never been approved by those whom it affected.

[33] *Ibid.*, II, pp. 259-260. Jean de Turre is probably to be identified with the son of the physician of Montpellier, Jourdain de Turre, who is noted by Wickersheimer as dedicating two of his works to his son in 1318: Wickersheimer, *Dictionnaire*, II, 497, 513-514.

[34] *Chart. univ. Paris.*, II, pp. 260-262; Arch. Nat. MM 266, pp. 18-19. Of the physicians named, Martin, Herman (Lombardus), Manfred, and Thomas (of Saint Georges), were all masters in the faculty of medicine, between 1310 and 1332: *Chart. univ. Paris.*, II, pp. 141, 350; 262, note 15; p. 394, note; Wickersheimer, *Dictionnaire*, II, 535, 766.

The various uses of the herbs camomile, or "camomilla" and melilot or "mellilotum" are noted in *The Herbal of Rufinus*, edited by L. Thorndike, Chicago University Press, 1945, pp. 71-72, 185-186.

[35] *Chart. univ. Paris.*, II, pp. 257-262, no. 813; Arch. Nat. MM 266, pp. 17-21. For the list of several other empirics condemned along with Jacqueline, see below.

[36] *Chart. univ. Paris.*, II, pp. 263-265, no. 814; Arch. Nat. MM 266, pp. 23-26, November 2, 1322.

62

It was merely an admonition by mandate of the venerable official of the bishop of Paris, an admonition, however, which was directed against ignorant, foolish, and unskilled persons merely simulating the medical art, yet totally ignorant of its precepts. Surely, it was argued, Jacqueline, an expert in the art of medicine and one who was well instructed in the precepts of medicine, could not be said to belong to this group. Moreover, if the university claimed that it was acting according to the law made some two hundred years earlier, the defense would direct attention to an even earlier law that states, " what touches all ought to be aproved by all." [37] Yet in this statute by which the faculty claimed to be proceeding, it does not appear that there was a summons of the masters, doctors, bachelors, and scholars of each faculty of the university then living at Paris, nor was there a summons of the bishop, archdeacon, dukes, barons, citizens, and burghers of Paris, whom such a decree also concerns and interests. Certainly none of these are named in the statute. In sum therefore, the defense argued, since those for whom the statute presumably was made had not been called, it was not valid, in their absence, and consequently it could not be binding on Jacqueline or on any other person.[38]

As a final argument, the defense counsel declared, it was better and more fitting that a wise and sagacious woman, experienced in the art of medicine should visit another woman, to examine her and to inquire into the hidden secrets of her being, than that a man should do this. For a man is not permitted to do these things, that is to inquire into her innermost secrets and to touch the various parts of her body. Indeed a man ought ever to avoid and shun the secrets of women and fly from their intimate association as much as he can. Besides, the defense counsel continued, it was often true that a woman would rather die than reveal the secrets of her infirmity to a man out of a sense of modesty and even of shame. For this reason many women have died in their illnesses since they were unwilling to have a physician who might learn their innermost secrets. In the case of Jacqueline, the court was reminded, members of both sexes had confided in her and she had been able to cure those whom other doctors could not. In conclusion the defense counsel asserted, the decree or statute invoked by the faculty of medicine could not be binding since it had been shown to be contrary to the public good.[39]

[37] For the use of this famous maxim, from the Roman Civil Code of Justinian, in the thirteenth and fourteenth centuries, see P. Kibre, *The Nations in the Mediaeval Universities* (The Mediaeval Academy of America), Cambridge, 1948, p. 39, note 64.

[38] *Chart. univ. Paris.*, II, pp. 263-265, no. 814; Arch. Nat. MM 266, p. 24.

[39] *Chart. univ. Paris.*, II, pp. 263-265, no. 814; Arch. Nat. MM 266, pp. 24-26.

Most of the above arguments the university members characterized as trifling. They answered the objection to the statute on the basis of its conflict with the earlier law, that what touches all ought to be approved by all, with the assertion that the statute in question was not made by the cathedral chapter of Paris, that it was not such a statute as would require that the persons named by the defense be called. The present dictum, the university insisted, provided a sufficient basis for the official of the bishop of Paris, the minister and executor of the law, to act upon. He could discern by this statute that such a person as the defendant was not qualified to practice the medical art. The final verdict against Jacqueline Félicie, issued on November 2, 1322, found her and several others named at the same time, guilty of willful disobedience. She and the others were prohibited by a solemn reiteration of the original sentence of excommunication from practicing medicine or from exercising the functions of a physician under the further penalty of a fine of sixty Parisian pounds.[40]

Despite the specific character of this condemnation, it is quite apparent that illegal practice by charlatans and empirics continued. In the search for a remedy the medical faculty turned to the pope for aid and humbly beseeched him to take some action. On June 21, 1325, Pope John XXII wrote to Stephen, bishop of Paris, to urge his cooperation in preventing those ignorant of the art of medicine from practicing in Paris or its suburbs. The pope stated that he had been informed in a petition drawn up by the masters and scholars of the university that persons ignorant of the medical art, old women particularly, and even more to be detested, soothsayers, as well as others, were presuming to practice medicine in the city and environs of Paris, and that these charlatans were causing many deaths. In complying with the university's petition, the pope further asked the bishop of Paris to make careful inquiries into the reports, and, if necessary, to endeavor to find out the truth by calling a council of men learned in medicine whose advice he should then follow.[44]

Whether from inaction of the bishop of Paris or because the bishop's efforts had no greater success in securing an elimination of illegal practice

[40] *Chart. univ. Paris.*, II, p. 267, no. 816; Arch. Nat. MM 266, p. 23. The list of other persons condemned at the same time as Jacqueline for practicing illegal medicine included several women: Domina Jacoba, Johanna Conversa, wife of John Liblous who was also condemned for illegal practice of medicine (cf. Wickersheimer, *Dictionnaire*, II, 505; *Chart. univ. Paris.*, II, pp. 256, 267); also Margarita de Ypra, surgeon, and Belota Judea. Others included were Stephanus Burgundus or Etienne Burgondus, empiric, and Master Jacob Lépelé.

[41] *Chart. univ. Paris.*, II, pp. 285-286, no. 844.

than the earlier efforts of the university itself, Pope John XXII again found it necessary, some five years later, on January 1, 1330, to address the new bishop of Paris, Hugh, on the subject of those illegally practicing medicine in the city and suburbs. His information regarding the presence of several such persons in the city had once again come from the university. He urged the bishop to make every effort to see that henceforth no one was permitted to practice medicine in the city or suburbs of Paris unless he was a master or was licensed in the art, or was otherwise known to be qualified by having been approved by a council consisting of the dean of the medical faculty and two of the masters then lecturing on medicine in the university. Those who should disobey this dictum must, he said, be subjected to ecclesiastical censure.[42]

Between 1330 and 1332 the medical faculty was involved in a dispute with the chancellor over the granting of licenses. In the course of the quarrel the faculty sought for and obtained the support of the pope, of the king, and also of the provost of Paris. The final settlement reaffirmed the faculty's right to determine the qualifications necessary for the licensing of candidates for medical teaching and practice. The chancellor would henceforth be obliged to confer the license on anyone whom the faculty declared worthy and qualified.[43]

Throughout the fourteenth century papal support for the faculty's supervision of medical practice continued. Clement VI, in 1340, threatened with excommunication not only those who should attempt to practice in Paris without the approval of the medical faculty but also those who should utilize the services of such physicians. Nevertheless illegal practice continued.[44] In 1347 (January 27), the dean and the faculty of medicine were obliged to petition the pope further for aid against those who were practicing illegally. Their petition again reported that there were at Paris men and women audaciously usurping the office of physician and engaging in the practice of medicine about which they knew little or nothing. To remedy this situation it was urged that the pope ask the bishop of Senlis, the conservator of the university's apostolic privileges, to use his authority to forbid anyone to practice medicine unless he was a master of the art or science of medicine or had at least been licensed in

[42] *Ibid.*, II, pp. 336-337, no. 900; and cf. no. 844 for a similar letter. In Arch. Nat. MM 266, p. 160, 'ad an. c. 1331,' are noted several illicit practitioners at Paris (*Chart. univ. Paris.*, II, p. 337, note).

[43] *Ibid.*, II, nos. 918-943, for the entire conflict. For the instrument of composition of the difficulties, see *ibid.*, II, pp. 397-399, no. 943.

[44] BN fonds franç. 22110, fol. 387r.

another university. He was also to announce to all transgressors that they would be punished by ecclesiastical censure.[45] Three years later, on April 2, 1350 (1351), the faculty was still trying through one of its representatives, Adam of Francovilla, at the papal court to obtain articles with the pope's signature against illegal practice.[46] Restrictions on student doctors were also tightened on February 3, 1375, by the measure requiring all bachelors in medicine or those not yet licensed to take an oath that they would not practice medicine nor visit the sick, unless they were accompanied by one of the masters in the faculty.[47]

The university made further efforts too to subject the apothecaries to specific regulation. In addition to the provisions relating to the dispensing of medicines contained in the statutes of 1271, the medical faculty had, on February 28, 1322, drawn up new articles, " in the public interest," which required that all apothecaries and dealers in drugs appear each year before the assembled faculty to take the oath that they were doing everything in their power to carry on effectively their work as apothecaries and herbalists. They must also swear that they were keeping on hand for easy reference a corrected copy of the *Antidotarium* of Nicholas of Salerno ;[48] that they were using true and accurate weights tested according to those used at the fairs; that they would not use for filling prescriptions any medicines that had been corrupted; and that if they could not obtain the simples called for in their recipes they would use no other substitutes than those provided for in the *Quid pro quo*.[49]

The ordinances provided also that the dean of the medical faculty and one apothecary chosen by the faculty would make periodic visits to the apothecary shops to look over the stocks of medicines. The apothecaries were prohibited from dispensing any medicinal laxatives or opiates which

[45] *Chart. univ. Paris.*, II, pp. 602-603, no. 1138.

[46] To defray the expenses incurred by Adam of Francovilla, the faculty was obliged to levy a tax on all its members: *Chart. univ. Paris.*, III, pp. 7-8, no. 1197; Arch. Nat. MM 266, p. 161.

[47] *Chart. univ. Paris.*, III, pp. 217-218, no. 1396.

[48] *Ibid.*, II, pp. 268-269, no. 817, and note. For Nicholas' Antidotarium, see also *ibid.*, I, p. 517, note 4. Nicholas probably flourished at Salerno in the twelfth century and is unknown except as author of the Antidotarium. See further for the work G. Sarton, *Introduction to the History of Science* (3 vols., Baltimore, 1927-48), II, 239-240.

[49] The Quid pro Quo (*Chart. univ. Paris.*, II, p. 569, note 6), which frequently appears with the Antidotarium of Nicholas, is probably by him. It gives an alphabetical list of medicinal simples or drugs with their substitutes. In the oath taken in 1422 by the apothecaries, they had to swear that they would not substitute one drug for another in the prescriptions except by the permission of the master who had given the original prescription; see below, note 51.

they had not first shown to the dean and the aforementioned apothecary, and had indicated the use to which they were to be put. They were further prohibited from selling or dispensing any laxative medicines, aborticides, poisons, or any other dangerous drugs, to any person without the advice of a physician who had been officially approved in the university of Paris, or in some other recognized university. Anyone who wished to become an apothecary must first read and swear to obey these regulations.[50]

The faculty ordinances relating to dispensers of drugs were later strengthened by royal mandate. On May 22, 1336, King Philip VI of France addressed the provost of Paris and his lieutenant to the effect that they must enforce the law requiring apothecaries to take the oath to obey the ordinances of the medical faculty. The apothecaries were also to be required to swear that they would take care to see that their subordinates and the herbalists took the same oath to uphold and observe the ordinances. The provost was asked to make certain that the regulation requiring the showing of the medicinal laxatives and opiates to the masters of the faculty of medicine were enforced, and that care was taken to ensure that the medicines were fresh and good and that they had not been permitted to become spoiled or soiled.[51]

Despite the foregoing measures, King John of France, in December of 1352, asserted that according to information received from the dean and masters of the faculty of medicine there were many unauthorized persons of both sexes dispensing drugs and medicines freely in Paris. Included in their number were old women, monks, rustics, apothecaries, and numerous herbalists, also students of the medical faculty not yet licensed,

[50] *Chart. univ. Paris.*, II, pp. 268-269, no. 817. For statutes of the corporation of herbalists (épiciers) at Paris, see *Les métiers et corporations de Paris*, ed. by Lespinasse, Paris, 1886, pp. 500, 503; *Chart. univ. Paris.*, II, 269, note 2.

[51] *Ibid.*, II, 269, note 2; p. 462, no. 1001; *Ordonn. des Rois*, II, p. 116. The mandate of Philip VI referred directly to the university statute of Febr. 1322; similarly King John's ordinance regarding the apothecaries in 1353, also agrees in large part with the faculty provisions of 1322: *Ordonn. des Rois*, II, 532. The earlier ordinances were also confirmed by Charles VI in 1390 (Aug. 3); and by Charles VII, on November 30, 1437: *Chart. univ. Paris.*, III, p. 534, no. 1586; IV, 601-602, no. 2515. See also the "Oaths required of Apothecaries at Paris," October 2, 1422, by the faculty of medicine: *Chart. univ. Paris.*, IV, pp. 406-407, no. 2196; translated by L. Thorndike, *University Records*, pp. 298-299. At this time (1422) the apothecaries were required to swear that they had on hand a corrected copy of the Synonyms (of Simon a Cordo of Genoa, physician to Pope Nicholas IV (d. 1292), and chaplain to Pope Boniface VIII (d. 1303): G. Sarton, *Introd.*, II, p. 1085), and of the Circa instans of Platearius, a pharmaceutical work, probably of the late twelfth century. See further Wickersheimer, *Commentaires*. Introduction.

The oldest statute regarding apothecaries at Montpellier, appears to date from the year 1340: *Cartulaire de l'université de Montpellier*, I, p. 344, no. 12.

or coming from other localities to practice in Paris. Such persons, although they were ignorant of the science of medicine, were unacquainted with the complexions and constitutions of men, and lacked knowledge of the virtues of medicines as well as of the time and method for administering them, were nevertheless administering them freely. The king found this a highly offensive proceeding, as well as a very dangerous one. For, his report continued, in such medicines, particularly laxatives, if administered unduly, lurks peril of death. Furthermore according to the reports, not only were these charlatans dispensing drugs about which they knew nothing, they were also applying clysters, and practicing phlebotomy, without calling in the aid of a qualified physician. Such shameful practices were resulting in " clandestine homicides and abortions on every hand and sometimes publicly." Accordingly, the king in his desire to provide for the welfare of his subjects, forbade anyone of either sex or of any condition whatsoever, " to administer any medicine, alterative, laxative, sirup, electuary, laxative pills, or clysters of any sort," for symptoms that he did not understand. No one was to administer opiates or offer medical advice or otherwise exercise the office of a physician in any way unless he was master or a licentiate in the science of medicine at the university of Paris, or in another university, unless he was acting under the advice and direction of a master of the university, or had been otherwise approved by the faculty of medicine as qualified to practice. The provost of the city of Paris was to have the power to enforce this edict by imposing pecuniary and other civil penalties upon those who should disobey it.[52]

In addition to the foregoing provisions, the king further decreed, in August 1353, that the pharmaceutical establishments of the city of Paris and of its environs must be visited twice each year, namely about Easter and at the feast of All Saints (November 1), by a commission made up of representatives of masters of the apothecary art together with two masters of medicine. Apothecaries were also prohibited from delivering any medicinal remedies without an express commission from a physician. Any apothecaries or pharmacists who violated the royal ordinances were to be punished severely.[53]

[52] *Chart. univ. Paris.*, III, pp. 16-17, no. 1211. The document is translated into English by L. Thorndike, *University Records*, pp. 235-236. See also *Chart. univ. Paris.*, II, p. 462, no. 1001; and *Les métiers et corporations*, ed. by Lespinasse, Paris, 1886, p. 504. For near deaths caused by illegal practitioners, see also *Chart. univ. Paris.*, II, p. 337, note.

[53] *Ibid.*, III, p. 20, no. 1215. The king was said to have confirmed certain ancient ordinances of the university (*Ordonn. des rois*, II, 532; and cf. *Chart, univ. Paris.*, II, p. 268).

It does not appear that the royal edicts were any more efficacious in stamping out charlatanism than were those of the university. On August 3, 1390, another royal ordinance indicated the continued persistence of illegal practice. Charles VI on that date reported to the provost of the city of Paris and to his other justices that the king's attention had been called to the fact that in Paris persons without approval or license were engaging in medical practice as well as in surgery. Such persons were said to be visiting patients and to be promising to effect cures which they were unable to accomplish. The king therefore demanded that the provost and other justices investigate these charges and take appropriate action against those who were found to be unqualified and who were practicing without the approval of the medical faculty.[54]

There was also at Paris, as in Naples and Salerno, an attempt made to regulate the practice of surgery, although this was at first primarily a municipal concern rather than that of the university.[55] The separation of manual surgeons from the medical faculty was rigorously maintained through the fourteenth and early fifteenth centuries.[56] The masters in medicine were, however, on occasion called in for consultation at the trials of unauthorized persons operating as surgeons. This is illustrated in the case of Perretta Petonne who, at the instance of the masters of the surgeons, was arrested in 1411 for operating as a surgeon although she had not been approved by either the physicians or surgeons. Her case was already before the Parlement in 1410. She had first been interrogated, on June 9 of that year, by masters in medicine who had tried to find out if she could read. Their conclusion was that she did not know an " a from a fagot," and furthermore that she did not know what were the

[54] *Ibid.*, III, pp. 534-535, no. 1586; *Ordonn. des rois*, VII, 353.

[55] As early as 1307 a municipal statute provided that barbers who practiced surgery were forbidden to do so unless they had been examined by six masters of surgery who had been named by the provost of Paris and who had been sworn in and made responsible for the loyalty and qualifications of the surgeons (BN fonds fr. 11709, fols. 14r, 13v; 86r-v). The ordinance was renewed in 1311 by Philip IV who put master Jean Pitard, his surgeon, in charge of the examining masters of surgery (*Chart. univ. Paris.*, II, p. 149, no. 692, and note) and by succeeding monarchs (*Chart. univ. Paris.*, III, p. 14, no. 1205; also *ibid.*, III, pp. 42, 70-71, 113; IV, pp. 423, 618). See also Wickersheimer, *Commentaires*, introduction pp. lxxvi *et seq.*

[56] Thus on June 9, 1408, the faculty of medicine in its congregation considered the case of Johannes de Pisis, a surgeon, who before his acceptance into the faculty had manually operated. This master was summoned before the faculty and was required to promise under oath that he would no longer operate manually in public surgery at Paris: *Chart. univ. Paris.*, IV, p. 156, no. 1853. Cf. E. Wickersheimer, *Commentaires*, pp. lxxvi, 5, 47.

properties of herbs in prohibited remedies, such as " ache " and " ysope."
At a second interrogation, on June 16, when the sick persons treated by
Perretta were summoned to testify, Perretta declared that she was working
" for God." She asserted that it was unjust that she should be molested
when several other women were engaged in the practice of surgery at
Paris, yet they were not being interrogated. The chief objection to
Perretta, as the learned editors of the *Chartularium* noted, was not her
sex, but the fact that she was practicing without the approval of the
commission of municipal surgeons.[57]

In 1436 the surgeons were admitted as actual scholars in the faculty
of medicine. They were allowed to attend lectures but could not proceed
to the degree. However, they were as scholars to enjoy all " the privileges,
franchises, liberties, and immunities conceded to the university." The
reasons set forth by the university for the admission of the surgeons to the
faculty of medicine, were that " in recent times," against the good of the
public, many unapproved, false, or fictitious surgeons, who were corrupting
and destroying the venerable science of surgery were making of it a
public horror and scandal to the detriment of the people. The reference
was to the struggle that was being carried on between the surgeons and
the inferior class of barbers. The latter were claiming that they could
operate surgically in certain cases although they had not been approved
by the commission of municipal surgeons.[58]

Some seven years later, in 1443, the surgeons and the medical faculty
also united to make common cause against a group of illicit medical practitioners called " cabusatores et cabusatrices." But not long thereafter, in
1446, a conflict broke out between the surgeons and the medical faculty
when the surgeons did not respond to the call to a faculty convocation.
The faculty had demanded that the surgeons take an oath in the presence
of the faculty that they would refrain from going outside their proper

[57] *Ibid.*, p. 60; *Chart. univ. Paris.*, IV, pp. 198-199, note 1, no. 1912. It would appear
that medical and surgical studies were not considered unsuitable for women. This is
illustrated by the plan of education outlined, in 1309, by Pierre Dubois. In his treatise
" On the Recovery of the Holy Land," Pierre Dubois stated that " to educate the girls
in medicine and surgery, it will be advisable that two girls more highly trained than
the others in medicine and surgery and their experiences remain to teach the others both
theory and practice ": selection translated by L. Thorndike, *University Records*, pp.
148-149. See further on women physicians in the middle ages, E. Nicaise, introduction
to his edition of *Guy de Chauliac*, pp. lxiii *et seq.*, p. 16.
[58] *Chart. univ. Paris.*, IV, pp. 594-595, no. 2496; Wickersheimer, *Commentaires*, p. 162.
For the litigation between the surgeons and barbers, see *Chart. univ. Paris.*, IV, pp. 442-
443, no. 2253; also *ibid.*, IV, pp. 675-676, no. 2621.

field of activity and that they would not prescribe digestive and laxative medicines or sedatives. This the surgeons refused to do.[59]

On January 11, 1494, the medical faculty opened its lectures to the corporation of the barbers. Up to that time the barbers had apparently taught each other. At one time a student in the medical faculty had acted as their teacher, but he had been obliged by the faculty to discontinue.[60] The surgeons requested that the faculty once again close its doors to the inferior barbers, and finally, in 1495-1496, reached an accord with the faculty. Not long afterward, however, in 1498, the medical faculty again complained that the surgeons were prescribing alterative and laxative medicines. It was not until 1506 that amicable relations were finally restored between the surgeons and the medical faculty.[61]

That the combined efforts of the medical faculty, the popes, the kings of France, as well as of the municipal magistrates, were unable to succeed in stamping out illegal practices in medicine, surgery, or in the sale and preparation of medicaments and drugs,[62] is amply illustrated by the continued reiteration of measures against these practices. In the first quarter of the fifteenth century, Henry V of England, as one of the first of his acts as regent of France, reaffirmed the statutes of the French monarchs against such evils. He threatened with imprisonment anyone found to be practicing without authorization or a license from the medical faculty of the university.[63] Nevertheless the university was obliged, from the year 1423 on, for some ten years, to carry on a long and wordy suit in the Parlement of Paris against a certain Jean de Domremi who designated himself physician, surgeon, and visitor of the surgeons of the kingdom, although apparently he had no official authorization whatever.[64]

Numerous other instances could be cited for the continuation of unauthorized and unlicensed medical practice both before and after 1500

[59] Wickersheimer, *Commentaires*, pp. 171, 179, 210.

[60] *Ibid.*, pp. 331-332; 353.

[61] *Ibid.*, pp. 365, 368, 390, 397, 403, 404, 474-478, 483.

[62] On December 7, 1437-1438 the medical faculty assembled to hear the response of the herbalists on the question of whether they would take the required oaths or not. The herbalists did not bother to appear and were declared, after they failed to heed a second summons, contumacious and hence subject to excommunication: Wickersheimer, *Commentaires*, p. 163.

[63] *Chart. univ. Paris.*, IV, p. 423, no. 2227; E. Nicaise, introduction to his edition of *Guy de Chauliac*, p. lxiii, cites a manuscript for the ordinance of Henry V in 1420.

[64] *Chart. univ. Paris.*, IV, pp. 424-428, nos. 2228-2231; *Journal de Clement de Fouquebergue, Greffier du Parlement de Paris, 1417-1435*, ed. by A. Tuetey (Société de l'histoire de France, 3 vols., Paris, 1903-1905), II, 168, 223, note 1, 224; *Wickersheimer, Commentaires*, pp. 129-149.

and even into our own time. The medical faculty of the university of Paris had thus been unsuccessful in its contest against such practice, and the university records of the fourteenth and fifteenth centuries reveal the obstacles encountered in the attempts to enforce the approved license requirements and to prosecute those who practiced without them. On occasion our sympathy may go out to such an empiric or natural healer as Jacqueline Félicie appears to have been. But there seems little doubt that the enforcement, by licensing, of specific requirements and qualifications was, then as now, in accord with the public interest. The continued instances of charlatanism, quackery, and illegal practice even into our own day illustrate the inherent difficulties of the problem. The efforts, therefore, of the medical faculty of the university of Paris in initiating in Paris the contest against these practices and in enlisting against them successively the aid of ecclesiastical, municipal, and royal authorities would appear worthy of our interest and earnest consideration.

LIST OF FREQUENTLY CITED WORKS

Chartularium universitatis Parisiensis, edited by H. Denifle and E. Chatelain, 4 vols., Paris, 1889-1897.

Conring[ius], H., *De antiquitatibus academicis dissertationes septem*, Gottingae, 1739.

Lesne, E., *Histoire de la propriété ecclésiastique en France*: Fasc. 50, Tome V, 1940: "Les écoles de la fin du VIIIe siècle à la fin du XIIe."

Migne, J. P. (editor), *Patrologiae cursus completus*, Series latina, 221 vols., Paris, 1844-1864.

Ordonnances des roys de France de la troisième race jusqu'en 1514, recueillies par ordre chronologique, 22 vols., Paris, 1723-1849.

Thorndike, L. (editor and translator), *University Records and Life in the Middle Ages* (Records of Civilization, Columbia University Press), New York, 1944.

Wickersheimer, E. (editor), *Commentaires de la faculté de médecine de l'université de Paris (1395-1516)*, Paris, 1915.

Wickersheimer, E., *Dictionnaire biographique des médecins en France au moyen âge*, 2 vols., Paris, 1936.

MANUSCRIPTS

Paris: Archives Nationales:
  M 70, no. 11 bis, Histoire de la faculté de Médecine, 1395-1434; no. 12, Chirurgiens, fols. 1r-3r, copied in the 17th century.
  MM 226, 17th cent.

 Bibliothèque Nationale:
  fonds français 11709, 14th-15th centuries.
  fonds français 22110, Actes concernant le pouvoir et la direction de l'université de Paris, fols. 3 et seq.

A SEVENTEENTH CENTURY ENGLISH MEDICAL LICENSE

JOHN H. RAACH

Anyone who is familiar today with the English medical system realizes the tremendous power and influence which the Royal College of Physicians exercises over the medical profession. Yet this power is a comparatively recent development confined almost entirely to the last century. To be sure, the College was founded in 1518 but for the first three centuries of its existence its authority and influence were felt only in London and " within seven miles of the same." [1] Even within the city of London itself the College shared the authority over the medical profession with the bishop of London, for, odd as it may seem to us today, the Church exercised a potent influence on regulating the medical profession from the sixteenth to the nineteenth centuries. [2]

Along with the development of England as a national state in the fourteenth and fifteenth centuries there occurred attempts to produce order in the social as well as the political fields. Just as there were powerful Lords and Barons contributing to political chaos, so there were many " uncunning and unapproved " [3] persons practicing medicine and leading to chaos in the medical field. The fact that people

---

[1] William Munk, *The Roll of the Royal College of Physicians* (London, 1878), I, 2.

[2] While ecclesiastical regulation of the medical profession actually counted for little in the latter part of the eighteenth and early nineteenth centuries, theoretically at least the Church was a legal licensing body for the profession until the Medical Act of 1858 (21 & 22 Victoria, c. 90) created the General Council of Medical Education and Registration of the United Kingdom, usually known as the General Medical Council.

[3] *Rotuli Parliamentorum*, IV, 158. I have made a thorough study of the early English attempts to regulate medicine and of the licensing system which evolved as a result; both have been elaborated and set forth in my doctoral dissertation, "The English Country Doctor in The Province of Canterbury, 1603-1643," submitted to Yale University in 1941.

recognized the need for some control of practitioners and sought to do something about it is highly significant. As early as 1421 a petition, which embodied ideas of medical control and sought some means to regulate medicine, was presented to parliament by the physicians themselves. Parliament failed to act upon the petition at that time and the subsequent disorders occasioned by the War of the Roses frustrated any further attempts to regulate medicine until the strong hand of the Tudors restored order to the country.

In 1511 parliament passed a medical licensing act which remained virtually unchanged [4] until 1858 and which sought to bring order to the medical profession and to furnish a legitimate and responsible authority for its supervision. The act provided that:

no person . . . take upon him to exercise and occupy as a Physician [or Surgeon] in any Diocese within this Realm, but if he be first examined and approved by the Bishop of the same Diocese, or he being out of the Diocese, by his Vicar-general; either of them calling to them such expert persons in the said faculties, as their discretion shall think convenient, and giving their letters testimonials under their seal to him that they shall so approve.[5]

To the Tudor mind nothing could be better suited for such duties than the universities and the Church, especially the latter with its elaborate hierarchy extending into every shire, hundred and parish. With life in rural sixteenth and seventeenth century England being confined almost entirely to ones immediate environs the provisions of the act proved to be a great boon to not only the State in its control of the professions, but to the individual practitioner who had neither the time nor the finance to travel to the distant capital or universities for a license. The Tudor state was not primarily concerned with the convenience of its citizens, but it so happened in the case of medical control that what was convenient to the citizen, likewise, happened to be convenient for the State.

Many licenses, no doubt, were granted according to the provisions of the act of 1511 during the remainder of the sixteenth century, but none of them appear to have survived. The earliest physician's license

[4] The archbishops had not been included as licensing authorities in the act 3 Henry VIII, c. 11. Sometime before 1604, however, they were permitted to license both physicians and surgeons.
[5] 3 Henry VIII, c. 11.

74

known is one of 1604 issued by the archdeacon of Bucks. to Richard Sandey.[6] The license is significant not only for being the earliest known physican's license,[7] but also for its revelation that one of the smallest ecclesiastical divisions—the archdeaconry—played an important role in the administration of the act. One might expect to find a license granted by the universities, by the archbishop of Canterbury or York, or by one of the bishops,[8] but scarcely by an archdeacon, and yet such are the vagaries of fate that the license of one of the lesser church dignitaries has survived while that of the other authorities have disappeared. Nonetheless, knowing as we do that legal forms then, as now, were all well standardized, we may then assume that this license represents the typical license issued by the Church to medical practitioners.

The original license, inscribed on velum, is 94" wide by 6¾" long and is in an excellent state of preservation as may be seen from the accompanying reprint of the photostatic copy. In transcribing it the abbreviations have been extended; capitalization and punctuation have not been changed.

WILLELMUS SMITHE legum doctor Comissarius ac Officialis Archidiaconiati Bucks. Diuersis et singulis Christi fidelibus provenientes litteras insequentur lecturas vel audituras, Salutem. AD vniuersitatis vero notitiam deduimus et dedui volumus [sic] per partes. Quod cum nos nuper ex fide et relacione nonullorum in arte medicina peritorum et aliorum subdignorum acceperimus quemdam Richardum Sandey clericum artium magistrum Rectorem de Linford magna Archidiaconiati predicti artis medicina peritum atque eandem artem iam diu non sine laudabili approbacione omnium vicinorum exercuisse

---

[6] The license is to be found in the Bodleian, Oxford, under the catalogue number of Ms. Ashmole Roll 5, Ashmole MSS. 1298.

[7] The only other physician's license of the seventeenth century known to exist is one issued by the bishop of Exeter in 1662. It is also to be found in the Bodleian catalogued as Ashmole MSS. 194.

[8] The best sources for university licenses are Joseph Foster, *Alumni Oxoniensis. The Members of the University of Oxford, 1500-1714* (Oxford, 1891), and John Venn and J. A. Venn, *Alumni Cantabrigiensis From the Earliest Times to 1751* (Cambridge. 1922). Each ecclesiastical diocese had its own nomenclature for the books in which it kept a record of the licenses granted. Of these the best sources which have survived to the present day are: the Registers of the archbishops of Canterbury, the Liber Licentiarum of the diocese of Canterbury, the Registers of the bishops of Chichester, the Registers of the Diocese of Exeter, and the Act Books of the archbishops of York.

multisque salutis corpores desperantibus illo faventibus subvenisse. Cuius dictus Richardus Sandey Licentiam et facultatem nostras ad publice exercendam artem medicina infra villam de Linford Magna predicta et alia loca vicina et adiacentia archidiaconiati predicti a nobis instanter petierit. Nos igitur eius honeste peticionem aumentes [*sic*] eidem Licentiam et facultatem nostras ad premissam artem medicina exercendam infra parochiam de Linford Magna predicta et alia loca vicina et adiacentia archidiaconiati predicti quantum a nobis est, aut huius regni Anglie statutis in ea parte salubriter editis et prouisis possumus et valemus tenore partium damus et concedimus. IN CUIUS rei testimonium Sigillum Offici nostri partibus apponi fecimus. DATUS vicesimo die mensis Decembris Anno Domini Millesimo Sex centimo Quarto.[9]

For the existence of this license we can be grateful to the acquisitive nature of Elias Ashmole, whose passion for collecting the unusual as well as the commonplace, resulted in the accumulation of a wealth of documents, curios and miscellany with which to bewilder and delight the modern scholar. Among Ashmole's acquaintances, if not among his intimate friends, was Sir Richard Napier, nephew and sole heir of Richard Sandey (alias Napier)[10] to whom the above license was given. It was through Sir Richard that Ashmole came into possession of the license, because Sir Richard bequeathed Ashmole his uncle's manuscript collections.[11] Thus, it is that the medical license of Richard Sandey managed to escape the ravages of time and the fate of its contemporaries.

Obviously this brief note cannot give a complete biographical sketch of Richard Sandey, but a few words about him will cast some light upon a certain type of seventeenth century country practitioner. Sandey was not a typical practitioner in view of the fact that he mingled astrology with his practice of medicine; but in an age when astrology was still widely believed in by a great number of country folk and at a time when medical training was still didactic and far from clinical, Sandey's mingling of the two can perhaps be excused. Sandey, like the rest of the youths of his day who went up to the English universities, received the usual sound foundation in the

[9] Ms. Ashmole Roll 5, Ashmole MSS. 1298.

[10] His father went by the alternate name of Sandey, although he was the eldest son of Sir Archibald Napier, 4th Laird of Merchiston and his third wife. *D. N. B.*

[11] *D. N. B.*

Classics.[12] He graduated with a B. A. from Exeter College, Oxford, in January 1584 and two years later received an M. A. from the same college. Although ordained when he left college, Sandey, was unlike many of his contemporaries in that he did not immediately obtain a church benefice and settle down to enjoy the fruits of his education. Instead he went to London where he studied and worked for some time with Simon Forman, one of the most noted astrologers of the period. Whether it was his inability to get along with Forman, or his need for money that compelled him to leave London is not known, but at any rate he was admitted to the rectory of Great Linford, Buckinghamshire, on March 12, 1589/90, and held that post until his death forty-four years later. Preaching apparently was not to his liking, for, according to Lilly, he broke down one day in the pulpit and ceased to preach after that time.[13] While he undoubtedly practiced both medicine and astrology prior to that eventful occasion, after that he made medicine his chief occupation the rest of his life.

How long he practiced before he took out a license is impossible to say, but that he did practice without such is attested to in the license. Indeed, according to the provisions of the act of 3 Henry VIII, c. 11, such a procedure was the usual thing.[14] People in that day were far more casual about demanding the legal stamp of approval on their physicians, and a legal license evidently meant much less than it does

[12] During his first year the student attended lectures on Grammar, which supplemented the Latin he had learned in the Grammar School, and Rhetoric, which included Aristotle, the Compends of Hermogenes, the Institutes of Quintilian and the Oratorical Treatises of Cicero. During the next three years the student was introduced to Logic, Geometry, Astronomy, and Moral Philosophy. Logic was based upon a study of Cicero and Aristotle; Geometry was based upon Euclid's Elements, the Comics of Apollonius, and all the books of Archimedes, in addition to this the Oxford professor was " to teach and expound arithmetic of all kinds both practical and speculative, land-surveying, or practical geometry, canonics or music and mechanics "; Astronomy was based largely on Ptolemy; Moral Philosophy was based on the *Nicomachean Ethics* of Aristotle, his *Politics* and *Economics*. G. R. M. Ward, *Oxford University Statues* (London, 1845), I, 20 f.

[13] William Lilly (1602-1681) was a famous seventeenth century astrologer who knew Napier well. He claimed that Napier kept a scholar after his breakdown to do the preaching for him. *D. N. B.*

[14] The Bishop . . . or . . . his Vicar-general; either of them calling to them such expert persons in the said faculties, . . . and giving their letters testimonials under their seal to him that they shall so approve. 3 Henry VIII, c. 11.

at the present time. In one respect the people were much more realistic in their requirements for medical practitioners, since their main concern seemed to be whether the physician could produce cures. That Richard Sandey complied with this requirement is also indicated in the license wherein he is described as having produced many cures.

In spite of the fact that Sandey mingled astrology with medicine and that he bordered on the fringe of quackery, nevertheless, he had an extensive practice as is indicated by his case books.[15] Among his patients were not only the local gentry and yeomen and their families as well as those of lesser social status, but also such notables as Emanuel Scrope, 11th baron Scrope of Bolton, and Earl of Sunderland. Sandey was apparently one of those doctors whose formal learning was not of the highest type, but whose common sense and practical knowledge allowed him to serve the society of his day in a beneficial way.

The license of Richard Sandey, therefore, is not only significant in being a rare document, and as revealing a type of character only occasionally found practicing in the country districts in that day,[16] but it is highly significant also in revealing one of the obscure pieces of mechanism whereby the act of 3 Henry VIII, c. 11 operated.

[15] In the Bodleian in the Ashmole collection there are many volumes containing the names of his patients. Actually they are the best records of a doctor's patients which can be found for the period 1600-1635. Only four other case books of the period may be found; among them is Shakespeare's son-in-law, John Hall, whose *Observations on Select English Bodies* (ed.) James Cooke (London, 1657) have been published. The other three case books are still in manuscript form and are those of John Hungerford, Sloane MSS. 461; James Rant, Cambridge University Library, Cambridge Dd. III, 21; and Reuben Robinson. Sloane MSS. 2369.

[16] Of the seven hundred and forty-one doctors who practiced in the country districts of the midlands and south of England in the period 1603-1643, Sandey is the only one who is definitely known to have practiced astrology along with medicine.

LIBERTY, LAISSEZ-FAIRE AND LICENSURE IN NINETEENTH CENTURY BRITAIN *

DAVID L. COWEN

The liberal political tradition in Great Britain, evident in the charters of liberties and the writings of John Locke, Jeremy Bentham, and John Stuart Mill, was joined by a liberal tradition in economics late in the 18th century. The work of Adam Smith and the classical economists who followed him, although not as doctrinaire as sometimes supposed, emphasized laissez-faire and free trade, ideas which are obviously difficult to separate from the political aspects of the liberal tradition. True, John Stuart Mill pointed out that the principle of individual liberty was not really involved in the doctrine of free trade (which found its justification on other grounds), but nevertheless he recognized that there might well be questions relating to interference in trade " which are essentially questions of liberty." It is interesting that his illustrations had pertinence to pharmacy. Mill saw no involvement of the ideas of liberty in the determination of how far " public control is admissible for the prevention of fraud by adulteration," but he did believe that the question of liberty was implicit in the restriction of the sale of poisons.[1]

Questions of liberty were involved not only in such matters as the sale of poisons and adulterated drugs, but also in matters pertaining to quarantine restrictions, sanitation requirements, restriction of the sale of nostrums, the regulation of madhouses, and the like. However, the idea of liberty as it influenced the development of the professions of medicine and pharmacy in Great Britain was manifest mainly in the attempts at limitation, by licensure and otherwise, of professional practice to qualified practitioners.

In the 19th century the tone for the debate on these issues had been set in an exchange of ideas between Adam Smith and William Cullen. Smith, in 1794, was undaunted by the hawking of medical degrees at Aberdeen and St. Andrew's, which, though he found " unhandsome," he believed did not cause the public to suffer. Rather he considered the development of the " exclusive and corporation spirit " in the professions " an intolerable nuisance." The absence of restrictions would keep the costs of

---

* Read at the forty-first annual meeting of the American Association for the History of Medicine, St. Louis, Missouri, April 18, 1968.
[1] John Stuart Mill, *On Liberty* (Atlantic Library Edition, Boston, 1921), pp. 133-134.

medical care low, and a practitioner's success would be a reflection of " his merit " rather than of any formal medical qualification.

Cullen's response, two years later, was to be the argument of the medical reformer for more than a century. " In the practice of medicine," he contended, " none of [the] reasons for unfettered competition are of any force. . . . The community are scarcely able to judge . . . of the merits of medical men. . . . The life and health of a great portion of mankind are in the hands of ignorant people. . . . The legislature should take especial care that the necessary art should, as far as possible, be rendered both safe and useful to society." [2]

It has been generally believed that the views of Adam Smith prevailed— in the entire political economy, and not merely in medicine. Lately, historians have tended to point out that the prevalence of laissez-faire was largely a myth and that state intervention was common enough in Victorian Britain in many aspects of life.[3] To a very appreciable extent this was true in medicine and pharmacy, but before we revise liberty and laissez-faire out of the history of medicine in the 19th century, it would be well to examine the situation a bit more intensively.

Let us first examine the case for the historical interpretation that minimizes the actual impact of liberal ideas on the development of the medical professions and which contends that state " interference " was not only achieved, but achieved with knowledge and forethought.

A good starting point is the Benthamites, once thought to be thoroughgoing individualists in the best tradition of Adam Smith. One glance at the neat bureaucratic arrangements in Bentham's *Constitutional Code* (1830-1841), where Bentham set up a Ministry of Health and a Ministry of Preventive Services to watch over such things as disease, contagion, mortality, and unhealthy employments, makes it obvious that the happiness of the greatest number required the manifold intervention of the state. The Health of Towns Act (1848) and Chadwick, of course, showed Benthamite influences, and the medical reformers, like Henry Warburton and Thomas Wakley, likewise came out of the Benthamite tradition.[4]

[2] Smith's letter to Cullen and Cullen's response in a graduation discourse are appended to J. R. McCulloch's editions of Smith's *An Inquiry into the Nature and Causes of the Wealth of Nations* (New edition, Edinburgh, 1863), pp. 582-586, 588-589.

[3] For example, see J. B. Brebner, " Laissez-Faire and State Intervention in Nineteenth Century Britain," in R. L. Schuyler and H. Ausubel, *The Making of English History* (New York: Dryden Press, [1952]), pp. 501-510.

[4] Sir George Clark, *A History of the Royal College of Physicians of London*, vol. II (Oxford: Clarendon Press, 1966), pp. 667-669; W. L. Burn, *The Age of Equipoise* (New York: Norton, 1965), p. 206, n.; W. J. Reader, *Professional Men* (London: Weidenfeld & Nicolson, 1966), p. 59.

Even if we judge only from the legislative record, it is quite safe to say that in the 19th century, " the majority (probably the great majority) of medical men " favored legislation restrictive of the practice of medicine.[5] Between 1834 and 1851 nine, between 1840 and 1858, seventeen, and between 1870 and 1881, twenty (private and unsuccessful) parliamentary bills have been counted that sought " medical reform." [6] Between 1813 and 1852, in addition, at least six attempts were made to regulate pharmacy. Parliamentary Select Committees and a Royal Commission studied the problem as well.[7] This activity was not without its effects. In 1815 the Apothecaries Act perpetuated the powers and interests of the established order and was more in the spirit of a Stuart patent than of the presumed liberal milieu in which it was born, as Holloway has pointed out.[8] Moreover, the Act contained a provision, albeit one that proved difficult to enforce, making it a punishable offense for one who was not certified to " act or practise as an apothecary." [9] This was a principle to which Smith would especially have taken exception, as he would have also to the whole concept of examination and certification set up in the Act. In 1852 the Pharmacy Act was passed, creating a national register—the chemists and druggists stole the thunder of the general practitioners—and making an attempt at sponsoring educational and examination requirements. Since pharmacy was considered a trade, and chemists and druggists tradesmen, this piece of legislation represents a more significant departure from hands-off doctrine than either the Apothecaries Act of 1815 or the Medical Act of 1858. That reform won out at this time was an indication that it would soon win on the broader medical front. When finally the Medical Act of 1858 was passed, although it was a typical Victorian compromise in attempting to establish something new (the General Council of Medical Education and Registration) without doing too much harm to the old (the 21 corporations in existence with some sort of examining and licensing powers), it sought to control education for, entry into, and discipline within, the medical profession. The Medical Council was the first body set up by Parliament with the

[5] Burn, op. cit., p. 202. Cf. Francis Cowper's statement in Commons, Hansard, Parliamentary Debates, vol. 150 (1858), col. 1408.
[6] Hansard, vol. 118 (1851), col. 112; Reader, op. cit., p. 66; Medical Acts Commission Report of the Royal Commissioners Appointed to Inquire into the Medical Acts (London, 1882), pp. xlvii-xlix.
[7] Select Committees: 1834, 1847, 1847-48, 1878-79, 1880, for medical profession; 1852, 1865 for pharmacy. Royal Commission: 1882.
[8] S. W. F. Holloway, " The Apothecaries' Act, 1815: A reinterpretation," M. Hist., 1966, 10: 221.
[9] 55 G. 3. c. 194, section 21, and Holloway, op. cit., p. 125.

intent of controlling a profession.[10] Its powers were to increase, by usage and statute (1886, 1950, 1956) as time went on.

There is more to the story than the legislation, however. One must wonder why such a plethora of Bills was necessary and why such a paucity of Acts was produced. While it is true, as will later be noted, that liberal ideas and traditions presented a constant obstacle, the stark reality that stares out of the parliamentary debates on medical reform was that the greater obstacles were the differences in interests, the selfishness, and the jealousies of the vested medical groups that had been created piecemeal and without plan over the centuries. For a long time none of the various establishments gave much indication of a willingness to surrender its prerogatives,[11] as evident at the very outset of the century with the collapse of Edward Harrison's plans for reform.[12] Moreover, it was not quite cricket to forcibly divest them of any of their powers: time and time again Parliament refused to act when one or another interested party opposed a bill. The rivalries that existed between physicians and surgeons or between apothecaries and pharmacists were the least of them. Involved were deeper problems: of the provinces versus London, of Scottish nationalism, of general practitioners versus the old trinity of physicians, surgeons, and midwives, of the democratization of the control of the Royal College of Surgeons and of the Medical Council, for example. It seemed impossible to bring these divergent interests under one umbrella.

Thomas Duncombe, Benthamite sponsor of one of the three bills before the Commons in 1858 and obviously a tired reformer, was so chagrined with this factionalism as to declare that the House of Commons "could not be a worse tribunal" to deal with medical reform; he would advise the House "to have nothing to do with the doctors." Indeed, he went on to say that he "should certainly never again attempt to legislate on the subject."[13] In 1882 the situation had not changed: only five members of the Royal Commission on the Medical Acts agreed in toto with the Commissioners' Report. Six expressed objections, in seven different dissents. Sir Lyon Playfair, in 1886, reminded the Commons that "the interests affected and the jealousies of different Medical Bodies" had been responsible for the failure of the many bills to pass.[14] What was

[10] Clark, op. cit., vol. II, p. 728. Clark has disregarded the earlier Pharmacy Act, which did apply similarly to the professional aspects of pharmacy.

[11] In the 1870's a more cooperative spirit was indicated by various gropings toward "conjoint" examinations. See the Royal Commissioners Report (1882), op. cit., ftn. 6 above, p. xxxvi.

[12] The Harrison story can be found in Clark, op. cit., vol. II, pp. 627 ff.

[13] Hansard, vol. 150 (1858), col. 1419.

[14] Hansard, vol. 305 (1886), cols. 236-237.

hammered out, to use a very apt phrase of Sir George Clark, came about "by a conjuncture of cross-purposes." [15]

Yet despite all of the attempts at legislation, despite the fact that traditional interests and rivalries were so significant, and despite some legislative success, the idea of liberty and laissez-faire cannot be disregarded as a powerful and ubiquitous force both in delaying legislation and in determining the content of that legislation.

Throughout the 19th century it is quite obvious that the advocates of liberty fought state intervention all the way. At times, perhaps, the resort to arguments of freedom was sheer ritual or oratory, but one cannot escape the pervasiveness of the ideas of liberty and the unwillingness and wariness with which medical legislation was approached. The underlying belief that the state should not meddle in medical matters continued to prevail.

John Mason Good, called by Clark "the morning star of medical reform," [16] thought the pending Apothecaries Bill (1814) was "founded in tyranny and oppression." [17] Sir James Graham was aware, when he introduced his Bill for the Better Regulation of Medical Practice in 1844, that "all interference by law had . . . been stigmatised," and he recalled Adam Smith's arguments in Smith's letter to Cullen.[18] His bill was noteworthy for his deliberate attempt to stay within the Smith tradition, but he did propose to set up a national Council. This was too much state interference for some, and the bill failed.

The story is told, whether apocryphal or not does not really matter, that Lord Palmerston advised a delegation of physicians that if they went home, agreed among themselves, and gained the confidence of their patients and neighbors, they would find that very few laws would be needed from Parliament.[19] In 1871 Herbert Spencer characteristically refused to accept honorary membership in the St. Andrew's Medical Graduates' Association because the legislative policy of the medical profession violated the principles he had "long publicly held respecting the functions of the State and the liberties of the subject." [20] And in 1883, T. H. Huxley was still insisting that the state should no more "interfere with

[15] Clark, *op. cit.*, ftn. 4 above, vol. II, p. 649.

[16] *Ibid.*, p. 623.

[17] Quoted by J. Bell and T. Redwood, *Historical Sketch of the Progress of Pharmacy in Great Britain* (London, 1880), p. 59.

[18] Hansard, vol. 76 (1844), col. 1896.

[19] L. D. Broughton, *A Plain Statement as to the Medical and Surgical College of the State of New Jersey*, 2nd ed. (New York, 1891), preliminary material.

[20] D. Duncan, *Life and Letters of Herbert Spencer* (New York: Appleton, 1908), vol. I, p. 202.

the profession of medicine than it does, say, with the profession of engineering." State intervention, he emphasized, was not justified on " any pretence of protecting the public and still less upon that of protecting the medical profession." [21] Even when it was finally determined, in 1886 after three years of struggle, to give the Medical Council " full power to enforce efficient examinations," this was done, the Commons was advised, " trusting to the Licensing Bodies in combination to do what they wished." [22]

One aspect of Smith's doctrines that recurs constantly is the opposition to monopoly. That the old corporations were monopolies had been pointed out as early as 1649, when Nicholas Culpeper castigated the College of Physicians for its monopolistic interference with THE LIBERTY OF THE SUBJECT (capitalization is Culpeper's).[23] Indeed, in some measure one might think of the whole medical reform movement as directed against monopolies, or, not unrelated, to the democratization of the control of existing corporations. The suggestions of Edward Harrison early in the century, the battles waged by the Provincial Medical and Surgical Association and the British Medical Association, and Wakley's tilting with the Surgeons all reflected,[24] as indeed did all of the legislative proposals, batterings at the bastions. The London and Dublin Apothecaries Companies came in for special criticism,[25] but the resort to the argument of free trade was reserved primarily for use against pharmacy legislation. Given the trade aspects of pharmacy, any effort to seek to establish qualifications for chemists and druggists had to be suspect in an age presumably devoted to free trade. The major obstacle to the Pharmacy Act of 1852, according to the later contention of Jacob Bell, the bill's sponsor, was that the law was " incompatible with the principles of free-trade." [26] Testimony before the Parliamentary Committee of 1847 and statements by Sir George Grey, the Home Secretary,[27] bear this out.

[21] T. H. Huxley, " The state and the medical profession," *Nineteenth Century*, 1884, *15*: 228-230.

[22] Hansard, vol. 305 (1886), col. 240.

[23] *The Physical Directory* (London, 1649), preface.

[24] For these struggles see Clark, *op. cit.*, ftn. 4 above, vol. II, *passim.*, and F. N. L. Poynter (ed.), *The Evolution of Medical Practice in Britain* (London: Pitman, 1961), especially F. N. L. Poynter, " The influence of government legislation on medical practice in Britain," Sir Zachary Cope, " The influence of the Royal College of Surgeons," and W. H. McMenemey, " The influence of medical societies."

[25] See Hansard, vol. 21 (1834), cols. 234, 235; vol. 76 (1844), col. 1904.

[26] Bell and Redwood, *op. cit.*, ftn. 17 above, pp. 211, 217.

[27] Burn, *op. cit.*, ftn. 4 above, p. 202 n.; Hansard, vol. 118 (1851), col. 117.

One particular aspect of the monopoly argument, however, is more basic to our problem. Any kind of qualification for any aspect of medical practice created a monopoly and was therefore contrary not simply to British ideas of laissez-faire, but to more fundamental concepts of British liberty. Even the absolutist, Thomas Hobbes, for whom the term " liberty of the subject " meant just that,[28] and for whom the only liberties were those few " praetermitted " by the sovereign, contended that among those liberties was that of choosing one's " own trade in life." [29] The right of anyone to practice medicine, and the corollary, the right of anyone to seek medical attention from anyone, was not simply an argument that was used to oppose medical reform, it became a principle of British medical legislation.

It is just at this point that Smith prevailed over Cullen. The resentment against the loosely-worded restrictive clause (Section 20) of the Apothecaries Act of 1815 and the equivocal success in attempts to enforce it,[30] abetted by the individualistic undertones to the thinking of some of the reformers, meant that in subsequent legislation short shrift was given to attempts to impose restrictive measures. Warburton, for example, differed from Wakley on this point and rejected restrictive measures in favor of definitive measures. (Restrictive measures limited practice to licensees and made it an offense to practice without a license; definitive measures regulated by definition—at least to the extent of making it an offense to use a title for which one had not qualified, but otherwise permitting medical activity.)[31]

The opposition to restrictive measures appears again and again and received its most significant expression in Sir James Graham's effort to assure the Commons that despite the fact that his Bill (1844) would establish a national register and Medical Council, it would sweep away all " exclusive privileges for practising medicine " and was indeed within the best tradition of British liberty. In presenting his Bill, Sir James remarked that:

[28] Any distinction between "individual liberty" and "liberty of the subject" seems to have disappeared. At least Sir George Clark (op. cit., vol. II, p. 660) uses the latter term in reference to the Royal College's refusal to suggest quarantine regulations in 1818, while in the pertinent document the actual words used by the Comitia were "individual Freedom." Royal College of Physicians Minutes, 6 November 1818, p. 45.

[29] The Leviathan, Part 2, Chap. 21 (W. G. Pogson Smith edition, Oxford: Clarendon Press, 1962, p. 163).

[30] See Holloway, op. cit., ftn. 8 above, pp. 225-226, 228-229.

[31] The classification of "restrictive" and "definitive" follows B. Spector, "The growth of medicine and the letter of the law," Bull. Hist. Med., 1952, 26: 516.

He proposed no restriction on private practice whatever; it would be open to any man to prescribe and administer medicine without any previous examination or proof of qualification. . . . A wise Legislature should offer to the public some certain and accredited guarantee of fitness, competency, skill, and knowledge of those practitioners who voluntarily submitted themselves to examination, and who, by examination had given proofs of their competency and skill. . . . He left it open to the public in their individual capacity to make their own choice of a medical attendant, even if they preferred an unregistered to a registered practitioner.

Fundamental to this system was to be the register, published annually, listing those practitioners who had duly qualified. Only those on the register were eligible for posts in government service, which imposed no inconsistency, for under such circumstances " the choice of the medical attendant did not rest with the patient or any member of his family." Those pretending to be registered would be guilty of a misdemeanor, and because " it amounted more nearly to a penalty than any other provision of the Bill," he offered, with " some hesitation," a provision that none but a registered practitioner was " entitled to recover at law for medicines, attendance, or advice." He meant it as a warning clause and hoped that it would be so understood.[82]

The disabilities of the unregistered practitioner were explained by Sir James when the Bill came up again in 1845. He still could not:

regard it as an offence for any person not professing to possess the required standard of an examination, to practise surgery or medicine, subject to the risk which he runs of a criminal prosecution, and, I believe also, of a civil action, if any injury shall result from his practice . . . if he does not pretend to be what he is not, I cannot see why we should make any new crime to make him amenable.

This, and the misdemeanor provision for assuming " the title of physician, of surgeon, or of apothecary or doctor," he thought went the " full length against empiricism." [83]

There was a fundamental strain of the idea of British liberty running through Sir James' argument. It was to appear later, in a more generalized form, in John Stuart Mill's essay *On Liberty*. The individual's liberty was so unassailable, Mill was to write, that though there might be " good reason for remonstrating with him, or persuading him, or entreating him," there could be none " for compelling him, or visiting him with evil if he do otherwise." [34]

Sir James was assailed from all sides. There were those who thought that his liberalism went too far. A *Punch* cartoon of January 11, 1845,

[82] Sir James' comments are from Hansard, vol. 76 (1844), cols. 1898-1899, 1903.
[83] Hansard, vol. 77 (1845), cols. 1214-1215.
[34] Mill, *On Liberty*, *op. cit.*, ftn. 1 above, p. 13.

for example, turned a chemist's shop into a grog shop, or vice versa, in a lampoon of the effect of Sir James' proposals. Theophilus Redwood was to claim (1880) that " Even chemists and druggists hardly viewed with satisfaction the extreme free trade principles upon which the measure was based." [35] There were also those,[36] like Wakley, who, although very much in favor of a register,[37] wanted to save the public " from becoming victims of a profligate, mercenary and extortionate set of men " and wanted the practice of the profession restricted to the qualified.[38] The verdict of historians that Graham failed because the " spirit of British liberty was affronted " and because it seemed to his contemporaries that the Government would be " assuming dangerously dictatorial powers " [39] is perhaps an oversimplification, but it is clear that the issues of liberty and laissez-faire played a substantial role in the legislative history.

Sir James' approach survived, however. A provision of the Pharmacy Bill of 1852, for example, which provided for restrictive licensing, was struck out because it " was wholly at variance with the views that prevailed in the Legislature and had been recognized by Government in bills . . . for regulating the practice of medicine." [40] More important, his views were incorporated into the Medical Act that finally did pass in 1858. That Act, as already described, set up a national Council and, on the basis of its stated purpose to make it " expedient that persons requiring medical aid shall be able to distinguish qualified from unqualified practitioners," established a national register.[41] Francis Cowper, chief sponsor of the Bill, was, as Sir James had been, " disposed jealously to guard the right of private individuals to consult whomever they pleased," [42] and the continued existence and activity of the unqualified was countenanced. The 1858 Act did, however, impose certain disabilities on the unregistered: he could not certify to statutory documents, he could not falsify anything pertaining to the Register, and he could not recover at law any charges for his activity. Most important, especially after the passage of National Health Insurance,[43] he might hold no position in government

[35] Bell and Redwood, op. cit., ftn. 17 above, p. 170.

[36] See Hansard, vol. 150 (1858), col. 1409.

[37] Dictionary of National Biography. The 1858 provisions were said to be almost entirely as Wakley had first proposed them.

[38] Hansard, vol. 76 (1844), col. 1907.

[39] Clark, op. cit., ftn. 4 above, vol. II, p. 710; Burn, op. cit., ftn. 4 above, p. 208.

[40] Bell and Redwood, op. cit., p. 217.

[41] The Act is found in 21 and 22 Victoria, c. 90.

[42] Hansard, vol. 149 (1858), col. 648.

[43] A. M. Carr-Saunders and P. M. Wilson, The Professions (Oxford: Clarendon Press, 1933), pp. 88-89.

88

service. (In addition, there were probably other disabilities under the common law, like liability to assault or manslaughter charges.) All of this might suggest a *de facto* if not a *de jure* elimination of the unqualified, but the continued dissatisfaction with this portion of the legislation indicates otherwise.[44]

Sir James' view prevailed again in the Pharmacy Act of 1868. Although restrictions were imposed against the keeping of open shop for the sale of poisons enumerated in the Act,[45] suggestions for general restrictive qualifications for chemists and druggists were beaten down.[46] Instead, the use of professional titles was forbidden to anyone not registered.[47]

The idea of definitive registration thus became an integral part of the regulation of the medical profession and something of a monument to the tenacity of the ideas of liberty and laissez-faire. Onslaughts against it in the legislature proved unsuccessful in 1870, 1877, and 1878.[48] The Royal Commission of 1882, acknowledging that " the assumption of medical titles by unregistered persons has constantly . . . excited much indignation," and that the pertinent section of the 1858 Act had " proved unsuccessful," nevertheless considered " it undesirable to attempt to prevent unregistered persons from practising." [49] In this respect, T. H. Huxley agreed with his colleagues on the Commission. " I think it is very much more wholesome for the public to take care of itself in this as in most other matters," he later wrote, " and am not such a fanatic for the liberty of the subject as to plead that interfering with the way in which man may choose to be killed or cured is a violation of that liberty, yet I do think it is far better to let everybody do as he likes." Huxley thought that it would be impossible to legislate the unqualified out of existence and deplored the " trade-unionism " he thought he detected in the activity of the profession. To the public he would say, " Practise medicine if you like—go to be practised upon by anybody." To the profession he would say, " Have a qualification or do not have a qualification if people don't mind it." [50]

The history of medical regulation follows closely the model of the " legislative-cum-administrative process " hypothecated by Oliver Mac-

[44] Poynter, *op. cit.*, ftn. 24 above, p. 13.
[45] 31 and 32 Vict., c. 121, sections 1, 15.
[46] Bell and Redwood, *op. cit.*, ftn. 17 above, pp. 327-328, 374.
[47] L. G. Matthews, *History of Pharmacy in Britain* (Edinburgh: Livingstone, 1962), p. 136.
[48] Royal Commissioners *Report* (1882), *op. cit.*, ftn. 6 above, pp. xxxvi, xlvii-xlviii.
[49] *Ibid.*, p. xiii.
[50] Huxley, *op. cit.*, ftn. 21 above, pp. 228-230.

Donagh.[51] Medicine was of course not alone in this process: factory, poor-laws, prison, education, and public health reforms all point up that the era of political reform was accompanied by much that was to foreshadow the welfare state.[52]

With especial regard to medicine, the impact of internecine wrangling on the legislation may perhaps have been greater than the arguments of liberty and laissez-faire, and the eventual establishment of the register and of a Medical Council of increasing prestige and power does suggest that consideration of social need had won out over the traditional spirit of freedom. It is true that the Act of 1886 did impose a triple qualification upon the medical profession, and that the Pharmacy and Poisons Act of 1933 was to impose membership in the British Pharmaceutical Society on every registered pharmacist, but the principle of definitive regulation remained, a significant survivor of the idea of laissez-faire and liberty. The principle still persists: the Medicines Act now under consideration exempts the herbalist from penalties so long as he sticks to his herbs and herbal decoctions and his "patient" is aware of what he is getting.[53] The shade of Nicholas Culpeper, champion of the liberty of the subject and idol of the herbalists of today, stands athwart the battlements holding both the State and modern pharmacodynamics at bay.

[51] O. MacDonagh, "The nineteenth century revolution of government: A reappraisal," Histor. J., 1958, 1: 58-61.
[52] See, D. Roberts, Victorian Origins of the British Welfare State (New Haven: Yale Univ. Press, 1960).
[53] I am indebted to Leslie G. Matthews, Esq. for his calling my attention to these aspects of both the 1933 Act and the pending Medicines Act referred to here.

AN EARLY NEW JERSEY MEDICAL LICENSE

JOSIAH C. TRENT

Before the Revolutionary War attempts by the colonies to regulate medical practice were for the most part ineffectual. Virginia in 1639 had adopted a law compelling the physician, if required by the debtor, to state the cost of his medicines under oath. In 1736 the same state enacted the first fee bill which was "An Act regulating the fees and Accounts of the Practicers of Physic." One rate was allowed for "Surgeons and Apothecaries who have served an apprenticeship to those trades" and a higher rate "to those persons who have studied physic in any University and taken any degree therein."[2] Chronologically these acts were much in advance of any in the more northern colonies although Massachusetts in 1649, with good intentions but poor results, passed a law aimed at protecting the populace from untrained practitioners of medicine.[1] Sixteen years later a law almost identical with the Massachusetts law was promulgated in New Jersey by the Duke of York.[5] Several other colonies and some of the larger cities in particular had adopted laws which granted partial recognition to the profession and some measure of protection to the people, but it was not until 1760 that any real beginning was made toward effectual control of the practice of physic. On June 10, 1760 New York passed a law which required the practitioners in the city of New York to obtain a license certifying their qualifications from his Majesty's Council, Judges of the Supreme Court, the King's attorney-general and the mayor of that city.[3] But even in this law there were many loop-holes, and in spite of the gradually increasing interest in medical legislation evinced by the colonies, quacks and charlatans flourished unchecked. Walsh[4] quotes the following passage from Smith's history of New York written shortly before the war:

Few physicians among us are eminent for their skill. Quacks abound like locusts in Egypt, and too many have recommended themselves to a full and profitable practice and subsistence. This is the less to be wondered at as the profession is under no kind of regulation. Loud as the call is, to our shame be it remembered, we have no law to protect the lives of the King's subjects from the malpractice of pretenders. Any man at his pleasure sets up for physician, apothecary and chirurgeon. No candidates are either examined or licensed or even sworn to fair practice.

It remained for New Jersey to enact the first significantly effective medical legislation in the colonies. In 1771 the newly formed state medical society (1766) petitioned the assembly for an act "regulating the practice of medicine." As a direct result of this action a law was passed on September 26, 1772 which was closely patterned after the New York law of 1760 but which was more specific and strict in its requirements.[6]   The law reads in part:

Whereas many ignorant and unskilful persons in Physic and Surgery, to gain a subsistence, do take upon themselves to administer Physic and practice Surgery, in the Colony of New Jersey, to the endangering of the Lives and Limbs of their Patients; and many of His Majesty's subjects who have been persuaded to become their patients have been Suffering thereby; for the Prevention of such Abuses for the future Be It Enacted by the Governor, Council and General Assembly and it is hereby Enacted by the Authority of the same, That from and after the Publication of this act, no person whatsoever shall practice as a Physician or Surgeon, within this Colony of New Jersey, before he shall have first been examined in Physic and Surgery, approved of, and admitted by any two of the judges of the Supreme Court, for the time being, taking to their Assistance for such Examination such proper Person or Persons, as they in their Discretion shall think fit, . . .[7]

The law thus provided for the licensing of physicians by judges of the Supreme Court after an examination before a board of medical men who were usually appointed by the Society.

I have in my possession what is thought to be one of the earliest licenses issued under the new law. It was issued to one Peter Turner who apparently has left no record of his accomplishments and signed by Frederick Smythe who served as Chief Justice of the Supreme Court of New Jersey from 1764 to 1776 and who thus was the last chief justice before the war. Although the license is foxed and torn in some places the writing is still legible and reads as follows:

> To all to whom   [these presents shall]
> come or may concern: [Know] ye
> That we whose names are hereunto ins-
> -scribed, in Pursuance of an act of the
> Governor, Council & General Assem-
> -bly of the Colony of   [New Jersey . . .]
> in the twelfth year of the Reign of our Sovereign
> Lord King George the third, entitled an Act
> to regulate the practice of Physic & Surgery
> within the Colony of New Jersey, have duly
> [examined] Peter Turner, Physician & Surgeon,

and having approved of his skill do admit
him as a Physician & Surgeon, to practice in
the said faculties throughout the Colony
of New Jersey,　　　In Testimony where[of we]
have hereunto subscribed [oure names and]
affixed oure seals to this Instrument, at
Perth Amboy, this Ninth day of April
Annoque Domini 1773

Fre: Smythe　　　　seal

According to Wickes [8] "the effect of the law upon the profession was immediate. It raised the standard of attainment and thus stimulated students to careful study and to improve the opportunities which were now beginning to offer themselves to students in medicine."

BIBLIOGRAPHY

1. Green, S. A.: *A Centennial Address Delivered in the Sanders Theatre at Cambridge, June 7, 1881, Before the Massachusetts Medical Society*, Groton, 1881, pp. 34-35.
2. Packard, F. R.: *History of Medicine in the United States*, New York, Hoeber, 1931, pp. 163-166.
3. Toner, J. M.: *Contributions to the Annals of Medical Progress and Medical Education in the United States before and during the War of Independence*, Washington, 1874, pp. 51-52.
4. Walsh, J. J.: *History of Medicine in New York*, National Americana Society, 1919, Vol. I, p. 75.
5. Wickes, S.: *History of Medicine and Medical Men in New Jersey*, Newark, Martin R. Dennis and Co., 1879, pp. 54-55.
6. *Id.*, pp. 55-56.
7. *Id.*, pp. 102-105.
8. *Id.*, p. 56.

EARLY MEDICAL LEGISLATION IN LOUISIANA
AND
A STATE MEDICAL BOARD EXAMINATION IN 1816

CHARLES I. SILIN, Ph. D.
Tulane University

The purpose of this paper is to present an early—if not the earliest—report of an oral examination given by a state board of medical examiners to a candidate for a license to practice medicine, and to publish the legislation which established the board and regulated the practice of medicine.

* * * * *

Five years after the Louisiana Purchase, the Legislature of the Territory of Orleans passed the first act establishing the procedure to be followed in order to obtain a license to practice. This measure, entitled " An Act Concerning Physicians, Surgeons, and Apothecaries," was signed by Governor W. C . C. Claiborne on March 23, 1808.[1] Its provisions are as follows:

> Be it enacted by the Legislative Council and House of Representatives of the Territory of Orleans, in General Assembly convened, That no person shall presume to practice, in the Territory of Orleans, as physician, surgeon or apothecary, without first exhibiting satisfactory proof of his having qualified himself as such, by previous studies, which shall be made to appear by a diploma of any university or school in which he may have pursued his studies. The candidate shall exhibit said diploma to the Mayor of the City of New Orleans, who shall fix on a day, and shall appoint four physicians or surgeons from among the oldest practitioners, whose duty it shall be publicly to examine the candidate, and to give him a certificate of admission, if he should be admitted; which certificate shall be signed by the four examiners, and by the Mayor, who shall cause the seal of the city to be affixed to the same.
>
> 2. And be it further enacted, That every physician, surgeon or apothecary, who shall sell, or cause to be sold, remedies or drugs, which shall be proved to have been, at the time of selling the same, injured, moulded,

---

[1] *Acts Passed at the First Session of the Second Legislature of the Territory of Orleans.* N. O.: Bradford and Anderson, 1808, pp. 24-30. The Sessions Laws of early Louisiana were published in both French and English, while the Journals appeared in French only.

discomposed, or sophisticated, shall, on conviction, forfeit and pay the sum of five hundred dollars, to the benefit of the hospital of the poor of New Orleans.

3. And be it further enacted, That no physician, surgeon or apothecary, shall sell, give, or in any way, directly or indirectly, part with any suspicious or dangerous remedy, but on application in writing of heads of families of good reputation. And it shall be the duty of said heads of families, in said application in writing, to state for what use said remedy is wanted, the day on which said remedy was delivered, and receive the name, the quality, and the quantity of said remedy. Said application in writing shall be the only means of defence allowed to the seller, in case said remedy should have been made use of with evil design; and should the seller prove unable to exhibit such a writing for his discharge, he shall be deprived of the exercise of his profession, and shall forfeit and pay the sum of one thousand dollars, to the benefit of the hospital of New Orleans.

4. And be it further enacted, That no salaries shall be exacted but by such physicians, surgeons, and apothecaries as shall have been examined and admitted in conformity with the provisions of this act, or who were residing in the territory of Orleans prior to the passage of said act. And the physicians applying for salaries, shall exhibit an account written in the language which is spoken by the debtor or his assign; and this account shall mention the year, the month and the day when the physician shall have been called for and employed; it shall define clearly the name and the characteristic symptoms of the disease, the detail of the remedy (whether simple or composed), the order in which said remedies were administered, how and with what drugs said remedy was composed; and the price claimed for every particular remedy, shall be added to every article of the account, which shall not be allowed but upon such conditions.

5. And be it further enacted, That the remedies thus administered by every physician and surgeon, shall be paid for at the rate of three hundred per cent. more than if the same had been bought at an apothecary's: provided, however, it be not in evidence that the remedies were useless, not convenient or too freely used for the mentioned disease; in which case the debtor may apply for a diminution of the account; and, in that case, a decision shall be had by three physicians or surgeons, two of whom shall be appointed by the debtor and one by the physician.

6. And be it further enacted, That verbal consultations, made at the house of the sick person, shall be charged four dollars, to be received by every consulting physician, not including the visit or journey; but in case of such consultations, the family physician shall not be entitled to the sum allowed to the other consulting physicians, he shall have a right only to the payment of his visit.

Visits made in the city shall be paid at the rate of four bits for each visit. Visits in the suburbs shall be paid at the rate of one dollar. But if the physician resides in the suburbs, the visit shall be paid no more than four bits.

Such visits only shall be paid as shall have been solicited. Every journey in the country shall be paid at the rate of four bits per league, both going and coming; Provided, all visits and journeys during the night shall be paid double, in the whole extent of the territory.

It is clear that the author of the Act of 1808 had before him like acts passed by legislatures of northern states, for some of the provisions are quite similar.[2] It will be noted, however, that the legislators neglected to provide any penalty for failure to comply with the licensing provisions of this act. Besides, the implication may be drawn from the first part of Section 4 that persons residing in the Territory prior to the passage of the act were not required to submit to an examination. The result was that numbers of quacks and charlatans continued to practice without a license.

This deplorable situation continued until 1816 when Representative Fortin,[3] who was a physician, introduced in the House " An Act prescribing the formalities to be observed in order to obtain the right of practising physic or the profession of apothecary within the State of Louisiana . . . ," which was passed over the opposition of the " American " members of the House,[4] and, after minor amendments in the Senate, was finally signed by Governor Claiborne on March 16, 1816.[5]

The new act omits all reference to fees, bills and drugs, leaving the door open to possible malpractice in the prescription and dis-

[2] Citations from statutes passed by northern legislatures may be found in Francis R. Packard, *History of Medicine in the United States,* 2 vols., N. Y.: Hoeber, 1931; Chap. III: " Early Medical Legislation."

[3] He is doubtless the same Fortin who is appointed a member of the Medical Board in 1819 and assumes office on July 21st of that year; cf. *Registre du Comité Médical de la Nouvelle-Orléans,* described below.

[4] The vote was 16 to 10. It is significant that the names in the " Yes " column are Creole and those in the " No " column are American; cf. *Journal de la Chambre des Représentans pendant la Seconde Session de la Seconde Législature de l'Etat de la Louisiane.* N. O.: P. K. Wagner, 1816, p. 46.

[5] *Acts Passed at the Second Session of the Second Legislature of the State of Louisiana.* N. O.: P. K. Wagner, 1816, pp. 84-86.

pensation of remedies and in the billing of patients. But it puts teeth into the requirement of certification by providing suitable penalties:

Sec. 1. Be it enacted by the Senate and House of Representatives of the State of Louisiana in general assembly convened; That from and after the first of August next, no individual shall have the right to practice physic or the profession of apothecary in any part of the State of Louisiana, without having previously undergone an examination, in the city of New Orleans, and obtained a certificate which shall be delivered to him by a medical board, in the manner hereafter prescribed.

Sec. 2. And be it further enacted; That it shall be the duty of the Governor, to appoint on the second Monday of April in every year, a medical board composed of four physicians and one apothecary, and to make said appointment known to the members composing the medical board, and to the mayor of New Orleans; the functions of the said board shall be to examine all the individuals who shall apply for the right of practicing physic or the profession of apothecary within the State of Louisiana.

Sec. 3. And be it further enacted; That every individual who shall intend to practice physic or exercise the profession of apothecary within this State, shall present to the mayor of New Orleans, a petition in which he shall state his intention and the wish to comply with the formalities prescribed by law, whereupon the mayor shall summon the medical board which shall be held to meet at the places pointed out in the summon; the board shall proceed to the examination and in the presence of the mayor and of two aldermen designated by him, and if a majority of the board are satisfied with the answers of the candidate, they shall grant him a certificate of examination and reception which certificate shall be signed by all the members of the board or a majority of them, and certified by the mayor; and it shall be the duty of individual thus received, to cause the said certificate to be recorded in the clerk's office of the parish in which he shall exercise his profession, in order to apply to it in case it should be necessary, provided always that every individual now practicing physic or the profession of apothecary and having complied with the formalities required by the act entitled " An act concerning physicians, surgeons and apothecaries," shall be authorised to continue the exercise of his profession, after having caused to be recorded in the clerk's office of the parish in which he practices, the certificate which the above recited act required him to obtain.

Sec. 4. And be it further enacted; That if any one shall practice physic or exercise the profession of apothecary in contravention of the law, the said person, shall incur a fine which shall not exceed one hundred dollars for the first offence, and should the offence be reiterated, such person for every new offence of the same description shall be subject to a fine at the discretion of the judge which shall not exceed two hundred dollars and to an imprisonment also at the discretion of the judge, which shall not exceed one year, and it shall be the duty of the attorney general of each district to prosecute the person so offending; provided that nothing in this section contained shall be made or construed to apply to any inhabitant or planter in the country, who on the application of any of his sick neighbours should procure them some alleviation or administer them any kind of physick.

Sec. 5. And be it further enacted; That the act entitled "An act concerning physicians, surgeons and apothecaries" past on the twenty third of March eighteen hundred and eight be and the same is hereby repealed.

In accordance with the Act of 1816, Governor Claiborne proceeded at once to appoint Doctors Trabuc, Gros, Conard, Spencer and Grandchamps as members of the "Medical Committee."[6] The Committee held its organization meeting on April 29, 1816, and elected Dr. Trabuc President, and Dr. Grandchamps, Secretary-Treasurer. It authorized the Secretary-Treasurer to purchase all articles necessary for the maintenance of his office, including a seal. It voted to impose an examination fee of fifty dollars of which ten was to pay for the Committee's expenses and the rest was to be divided among the members. It also decided that all candidates had to submit documentary proof that they had reached the age of 21.

Dr. Grandchamps started and his successors continued a *Registre du Comité Médical de la Nouvelle-Orléans* which was most meticulously kept up until August, 1854, and in which one finds recorded the activities of the Committee and the names of the thousands of physicians and surgeons to whom it granted license to practice.[7]

Although the Committee was established for the sole purpose of examining and licensing candidates, in the absence of regularly established agencies usually staffed by medically trained men it at once assumed functions and prerogatives of a scientific society, a

[6] It is interesting to note that Doctors Trabuc and Gros were also President and Vice-President of the "Medical Society of New Orleans" which was incorporated on February 16, 1818; cf. *Acts Passed at the Second Session of the Third Legislature of the State of Louisiana.* N. O.: J. C. de St. Romes, 1818, pp. 20-24.

[7] This precious document reposes, in an excellent state of preservation, in the library of Tulane University's School of Medicine.

medico-literary society, a board of sanitation, a board of public health, etc.[8] But the bulk of its work consisted of examining candidates. Between April 29 and July 24 it examined 26 candidates[9] of whom 19 were in Medicine and Surgery, 1 in Surgery alone, and 6 in Pharmacy. Of these, 21 passed without qualification, 4 were allowed probationary periods of practice of one year or six months, and one failed twice in one week and was told to try again in six months.[10]

One of these examinations, that given to Matthew Creighton of Attakapas, was reported by the examinee in a contemporary newspaper, and has remained hitherto unnoticed. In addition to the intrinsic interest of this report, it is also valuable as a possible illustration of what was being done to carry out the statutory provisions of the time. It may be well, however, to complete first the trend of legislation.

*　　*　　*　　*　　*

Squire Lea was the fourth candidate to appear before the Medical Committee, passing his examination of May 9th. When the Third Legislature convened on November 18th, Dr. Squire Lea was seated as a Representative from Feliciana County and became at once one of the most important members of the House.[11] He was interested not only in practical politics but also in the improvement of education and in the elevation of the medical profession, in both of which fields he sponsored new legislation.

On December 5, 1816, on Dr. Squire Lea's motion, the House re-

[8] In its first four months of existence, the Committee enters into scientific correspondence with the Medical Society of Marseilles, advises the City Council on means for preventing spread of contagious diseases following a flood due to a break in the levee, devises a method for handling a shipload of Negro slaves among whom smallpox has broken out, issues permits for burials, writes a testimonial letter on the sanitary state of the city's Hospital, etc., etc.

[9] One, Dr. Joseph Forster, native of Bavaria, was admitted by courtesy without an examination. Cf. *Registre*, 6 juin 1816.

[10] Auguste Provosty failed on June 6th and 12th; he passed at his third trial on Dec. 12th.

[11] He was, for example, named chairman of the permanent " comité de revision et des affaires non-terminées," and elected delegate to the electoral college; cf. *Journal de la Chambre des Représentans durant la Première Session de la Troisième Législature de l'Etat de la Louisiane*. N. O.: J. C. de St. Romes, 1817, pp. 5, 11.

solved to appoint a committee to inquire into the effects of the Act of March 16, 1816, with authority to address the President of the Medical Committee for the purpose of obtaining information necessary for the proper judgment as to the efficacy with which the statute was being administered.[12]

A few days later, Chairman Squire Lea wrote to President Trabuc asking for a written statement as to the activities of the Medical Committee. After due deliberation, the Medical Committee framed their answer.[13] In it they described the measures adopted at their organization meeting, which we noted above. In the matter of the $50 fee, however, the letter stated that the examination lasts for three hours, it glossed over the disposition of the money in vague terms, and added an " N. B." brimming with guilty conscience that diplomas had been furnished free to all those who appeared to be unable to pay for them, " et le nombre en est assez grand! "

The Committee went on to state that many pharmacists refuse to submit to an examination on the false pretext that they are druggists selling only simple medicines. It asked for legislation that would force them to come before the Committee and that would also authorize the Committee to inspect their pharmacies twice a year.

It asked for strong legislation providing for the prosecution of delinquents in the medical and surgical practice, crying that it is high time Louisiana were rid of " ces nombreux charlatans, ces ignorans étrangers à un art qu'ils exercent avec autant d'impudence que d'incapacité. . . ."

Further, it urged the necessity of establishing in New Orleans a Board of Health, suggesting that the Medical Committee would itself be glad to assume the functions of such a board, in which case it would establish a sanitary code modelled after those in Boston, New York and Philadelphia. It also hoped for a state Vaccination Bureau where children of the poor might be vaccinated by a doctor salaried by the State and working under the supervision of the Medical Committee.

But Dr. Squire Lea disregarded these suggestions and recommendations. He was less interested in increasing the powers of the

[12] *Ibid.*, p. 17. [13] *Registre*, pp. 13-15.

old-timers on the Medical Committee than he was in improving the administration of the Act of 1816. In his report to the House, on January 10, 1817,[14] he recommended that the powers of the Medical Committee be limited strictly to the examining and licensing of physicians and surgeons, even omitting apothecaries. He even advised that the Legislature limit the Committee's jurisdiction to the eastern part of the state, setting up a second Medical Board for the western half. And to cap the climax, he recommended that the examination fee be reduced to $20. These recommendations were incorporated in a new act which was passed and signed by the new Governor, James Villeré, on February 18, 1817:[15]

> An Act supplementary to an act entitled: "An Act prescribing the formalities to be observed in order to obtain the right of practicing physic, or the profession of apothecary within the State of Louisiana, and for other purposes."
>
> Section 1. Be it enacted by the Senate and House of Representatives of the State of Louisiana in general Assembly convened, That for the convenience of the citizens of this state, there shall be appointed in and for each of the judicial districts of the supreme court of this state, a medical board, consisting of physicians eminent for their medical skill and science; the board for the eastern district shall hold their sessions in New Orleans, and be composed of five members; the board for the western district shall hold their sessions at Opelousas, and the town of Alexandria, Rapides, and shall be composed of six members.
>
> Sect. 2. And be it further enacted, That the board at present organized in New Orleans shall constitute the board for the eastern district of this state, and that Alfred Thruston, Ramus Davis, Ive Devy, Daniel Yeizer, John Rippey, and James Carman, shall be, and are hereby constituted members of the western board of this state; three of the members of either board shall constitute a quorum to do business, and all vacancies occurring hereafter in either board, shall be filled by a commission from the governor, (with the advice and consent of the senate) as members of the medical board for the eastern or western district of the state of Louisiana, as the case may be; provided however, that no member shall

[14] Journal of this session, cited above, note 11, p. 37.
[15] *Acts Passed at the First Session of the Third Legislature of the State of Louisiana.* N. O.: J. C. de St. Romes, 1817, pp. 90-94. A year later, the Legislature will enact a complete and well considered measure entitled "An Act to establish a Board of Health and Health Office, and to prevent the introduction of Malignant, Pestilential and Infectious Diseases into the City of New Orleans"; cf. *Acts Passed at the Second Session of the Third Legislature of the State of Louisiana.* N. O.: J. C. de St. Romes, 1818, pp. 124-152.

be appointed for either board who has not obtained a certificate to practice the profession of apothecary or surgery under some law of this state; provided that the apothecary making part of the board of New Orleans, shall only take part to the examination of apothecaries to be licenced by virtue of the act now in force.

Sect. 3. And be it further enacted, That the members of each board, shall choose from among their own number a president, who shall preside at their respective meetings, they shall also appoint a clerk, who shall keep a correct journal of all the proceedings of the board, which shall contain a registry of the names of the different applicants they may have admitted, in virtue of this act, to the practice of physic and surgery, and the majority of either board agreeing to the admission of an applicant after his examination, shall be authorised to issue a certificate of such examination and admission, for which they may demand and receive the sum of twenty dollars to be appropriated as the board may direct.

Sect. 4. And be it further enacted, That the powers of each board shall be confined to the admission to the right of practicing physic and surgery of such applicants as reside within their respective districts; provided that the persons thus once admitted, shall be entitled to practice as physicians or surgeons, as the case may be, throughout the state.

Sect. 5. And be it further enacted, That all persons who may have practiced medicine in the State of Louisiana for and during the space of ten years antecedent to the date of the act to which this is a supplement, are hereby permitted to practice physic in the state without being obliged to obtain a licence as required for other physicians by the laws of this state.

Sect. 6. And be it further enacted, That so much of the act to which this is a supplement as is in opposition to the provisions of this act, be, and the same is hereby repealed.

*   *   *   *   *

On July 24, 1816, Matthew Creighton of Attakapas failed his examination before the Medical Committee at New Orleans,[16] being the 26th candidate to appear before them under the Act of 1816, and the 4th to be given a probationary period. Shortly thereafter, Creighton wrote out what purported to be an accurate account of the examination, and sent his transcription to the editor of the bilingual *Louisiana Courier*, published at New Orleans. His ac-

[16] Alfred Thruston, also from Attakapas, passed on the same day; though he had only recently come to Louisiana from Virginia, he was the first man named for membership on the Medical Committee for the western half of the state, as provided in Section 2 of the Act of 1817.

count appeared in that paper on August 23, 1816, in both English and French.

This aroused the indignation of the Medical Committee who instructed their Secretary to write to the paper as follows:

New Orleans, Aug. 31, 1816

Mr. Editor,

The piece inserted in No. 1393 of your paper (23d August), entitled " A Faithful Statement of an Examination by the Louisiana Medical Board," &c., is of the fabric of Mr. Matthew Creighton, physician at Attakapas. That gentleman having undergone the examination prescribed by law, and not having answered in a satisfactory manner to the questions laid to him by the Medical Board, was referred to a new examination. The Board allowed him one year to prepare for it.—Instead of availing himself of this indulgence, he has amused himself with writing a long series of questions and answers which he addressed to you for insertion; but, with the exception of a few of the latter which attest the ignorance of that pretending physician, all is a mere invention. The Board have thought it necessary to give this information to the public, who may see in that extraordinary piece the work of a man endeavoring to throw ridicule upon an useful institution, the members of which are too well known to find themselves within the reach of such shaft, and who shall always make it their duty to exercise with zeal and impartiality the functions confided to them by government.

Please to insert the above in your next paper, and to accept the sentiments with which I have the honor to be, &c.

By order of the Medical Board,

GRANDCHAMPS,
Secretary.

Obviously, Creighton's version of the examination must be regarded with a certain amount of reserve. Under the best of circumstances, no candidate can reproduce from memory a complete and accurate account of a long oral examination to which he has been subjected. Furthermore, when he has been failed by the examining board, he becomes *ipso facto* an unreliable witness as to the conduct of the examination. And when, besides, the board officially declares that the report is a fabric of his own imagination, then one must certainly be cautious in accepting his account.

One cannot, however, throw the whole thing out as a hoax unworthy of serious attention. The Committee's assertion that the report is an attempt to make them appear ridiculous does not seem substantiated by the account itself. The account does not show that the questions asked were foolish, that the answers accepted were grossly erroneous, or that the remarks made by the members of the Committee indicated a gross lack of knowledge on their part. On the contrary, ridicule falls rather upon the candidate himself who is repeatedly made to falter and to fail.

The secretary of the Committee admits that Creighton is accurately reproducing some of his erroneous answers. By implication, then, the secretary is also admitting that some of the questions are also accurately reproduced. Would the historian therefore not be on safe ground in entertaining the possibility that the whole account is as accurate as imperfect memory will permit? It is quite possible that the Committee, feeling that medicine is an esoteric science the mysteries of which should not be spread before the laity, regarded Creighton's violation of the confidence of its procedure as an act of *lèse-majesté,* and that, feeling the necessity of showing their displeasure and hoping thereby to preclude recurrences of such an unwise act in the future, they unwarrantedly branded the whole thing as pure invention unworthy of a real physician.

Aside from these considerations, the examination remains important because the Committee disclaims it only in part. We therefore feel no hesitancy in submitting the English text of the examination as an item of great interest to students of the history of medicine in the United States:

A FAITHFUL STATEMENT OF AN EXAMINATION BY THE
LOUISIANA MEDICAL BOARD, HELD AT N. ORLEANS,
THE 24TH JULY, 1816.

Question. What are the bones of anatomy? —Answer. Do you wish me to name every bone in order?

Q. What are the bones of the skull? —A. Os frontis, two parietal bones, os occipitis, two temporal bones. (Much talking.)

Q. What number of bones belong to the skull? —A. Six. (The board then said no; there are eight—and said it was of the greatest importance to know these bones.)

Q.What are the bones of the thorax? —A. Sternum, the ribs, and the vertebra.

Q. How many vertebra are there? —A. Twenty-four.

Q. How do you divide them? —A. Seven cervical, twelve dorsal, and five lumbar.

Q. What are the bones of the pelvis? —A. Os sacrum, os coccygis, and two ossa innominata.

Q. How many bones are there in the ossa innominata? —A. In the adult one, in the young subject three.

Q. What do you call the thigh bone? —A. Os femoris.

Q. How many bones are there in the leg? —A. Two.

Q. What are their names? —A. Tibia & fibula.

Q. Is there not another bone in the leg? —A. No, none that I know of.

(The board articulated rotula.) —A. Ah! the patella is on the articulation of the knee: not in the leg.

Q. What are the bones of the foot? —A. Tarsus, metatarsus, and toes.

Q. How many bones are there of the tarsus? —A. Seven.

Q. What are their names? —A. I do not remember their names.

Q. How many bones are there in the metatarsus? —A. Five.

Q. What are the bones of the shoulder? —A. Clavicula and scapula.

Q. What is the name of the arm bone? A. Os humeri.

Q. How many bones are there in the fore arm? —A. Two.

Q. What are their names? —A. Radius & ulna.

Q. How many bones of the carpus? —A. Eight.

Q. What are their names? —A. I do not remember their names.

Q. Is there not a little bone lays under the scapula!!! —A. No; none that I know of.

Q. Is there no other bone? —A. None other.

Q. What! no bone? (putting his hand to his throat.) —A. Do you mean, sir, the larynx or pharynx? (From the board, No.)

Q. Is there not a bone here? (putting his hand again to his throat.) —A. None that I can recollect. (A significant shrug from the board.)

Q. What are the bones made of? —A. Do you mean their component parts?

Q. Yes, their component parts. —A. Phosphorie——I do not know, sir. (The board said that it was very necessary to know the composition of bones, to be able to treat diseases!!!)

Q. What is the substance of the bones? —A. I do not understand you, sir.

Q. Are the bones hard all through? —A. The ends of some bones have little cells for the medullary juice.

Q. What would you do for a puking of blood! —A. From the stomach, sir?

Q. Yes, from the stomach. —A. What is the state of the patient?

Q. He has a puking of blood from the stomach. —A. If it was a recent attack from plethora, or a blow, I would bleed him from the arm, and give him an astringent dose. (I was then told that the blood should be taken from the foot.)

Q. What dose would you give? —A. Common salt or gum kino.

Q. What other medicine would you give? —A. If the indication was such, I would give ipecacuanha.

Q. What would you give ipecac. for? —A. To lessen arterial action.

Q. What are the causes of a puking of blood? —A. Plethora, blow on the stomach—poisonous ingestion——.

Q. Are there no other causes? —A.—Perhaps obstructed menstruation. (A nod of approbation from the board.)

Q. What are the symptoms? —A. A sense of weight and obtuse pain in the region of the stomach; a pricking in the stomach.

Q. Are there no other symptoms? —A. Yes, sir; —a—a—flushing of the face. (I was then told from the board that the face was pale.)

Q. What is the difference of blood from the stomach and blood from the lungs? —A. The one being more black and coagulated than the other.

Q. Which would be the more black? —A. That from the stomach.

Q. Suppose the patient passed a little blood downwards, what would you do!! —A. Does the gentleman mean a passive hamorrhagae?

(From the board) Yes. —A. I would give tonics.

Q. What tonics? —A. Bark.

Q. What drink would you give? —A. Water.

Q. Would you give any acids? —A. Yes.

Q. What acid would you give? —A. Sulphuric acid.

Q. Is there nothing else? —A. I now recollect of none other. (I was then told from the board, that blisters should be put on the thorax some distance from the stomach in order to divert the disease!!)

Q. How many tumours are there? —A. There are a great many, more than I can recollect.

Q. Can you recollect any? —A. There are encysted tumours, inflammatory tumours, sarcomatous tumours, and a—a—.

Q. How many tumours are there in the groin? —A. There is a hernia, a—a—.

Q. Are there no other tumours in the groin? —A. Is it a strangulated hernia, sir, you ask me for?

Q. The gentleman asks if there are no other tumours in the groin? —A. There is a—a—bubo.

Q. How do you distinguish a hernia from a bubo? —A. In a strangulated hernia the patient feels pain all over the belly, is sick, he can seldom stand still even for a short time, he will either go forward or backwards.

Q. How do you distinguish a bubo from a hernia? —A. A bubo has an inflammatory appearance, examine if there was syphilis lurking in the system, it has a round firm base, a—a—.

Q. You say, that in a hernia the patient can't stand still? —A. Yes: he will either go backwards or forwards, pain and sickness accompanying. (I was then told from the board that a hernia gave no pain, that it had a hard feel as a bubo.)

Q. How does a bubo progress and terminate? —A. It progresses either fast or slow, and terminates in resolution or ulcer.

Q. Do you know what a whitlow is? —A. There is a sensation of heat and pain in the end of the finger, it becomes more tender and swells, and ends like inflammation.

Q. Does a whitlow extend to the periostum & to the joint? —A. Yes.

Q. What would you do·with it then? —A. I would lay it open as far as the sinus went.

Q. Where would you make the incision? —A. At the most depending part.

Q. Would you make the incision in front of the finger? —A. Yes, sir. (The board shook their heads and told me that the incision should be a lateral one, or the theca of the flexor tendon would be wounded and the finger made stiff.)

Q. What treatment would be best after the finger was opened? —A. Apply an emollient poultice, afterwards a simple pledget.

Q. What would be your general treatment, i. e. internal, or treatment of the system? —A. At the commencement, sir?

Q. Yes, at the commencement. —A. The treatment should be entirely antiphlogistic.

Q. After it is cured up or got well, what part of the body or where would it break out again!!! —A. I do not know where it would break out again.

Q. What is the cause of whitlow? —A. It often originates from bruises, change of temperament, a—a—from pricks of needles.

Q. What is pink-root good for? —A. It is given as an anthelmintic.

Q. What else is it good for? —A. I do not remember anything else.

Q. What is a better anthelmintic? —A. Calomel.

Q. How would you give the pink-root? —A. In infusion.

Q. How? —A. Make a tea.

Q. What is calomel good for? —A. It's a purgative, it excites ptyalism, it's antivenereal, it's an anthelmintic, it's good in chronic inflammation, it's—it's—it's—.

Q. What else is it good for? —A. It's—it's—it's———I remember nothing else.

Q. How would you check its effects on the system? —A. Do you mean a profuse ptyalism?

Q. Yes. —A. Stop giving any more, give an astringent gargle, with laxatives, or sulphuret of kali.

Q. What is the dose of calomel for a child 4 years old!!! —A. (Indignation—indignation—indignation—) 4 grs. is the proportion if 16 are given to an adult.

MALPRACTICE SUITS IN AMERICAN MEDICINE
BEFORE THE CIVIL WAR *

CHESTER R. BURNS **

Numerous court actions involving medical practitioners occurred in the United States before the Civil War. Problems with medical licensure, admission and expulsion prerogatives of a medical society, and matters of compensation were subjected to judicial review.[1] The majority of these court actions, though, involved affairs of forensic medicine and accusations of malpractice. In this paper, attention is focused on malpractice claims, as foreboding to doctors then as now.

There are no reliable statistics for the total number of medical malpractice actions initiated before the Civil War. No one has systematically tabulated cases adjudicated in local courts without appeal.[2] To provide

* This is a revised version of the paper presented on April 20, 1968, at the forty-first annual meeting of the American Association for the History of Medicine, St. Louis, Missouri.

** This investigation was supported by U. S. Public Health Service Training Grant numbers 5 TO1 LM00105-08 and 5 TO1 LM00105-09 from the National Library of Medicine.

[1] Some cases illustrating these court actions are cited in *Century Edition of the American Digest, 1658-1896*. St. Paul: West Pub. Co., 1903, vol. 39, " Physicians and Surgeons," sections 5-6, 13, 50-62.

[2] Smith and Sandor prepared general surveys of malpractice cases in American medicine. Hubert W. Smith, "Legal responsibility for medical malpractice. IV. Malpractice claims in the United States and a proposed formula for testing their legal sufficiency," *J. A. M. A.*, 1941, *116*: 2670-2679. Andrew A. Sandor, "The history of professional liability suits in the United States," *J. A. M. A.*, 1957, *163*: 459-466. Smith located twenty-three cases for the period, 1794-1860. But, as Sandor observes, Smith made no distinction as to type of practitioner. Thus, for example, he included a case involving a veterinarian (1856 Indiana, Conner v. Winton). Sandor located 224 cases for the period 1794-1900 but offered no further chronological subdivision. Neither Smith nor Sandor gave complete citations to the cases used for their tables; nor did they offer detailed analyses of their tabulated cases.

Randomly, I have located ten non-appeal examples for the pre-Civil War period. References to these are as follows: John J. Elwell, *A Medico-Legal Treatise on Malpractice and Medical Evidence, comprising the Elements of Medical Jurisprudence*. New York: John S. Voorhies, 1860, pp. 115-117, 146-162, 163-168; *Buffalo M. J. and Month. Rev.*, 1847, *3*: 145-148, 196-197, 220-225, 447-448; John C. Warren, *A Letter to the Hon. Isaac Parker, Chief Justice of the Supreme Court of the State of Massachusetts, Containing Remarks on the Dislocation of the Hip Joint, Occasioned by the Publication of a Trial which took place at Machias, in the State of Maine, June, 1824.* Cambridge: Printed by Hilliard and Metcalf, 1826; Azariah B. Shipman, *A Report of the Facts and Circumstances relating to a Case of Compound Fracture, and Prosecu-*

108

some quantitative perspective, a survey of trial court records in particular states would be informative, but, practically speaking, impossible to a prospective surveyor.[3] The following report is limited to an analysis of twenty-seven malpractice suits that were adjudicated as appeals in various state supreme courts between 1794 and 1861, their distribution among sixteen states from Maine to California and Wisconsin to North Carolina indicating no regional monopoly.[4]

These appeals offer no evidence of extensive judicial bias for or against medical practitioners. Of seven trial court decisions for physicians, the state courts sustained two (J, AA), reversed one (G), and granted new trials in four cases (D, K, P, V). Of twenty lower court decisions for plaintiffs, the higher courts sustained eight (A, B, C, H, S, T, U, X), reversed six (E, I, L, Q, R, Z), and granted new trials in six cases (F, M, N, O, W, Y). Each of these six categories will now be illustrated by a representative case.

In the late 1850's, the Lee District Court of Iowa had not allowed the plaintiff, Mr. Piles, to recover damages for alleged negligent treatment of a fractured leg (AA). The plaintiff believed that shortening of his leg had been caused by the defendant's negligence. In October of 1860, the claims of Piles vs. Hughes were presented before the Supreme Court of Iowa. According to a defense witness, the limb had been measured at the time of discharge, and the plaintiff had agreed with the reasons

tion for Mal-practice, in which William Smith was plaintiff, and Drs. Goodyear and Hyde were defendants, at Cortland Village, Cortland Co., N.Y., March 1841. Cortland-ville: S. Haight, 1841; and *St. Louis M. and S. J.*, 1846, *3*: 529-563.

[3] However, for the colonial period, an examination of published court records might be rewarding. The available records are evaluated by Michael G. Kamman, "Colonial court records and the study of early American history: a bibliographical review," *Am. Hist. Rev.*, 1965, *70*: 732-739.

[4] My list of appeal reports was compiled from *Century Edition of the American Digest, 1658-1896, op. cit.*, sections 35, 37, 38; Smith, *op. cit.*, pp. 2672-2673; and Sandor, *op. cit.*, pp. 461-463. Some cases cited in these sources were not included in my study for specific reasons. Sumner v. Utley (1828 Connecticut) involved a suit for slander initiated by a physician against a patient. The phrases of slander included malpractice accusations, but the patient had not initiated a malpractice suit *per se*. Piper v. Menifee (1851 Kentucky) and Graham v. Gautier (1858 Texas) were suits initiated by physicians for fees. The patient-defendants rebutted with malpractice accusations.

Some guidelines for my approach were suggested by Stetler in his cautious and informative analysis of 605 decisions occurring between 1935 and 1955. C. Joseph Stetler, "The history of reported medical professional liability cases," *Temple Law Quart.*, 1956-57, *30*: 366-383.

In an appendix, the twenty-seven appeals selected for analysis are listed according to date and state, commonly used legal citation to the state reports, and a more complete citation to these reports. In the appendix, each appeal is preceded by an alphabet letter that is used for textual and footnotes references.

given by the defendant to explain the shortening. The plaintiff's lawyer argued that the district court had instructed the jury improperly. The court should have asked the jury to evaluate the defendant's actions by criteria of extraordinary skill, since, claimed the lawyer, the defendant had presented himself as a physician and surgeon of extraordinary skill. The supreme court justices maintained that no evidence had been given to show that the defendant ever professed extraordinary skill. They also ruled that shortening of a leg after recovery from a fracture was not *prima facie* evidence of negligence or unskillfulness on the part of the surgeon. For these reasons, the Iowa Supreme Court upheld the lower court decision in favor of the physician.

The following 1845 Pennsylvania judgment is the only example, among the twenty-seven appeals, of a higher court reversing a lower court decision favorable to physicians. The Common Pleas Court of Northampton County, Pennsylvania, had rendered a verdict in favor of two physician-brothers who were sued for malpractice by Henry Mertz (G). Mertz believed that the defendants had improperly treated his injured leg, thereby necessitating amputation. The Pennsylvania Supreme Court, adducing three reasons, reversed this decision and awarded damages to the plaintiff. First, medical witnesses had refused to answer questions about the nature of remedies employed by the defendant. Second, medical colleagues had excluded the defendants from a consultation regarding the treatment of the plaintiff's gangrenous leg. Such exclusion indicated that these colleagues were biased towards the defendants. Third, a jury should not make a malpractice decision on the basis of testimony which upheld only the general skill and reputation of physicians. Each case should be evaluated according to the skill manifested in the particular circumstances.

The state courts granted four new trials after evaluating lower court decisions for physicians, one having occurred in Wisconsin (P). During the October 1853 term of the Racine, Wisconsin, Circuit Court, Benjamin Reynolds testified that the defendant had been retained to " set, dress, take care of, manage, and cure a certain broken bone " of his thigh.[5] For a mutually acceptable sum of money, the defendant agreed to " set, dress, take care of, and manage the broken bone " with "due and proper care, skill, and diligence." [6] The plaintiff accused the defendant of managing the broken bone in a " careless, unskillful, negligent, undue, and improper manner." [7] The bone became " crooked, weak, shortened, and useless," thereby making the plaintiff a cripple.[8] Counsel for the plaintiff introduced evidence which proved the injury, showed that the

[5] P, p. 416.   [6] **P, p. 417.**   [7] *Ibid.*   [8] *Ibid.*

defendant had been called " doctor," and signified that this " doctor " had treated the plaintiff's injured leg. Additional testimony disclosed that the precise place of the fracture had not been discovered until the plaintiff had consulted with other physicians, despite attendance by the defendant for several weeks. Specifying two reasons, defense counsel moved for a dismissal. First, no evidence had been presented which proved that the defendant was a physician and surgeon. Second, there was no proof that the defendant agreed to a special contract for cure. The circuit court judge refused to allow testimony regarding the nature of the defendant's profession. He also refused to allow a deletion of the word " cure " from the plaintiff's original declaration. A verdict was given in favor of the practitioner. At the time of appeal, a new trial was granted by the Supreme Court of Wisconsin. Although the original declaration did not contain any special agreement for cure, the lower court had made an error in not allowing presentation of evidence regarding the professional status of the defendant.

Eight lower court decisions for plaintiffs were sustained, as exemplified by the following. In 1843, a Maine practitioner decided that amputation was necessary to arrest thigh bone disease in one of his patients (H). After surgery, a portion of the femoral stump protruded from the muscular parts. Four years later, the plaintiff sued the surgeon and received a favorable verdict worth $2025. A motion for a new trial was presented before the Maine Supreme Court in 1848. Counsel for the defendant disclosed that the protruding portion of the femur was removed during a second operation. The plaintiff's lawyers declared that the defendant had made an error of judgment in not removing more of the diseased limb at the time of the first operation. Damages had not been awarded because the doctor failed to amputate the limb at the hip, a procedure eventually performed by another surgeon. Damages had been awarded because the defendant had allowed a portion of the femur to protrude after the first operation. As a result of this error, the plaintiff had experienced protracted suffering, increased expense, and extensive loss of time. The supreme court judge denied the motion for a new trial.

Reversal of a lower court verdict for a plaintiff is exemplified by an 1853 California lawsuit (L). The Tenth Judicial District Court of Yuba County had awarded a verdict to the plaintiff in a malpractice suit concerning amputation of his arm. The presiding judge of the district court had given the following instructions to the jury. " That if the jury believe, from the evidence, that the defendants were guilty of negligence, carelessness, or inattention, in their treatment of the plaintiff's wounds, by which the plaintiff was caused great *bodily pain and suffering*, the plaintiff is entitled to a verdict." [9] The California Supreme Court declared these instructions to be in error and reversed the lower court decision. The defendants had not been sued for causing bodily pain and suffering by their negligence. They had been sued for malpractice which resulted in the amputation of an arm. If the amputation had not been caused by a malpractice of the defendants, then they were entitled to a favorable verdict.

The following 1853 New Hampshire example is one of the six new trials granted by state courts after evaluating trial court decisions for plaintiffs. In the early 1850's, a jury of the Strafford County Court returned a verdict for the plaintiff, who had made malpractice accusations against a physician (O). The defendant had been employed to " treat, set, cure, and heal" the right ankle and foot of the plaintiff, which had been " dislocated, put out of joint, disruptured, broken, fractured, wounded, and bruised." [10] Because of negligent and unskillful treatment, the ankle and foot of the plaintiff had been " greatly inflamed, swollen and festering . . . for the space of eighteen months," eventually becoming " stiff, set, immoveable and fixed in an unnatural position." [11] Henceforth, the plaintiff was unable to walk without the aid of canes or crutches. It was also alleged that the ankle and foot of the plaintiff had become " greatly inflamed, virulent, corrupt and festering, and a mass of gathering putrid sores " because of the carelessness, negligence, and unskillfulness of the defendant. During the county court proceedings, counsel for the plaintiff contended that the defendant had failed to place the plaintiff's foot in a position at right angles with his leg. The limb had become useless for walking because the forward part of the foot had been depressed at an angle of about thirty or forty degrees during convalescence. Counsel for the plaintiff also introduced medical witnesses who testified that the course of treatment pursued by the defendant differed from that used by other practitioners. Defense counsel rebutted with testimony showing that means had been used to keep the foot at right angles to the leg. Witnesses also testified that the defendant had received a regular medical education.

These arguments were reviewed in appeal proceedings held during the December 1853 term of the Supreme Court of New Hampshire. The physician's lawyer asserted that the testimony regarding prolonged in-

[9] L, p. 190.
[10] O, p. 460.
[11] O, p. 461.

flammation and eventual immobility of the plaintiff's foot did not prove malpractice. Medical witnesses testified that "the swelling, festering, inflammation and sores were a necessary and unavoidable consequence of the severe injury and fracture the plaintiff had received," and would have accompanied the best possible surgical and medical treatment.[12] The plaintiff's lawyer asserted that the original declaration was adequate for sustaining the litigation. Perhaps a trifle unsure, he concluded by citing the 1845 Pennsylvania decision and reminding the court that a formal medical education did not mean that knowledge received as a result of such education had been appropriately used in a particular case. In an especially informative and carefully reasoned statement, Justice Bell presented the opinion of the New Hampshire Supreme Court. A malpractice verdict could be justified if it was proven that a physician fraudulently undertook to act as a physician without the education, knowledge, and skill which entitled medical practitioners to be so qualified; or, that having such knowledge and skill, a physician neglected to apply them with the care and diligence necessary for a particular case. In this 1853 suit of Leighton vs. Sargent, it was ruled that counsel for the plaintiff had not proven either point. Was the defendant ignorant or had he acted from negligence and carelessness? Evidence had been given that the defendant was not ignorant. Had the defendant adopted his course of treatment from negligence and lack of ordinary care, or from a mere error of judgment for which he was not liable? Since neither had been satisfactorily proven, a new trial was granted.

As indicated by these six examples, and corroborated by the other twenty-one, most malpractice claims originated with patients who believed that they had received improper treatment of their injuries or diseases. Fractures (E, F, J, M, O, P, Q, S, T, U, Y, AA), amputations (A, G, H, L), and dislocations (Z) comprised two-thirds of the ailments reported in these appeals.[13] Injured or diseased limbs of friends and relatives had returned to normal shape and function after surgical treatment. Why were theirs shortened or useless or absent? To them, the only apparent variable was medical care, and its unskillful application was surely responsible for their unfortunate conditions. Since these conditions—shortened

[12] O, pp. 464-465.
[13] Of those remaining, five involved deliveries (B, D, I, R, V), two involved drugs (K, N), one involved smallpox inoculation (C), and two were not specified (W, X). In 1860, Elwell stated that nine-tenths of all malpractice cases involved amputations, fractures, or dislocations. Elwell, *op. cit.*, p. 55. Stephen Smith believed that only two-thirds of malpractice suits involved these surgical problems. See Smith's review of Elwell's book in *Am. J. M. Sc.*, 1860, n. s. *40*: 162.

legs, amputated limbs, misshapen appendages, occasionally death—were irremediable, recompense was necessary, especially for injuries which prevented livelihood or family support.

Had the patients actually received improper medical treatment? It was probably not difficult to decide that a grocer (formerly dancing and fencing master) without a medical education was guilty of injuring both mother and infant during a delivery (B). But, if proven, did abandonment of a patient constitute malpractice (E)? Or, was a patient who did not obey the doctor's prescriptions entitled to recover for malpractice claims (G, J, S)? Or, was a physician guilty of malpractice when he treated a slave without the consent of his master (K)? These and other similarly difficult questions were considered by the doctors, lawyers, judges, and juries who examined the claims of each lawsuit.

Doctors provided presumably expert testimony to guide the thinking of the legal officials and the laymen who served on the juries. They were asked about the educational background and general reputation of the defendants and about their professional relationship to the defendants (G, P). They were requested to confirm the nature of the injury or disease, to evaluate the form of treatment employed by the defendant, and to state their opinion about the presence or absence of malpractice in a particular case (I, N). As seen in the 1845 Pennsylvania decision, refusal to answer legitimate questions could be as incriminating as positive statements. This testimony by physicians was seldom unimportant, often crucial.[14]

Lawyers provided logical analyses and rhetorical flourishes. The quest for logical accuracy is well-illustrated by the Maine lawyers who successfully argued that the surgeon was sued because he left a protruding portion of the femoral stump, not because he failed to remove more of the diseased limb. The linguistic displays were persuasive. Referring to the grocer who had been accused of midwifery malpractice, counsel for plaintiff proclaimed that a practitioner who acted without proper qualifications manifested " extreme depravity " and a " general hostility towards the human race." [15] The injury to the ankle and foot of the New Hampshire citizen must have seemed enormous when it was described as " dislocated, put out of joint, disruptured, broken, fractured, wounded, and bruised." Blends of logic and rhetoric were not infrequent. In the 1860 Iowa case, the issue of extraordinary versus ordinary skill, although

[14] A physician could even be an accuser. In one of the appeals, the plaintiff was a practicing surgeon who won a verdict of $1000 against the surgeon who had improperly treated his fractured arm (T).

[15] B, p. 265.

logically relevant to a definition of malpractice, was spontaneously introduced to confound the listeners.

The judges were compelled to respond to the crosscurrents produced
by the encounters of two professions and injured citizens. They repri-
manded counselors, censured their trial court colleagues, and delivered
conditional verdicts. In the 1848 Maine case, defense counsel had based
the motion for a new trial on reasons of excessive damages and discovery
of new evidence. The Maine Supreme Court told defense counsel that
use of ordinary diligence during the lower court proceedings would have
produced the so-called " new " evidence, which was not allowed in the
appeal hearing. Several state justices censured their lower court colleagues for inaccurately instructing juries. As seen in the 1853 California
decision, a few words in a judge's instructions were responsible for a
reversal. In the Kentucky suit involving treatment of a slave, a new trial
was awarded because the judge of the Fleming Circuit Court, in instructing the jury, altered the arguments of the plaintiff's counsel. In an 1853
session of the Common Pleas Court of Beaver County, Pennsylvania, the
presiding judge had charged the jury: " That the defendant was bound
to bring to his aid the skill necessary for a surgeon to set the leg so as
to make it straight and of equal length with the other, when healed; and
if he did not, he was accountable in damages, just as a stonemason or
bricklayer would be in building a wall of poor materials, and the wall fell
down; or if they built a chimney, and it would smoke, by reason of a
want of skill in its construction. . . ." [16] The Supreme Court of Pennsylvania labeled the analogy of surgery to stonemasonry as inaccurate and
misleading to a jury. In some cases, the lower court judges were censured for refusing to hear testimony. In Twombly vs. Leach, the Middle-
sex County, Massachusetts, Court judge allowed counsel for the plaintiff
to ask medical witnesses if it was good practice to say " you open a thumb
to cut off a nerve because it is already partly cut off ? " [17] Subsequently,
the judge did not allow defense counsel to ask these same doctors if they
saw any evidence of malpractice committed by Leach. The judge was
reproved by the Massachusetts Supreme Court for not allowing this
inquiry.[18] The conditional verdicts concerned money. Although denying
a new trial in the 1848 Maine case involving the protruding femur, the

---

[16] M, p. 120.

[17] N, p. 403. They stated that it was not good practice.

[18] It was also considered necessary for a trial court judge to state his opinion to a jury.
In 1860, a new trial was granted by the Supreme Court of North Carolina because a
lower court left " it to the jury to decide the question of skill and care in a surgeon's
treatment of his patient, without the aid of the court's opinion. . . ." (W, p. 298).

supreme court judge stipulated that the plaintiff had to reduce the sum of damages by $500 because " surgeons should not be deterred from the pursuit of their profession, by intemperate and extravagant verdicts." [19] One judgment was to be removed from the record if the court costs were paid in sixty days (D).

The judges exhibited varying attitudes towards doctors and medicine. One judge believed that the number of unqualified practitioners would be reduced if patients were encouraged to make malpractice accusations more frequently (M). The justices were especially sensitive to the distinction between medical and legal judgments. When the Pennsylvania Supreme Court discussed proper methods of treating fractures, various texts of surgery were quoted by two of the three justices. The third justice emphatically declared that questions of surgery had not been adjudicated. " But when we decide the legal point we are done with it. We are not authority on the questions of surgery." [20] Sometimes the judges forgot this point. In 1856, the presiding judge of the Washington County, Pennsylvania, Court of Common Pleas expressed astonishment at the inability of the defendant to diagnose the nature of a hip injury (S). How could there have been any doubt, inquired the judge, since the injury was promptly diagnosed by the surgeon who had appeared as a witness during the trial (held six years after the accident). In 1853, the Pennsylvania Supreme Court expected doctors to be equipped with the latest knowledge, " to be up to the improvements of the day." [21]

The actions of jurors were decisive in some appeals. A conversation between a juror and a defense witness constituted one reason for not allowing a new trial in the 1812 case involving the Connecticut grocer-midwife. A remarkable influence of juror behavior occurred in the New Hampshire suit of Leighton vs. Sargent. As previously described, a new trial had been granted in 1853. A Strafford County Court jury again returned a verdict for the plaintiff. At the request of a juror complaining of illness, brandy was brought into the jury room while this verdict was being decided. Thus, in a second appeal to the New Hampshire Supreme Court, the defendant was acquitted; " for the cause that brandy was furnished to the jury, and drank [sic] by several of them while deliberating upon the cause, after retiring to form their verdict, we think the verdict must be set aside." [22]

[19] H, p. 101. $1525 was still the largest award specified in these appeals. Others were $50 (I), 40 pounds (A), $500 (W), $900 (Y), and $1000 (T).
[20] M, p. 135.
[21] M, p. 128.
[22] Q, p. 137.

Final decisions were based on medical evidence, legal maxims, or both.
Of the six cases described earlier, medical evidence was decisive in the
1845 Pennsylvania, 1848 Maine, and 1853 New Hampshire decisions.
With widespread differences of opinion about medical treatment, it was
difficult, but not impossible, to obtain consistent or reliable medical evidence. A legitimate practitioner, aware of uncertainties and differences,
was reluctant to point an accusing finger towards a professional colleague.
In view of these scientific disagreements, it was important to maintain
cordial relationships with other physicians who might be called to testify
at one's malpractice trial. In determining final decisions, points of law
were as important as medical evidence. New trials were granted exclusively on points of law (D, Y). The exact words of the declaration or
of the judge were decisive, as seen in the 1853 California and 1854
Wisconsin illustrations. Several appeal verdicts were determined according to errors made by lower court judges in instructing juries (K, L, M,
W) or in refusing to allow testimony (N, P). One appeal involved the
question of who could sue in case of the death of the injured party (X).
Another involved the right of an injured party to sue a deceased surgeon
(Z). One enterprising New Yorker, having already won damages as
husband of the plaintiff, again sued a physician, this time as the admin-
istrator of his wife's estate (R).[23] In four appeals, including the 1860
Iowa case, legal and medical points were equally significant in determining the verdicts (N, S, V, AA). Final decisions were primarily
determined by points of medicine in ten cases, and points of law in
thirteen cases.[24]

Certain recurring judicial opinions may be viewed as fundamental legal
principles about medical malpractice announced by the state justices
before the Civil War.[25] These can be arranged in five groups, of which
the first dealt with education and knowledge.

A medical practitioner was held legally responsible for what he professed he was able to do. If he was unable to perform what he professed
he could do, he was practicing fraudulently. If a practitioner declared
himself to be a member of the medical profession, he was held liable for
lack of suitable education and training. In 1856, a justice of the Tennessee
Supreme Court declared that a physician " contracts with those who employ

[23] He was unsuccessful.
[24] Points of medicine: A, B, E, G, H, I, J, O, T, U. Points of law: C, D, F, K, L, M, P, Q, R, W, X, Y, Z.
[25] No attempt has been made to evaluate British precedents for these principles. For two oft-cited British cases, see Elwell, *op. cit.*, pp. 110-115.

him that he has such skill, science, and information as will enable him properly and judiciously to perform the duties of his calling." [26]

The second group consisted of opinions about the nature of skill. Ordinary, not extraordinary, skill was all that was required by law. Ordinary skill involved the exercise of a reasonable, fair, and competent degree of skill. In 1860, a judge of the Illinois Supreme Court succinctly expressed this opinion. " The principle is plain and of uniform application, that when a person assumes the profession of physician and surgeon, he must, in its exercise, be held to employ a reasonable amount of care and skill. For anything short of that degree of skill in his practice, the law will hold him responsible for any injury which may result from its absence. While he is not required to possess the highest order of qualification, to which some men attain, still he must possess and exercise that degree of skill which is ordinarily possessed by members of the profession." [27]

The nature of care was considered in a third class of opinions. The judges asserted that physicians contract to use reasonable and ordinary care in the application of their knowledge and skill. Extraordinary care was not legally required. In 1860, for example, a Georgia Supreme Court justice observed that " a physician called on to deliver a woman in labor does not undertake that he will, at all events, safely deliver the woman of her child, without injury to the mother or child, but he undertakes that he will bring to the work a fair, reasonable, and competent degree of care and skill in reference to the operation to be performed." [28]

A fourth category of recurring judicial opinions dealt with mistakes. Where there were reasonable grounds for diagnostic doubts and differences of opinion about treatment, the physician who exercised his best judgment was not responsible for errors of judgment or mistakes. Errors of judgment were not to be excused where what was well known and clearly indicated was not used in treatment. Generally though, as Justice Bell asserted in the 1853 New Hampshire decision, freedom from errors of judgment is never a part of a contract with a professional man.

The fifth group comprised opinions about cure. A physician was not legally required to guarantee or insure a cure. Separate and special contracts were necessary for cure warranties. That is, law would not prevent the writing of cure contracts, but law would not support any

[26] T, column 67. None of the state justices defined the nature of a " suitable " education. Presumably they believed that physicians should do this.

[27] U, p. 385. Incidentally, Abraham Lincoln was the attorney for the defendant in this case. Sandor, *op. cit.*, p. 465.

[28] V, p. 243.

compensation claims if absolute cure did not occur. Furthermore, law would not support malpractice defense by a physician if absolute cure had been promised.

Between 1845 and 1861, physicians were truly alarmed at the increase of malpractice claims.[29] " Legal prosecutions for malpractice in surgery occur so often that even a respectable surgeon may well fear for the results of his surgical practice," reported Alden March in 1847.[30] While a student in Philadelphia and Baltimore, and a practitioner in Philadelphia and New York City (1822-1839 inclusive), James Webster had not known of a medical malpractice suit. But in an 1850 lecture introductory to an anatomy course at Geneva Medical College, Webster discussed the " frequency of suits for malpractice." [31] An 1850 communication to the Massachusetts Medical Society referred to the " alarmingly frequent " prosecutions for malpractice.[32] In 1856, one surgeon was informed of four cases in four different Ohio counties in one week.[33] It was believed that some practitioners were stopping their surgical practices because of the threat of malpractice.[34]

Means of alleviating this threat were offered. Webster wanted doctors to protect themselves by having witnesses, especially when surgically treating the poor. With bountiful *esprit de corps*, the Massachusetts Medical Society recommended that a disinterested physician be engaged to adjudicate a threat of malpractice by a disgruntled patient.[35] Trained as a physician and lawyer, John Elwell believed that elevating the standard of medico-legal knowledge in both professions, legal and medical, would reduce the number of malpractice charges. Stephen Smith dissented. He thought that malpractice claims were frequently caused by the contradictory nature of medical testimony, which confused judges and juries. Since physicians were legally required to exercise only average skill and care, Smith desired a consensus of medical opinion based on the average knowledge and experience of the profession.[36] Frank Hamilton's

[29] Twenty-one of the twenty-seven appeals occurred in this period.

[30] *Buffalo M. J. and Month. Rev.*, 1847, 3: 225.

[31] James Webster, *Introductory to the Course on Anatomy, in Geneva Medical College, March 7, 1850*. Geneva: Volkenburgh, 1850.

[32] Walter L. Burrage, *A History of the Massachusetts Medical Society*. Norwood, Mass.: Privately Printed, 1923, p. 447.

[33] Elwell, *op. cit.*, p. 55.

[34] Elwell, *op. cit.*, p. 82. Daniel Drake believed that fewer medical school graduates practiced surgery because of the threat of legal penalties. Daniel Drake, *Practical Essays on Medical Education and the Medical Profession in the United States*. Reprint of the 1832 edition. Baltimore: Johns Hopkins Press, 1952, p. 87.

[35] Burrage, *op. cit.*, p. 449.

[36] Smith also objected to the view, expressed by some judges, that criteria of ordinary

analysis of cases of deformities after fracture dispelled the myth that properly treated broken bones would perfectly unite. Of 67 cases of fracture of the humerus, only 34 resulted in perfect cure, though all were treated by good surgeons. Of 38 cases of fracture of the radius, some 25 remained imperfect after satisfactory treatment. These and similar statistics for other bones showed both courts and patients that appropriate medical care was not the only variable involved in the recovery of normal shape and function.[37]

Inconsistencies between legislative actions and judicial decisions provoked complaints by some physicians. The strongest complaint concerned sectarian practitioners who were approved by legislators and condemned by judges. State legislators ignored or repealed regulations about medical education during the pre-Civil War period.[38] In contradistinction, the state supreme court justices, as noted with the first group of recurring opinions, championed a regular medical education.[39] Only one appeal definitely involved an uneducated doctor (B). But irregular practitioners were undoubtedly seen more frequently in the county and circuit courts. Two of the four cases reported in the *Buffalo Medical Journal* for 1847 involved unqualified practitioners. Webster mentioned one self-styled doctor who had testified that the arterial and venous circulations were on opposite sides of the body.[40] John Ordronaux proclaimed that " the quack, the pill-vender, the life-elixir compounder, the panacea concocter . . . may permanently injure health, or even steal the breath from man's nostrils " without being charged with misdemeanor or felony.[41]

skill should be different for rural and city doctors. There were some rules of practice which should give the same ordinary degree of success in both city and village.

[37] Elwell, *op. cit.*, pp. 86-104, gives a synopsis of Hamilton's reports, which originally appeared in volumes 8, 9, and 10 of the *Transactions of the American Medical Association*.

[38] Richard H. Shryock, *Medical Licensing in America, 1650-1965*. Baltimore: Johns Hopkins Press, 1967, p. 27 ff.

[39] Justice Greene of the Iowa State Supreme Court was an important exception (I). In this case involving a botanic doctor, Greene noted that the law was not partial towards regular medicine; nor was regular medicine recognized as the exclusive standard in medical science. A physician was expected to practice according to his professed system.

[40] An irregular practitioner was the defendant in the only trial for criminal malpractice reported before 1861. In 1809, Samuel Thompson was acquitted of murdering Ezra Lovett, to whom Thompson had given repeated doses of lobelia for treatment of a cold. "It is to be exceedingly lamented," said the judge, "that people are so easily persuaded to put confidence in these itinerant quacks, and to trust their lives to strangers without knowledge or experience." Dudley Atkins Tyng, *Reports of Cases Argued and Determined in the Supreme Judicial Court of the Commonwealth of Massachusetts*. Newburyport: Edward Little, 1811, vol. VI, p. 142.

[41] Review of Elwell's 1860 text by John Ordronaux, *New York J. Med.*, 1860, 8: 400.

He insistently urged legislators to make malpractice at the hands of an empiric a felony. Complaint was also voiced about the legal inconsistency of expecting surgeons to be responsible for accurate anatomical knowledge while withholding the means for obtaining that knowledge.[42]

Between 1810 and 1855, several American physicians—Rush, Beck, Griffith, Williams, Ray, Howard, Stillé—had written essays or monographs dealing with problems of medical jurisprudence and forensic medicine. None of them discussed malpractice. On the eve of the Civil War, physicians interested in medical jurisprudence could no longer ignore malpractice claims. In 1860, Elwell published the first systematic discussion of malpractice by an American. Elwell fully recognized that malpractice claims had become an enduring component of the American medical experience.

APPENDIX

A. 1794 Connecticut. 2 ROOT 90. Jesse Root, *Reports of Cases Adjudged in the Superior Court and in the Supreme Court of Errors in the State of Connecticut, 1793 to 1798.* n. p., 1802, vol. II, pp. 90-92.

B. 1812 Connecticut. 5 DAY 260. Thomas Day, *Reports of Cases Argued and Determined in the Supreme Court of Errors of the State of Connecticut.* Hartford: Peter B. Gleason, 1823, vol. V, pp. 260-274.

C. 1832 Connecticut. 9 DAY 209. Thomas Day, *Reports of Cases Argued and Determined in the Supreme Court of Errors of the State of Connecticut.* Second edition. New York: Banks, Gould & Co., 1853, vol. IX, pp. 209-216.

D. 1833 Ohio. WRIGHT 351. John C. Wright, *Reports of Cases at Law and in Chancery, Decided by the Supreme Court of Ohio.* Columbus: Isaac Whiting, 1835, pp. 351-353.

E. 1834 Pennsylvania. 3 WATTS 255. Frederick Watts, *Reports of Cases Argued and Determined in the Supreme Court of Pennsylvania.* Philadelphia: James Kay, 1836, vol. III, pp. 255-258.

F. 1836 Ohio. 7 OHIO (7 HAM) 123, pt. 2. Charles Hammond, *Cases Decided by the Supreme Court of Ohio in Bank, at December Term, 1835.* Cincinnati: Corey and Webster, 1836, vol. VII, pt. 2, pp. 123-125.

G. 1845 Pennsylvania. 8 WATTS 376. Frederick Watts and Henry J. Sergeant, *Reports of Cases Adjudged in the Supreme Court of Pennsylvania.* Philadelphia: James Kay, 1846, vol. VIII, pp. 376-378.

H. 1848 Maine. 28 ME (15 SHEP) 97. John Shepley, *Reports of Cases Determined in the Supreme Judicial Court of the State of Maine.* Hallowell: Masters, Smith and Long, 1850, vol. XV, pp. 97-101.

[42] Elwell, *op. cit.*, p. 54. Also, John F. Townsend, *Relations between the Professions of Law and Medicine.* Albany, 1854, p. 4.

I. 1848 Iowa. 1 G. GREENE 441. George Greene, *Reports of Cases in Law and Equity Determined in the Supreme Court of the State of Iowa.* Dubuque, Iowa: S. Hoyt, 1849, vol. I, pp. 441-445.

J. 1852 Massachusetts. 63 MASS (9 CUSH) 505. Luther S. Cushing, *Reports of Cases Argued and Determined in the Supreme Judicial Court of Massachusetts.* Boston: Little, Brown & Co., 1856, vol. IX, pp. 505-508.

K. 1852 Kentucky. 52 KY (13 B. MON) 188. Ben. Monroe, *Reports of Cases at Common Law and In Equity, Decided in the Court of Appeals of Kentucky.* Frankfort: A. G. Hodges, 1853, vol. XIII, pp. 188-190.

L. 1853 California. 3 CAL 190. H. P. Hepburn, *Reports of Cases Determined in the Supreme Court of the State of California.* San Francisco: Bancroft-Whitney, 1888, vol. III, pp. 190-191. Reprint of the 1855 edition.

M. 1853 Pennsylvania. 22 PA (10 HARRIS) 261. George W. Harris, *Pennsylvania State Reports.* Philadelphia: Kay, 1855, vol. XXII, pp. 261-274. Quoted from Elwell, *op. cit.*, pp. 118-138.

N. 1853 Massachusetts. 65 MASS (11 CUSH) 397. Luther S. Cushing, *Reports of Cases Argued and Determined in the Supreme Judicial Court of Massachusetts.* Boston: Little, Brown & Co., 1857, vol. XI, pp. 397-406.

O. 1853 New Hampshire. 27 N. H. (7 FOST) 460. William L. Foster, *Reports of Cases Argued and Determined in the Superior Court of Judicature of New Hampshire.* Concord: G. Parker Lyon, 1855, vol. VII, pp. 460-476.

P. 1854 Wisconsin. 3 WISC 416. Abram D. Smith, *Reports of Cases Argued and Determined in the Supreme Court of the State of Wisconsin, at the June Term, 1854.* Milwaukee: Rufus King, 1856, vol. III, pp. 416-423.

Q. 1855 New Hampshire. 31 N. H. (11 FOST) 119. William L. Foster, *Reports of Cases Argued and Determined in the Superior Court of Judicature of New Hampshire.* Concord: G. Parker Lyon, 1857, vol. XI, pp. 119-138.

R. 1855 New York. 12 HOWARD PR 323. Nathan Howard, Jr., *Practice Reports in the Supreme Court and Court of Appeals of the State of New York.* Albany: William Gould, 1877, vol. XII, pp. 323-325.

S. 1856 Pennsylvania. GRANT 355. Benjamin Grant, *Reports of Cases Argued and Adjudged in the Supreme Court of Pennsylvania.* Philadelphia: H. P. & R. H. Small, 1859, pp. 355-359.

T. 1856 Tennessee. 36 TENN (4 SNEE) 65. John T. L. Snee, *Reports of Cases Argued and Determined in the Supreme Court of Tennessee.* New edition by William Cooper. Second edition of Cooper edition by Robert T. Shannon. Louisville: Fetter, 1903, vol. IV, columns 65-68.

U. 1860 Illinois. 23 ILL (PECK) 385. E. Peck, *Reports of Cases Determined in the Supreme Court of the State of Illinois, at April Term, 1859, November Term, 1859, and January Term, 1860.* Chicago: E. B. Myers, 1862, vol. XXIII, pp. 385-387.

V. 1860 Georgia. 30 GA 241. B. Y. Martin, *Reports of Cases in Law and Equity Argued and Determined in the Supreme Court of Georgia.* Macon: J. W. Burke, 1871, vol. XXX, pp. 241-248.

122

W. 1860 North Carolina. 52 N. C. 297. Hamilton C. Jones, *Cases Argued and Determined in the Supreme Court of North Carolina.* Second edition by Walter Clark. Raleigh: Mitchell, 1920, vol. LII, pp. 297-298.

X. 1860 Indiana. 14 IND 595. Gordon Tanner, *Reports of Cases Argued and Determined in the Supreme Court of Judicature of the State of Indiana.* Indianapolis: Merrill, 1861, vol. XIV, pp. 595-600.

Y. 1860 New York. 31 BARB 534. Oliver L. Barbour, *Reports of Cases in Law and Equity Determined in the Supreme Court of the State of New York.* Albany: W. C. Little, 1860, vol. XXXI, pp. 534-540.

Z. 1860 Ohio. 2 OHIO DEC 268. *Reprint of Ohio Cases Published in Five Volumes Western Law Monthly, 1859-1863.* Norwalk: Laning, 1896, vol. II, pp. 268-272.

AA. 1860 Iowa. 10 IOWA 579. Tho. F. Withrow, *Reports of Cases in Law and Equity Determined in the Supreme Court of the State of Iowa.* Chicago: T. H. Flood, vol. X, pp. 579-583.

THE PARISH DOCTOR: ENGLAND'S POOR LAW MEDICAL OFFICERS AND MEDICAL REFORM, 1870-1900 [1]

JEANNE L. BRAND

While sickness and poverty have been familiar partners throughout the centuries, state responsibility for caring for the sick poor has developed grudgingly and slowly in modern society. Nineteenth century England, wrestling with the evils accompanying industrialism, with new concentrations of population in crowded, dirty cities, all levels of society mutually vulnerable before the sweeping cholera epidemics, had moved by mid-century away from the policy of supplying only minimum relief to the poor. Occasionally, in fact, the healthy destitute who were assisted under the poor law were in a more favorable condition than their working class competitors. But the gap between legal provision for medical care to the poor and provision for adequate care (even by nineteenth century standards) was still wide by 1871 when the Poor Law Board was merged in the new Local Government Board. Reformers like Doctors Neill Arnott, James Kay Shuttleworth, Southwood Smith and Henry Wyldbore Rumsey, supported by the influential medical journal, the *Lancet*, and

[1] Presented in part to the 32nd Annual Meeting of the American Association for the History of Medicine, Cleveland, Ohio, May 8, 1959. This article is abstracted from one chapter of a dissertation: "Doctors and the State: A Study of the British Medical Profession and State Intervention in Public Health, 1870-1911," which was submitted to the University of London for the Ph. D. degree, 1953.

by the Workhouse Infirmary Association, had enlarged the concept of state responsibility for curative treatment. Nevertheless, medical care to the poor was still hedged within a pervasive atmosphere of deterrence.

This dichotomy was reflected in the respective attitudes of the central poor law authorities and the local Boards of Guardians. The central government authorities from 1847 to 1871 began to bring administrative pressure to bear upon Guardians to improve medical services to the poor. Time and again, however, the Boards of Guardians blandly resisted these overtures and continued to curtail medical relief to save the ratepayer's pocket. The Guardians' actions stemmed from the nineteenth (and in part the twentieth) century view of the pauper, even the sick pauper primarily as a malingerer, draining the substantial members of the community, and therefore to be discouraged from applying for any public assistance. The harsh Poor Law Act of 1834 had been expressly designed to make the acceptance of relief so disagreeable as to exclude all but the literally homeless and starving.

Actively opposing the application of " deterrence " in poor law treatment were the leaders of the humanitarian movement. Dr. Joseph Rogers, President of the Poor Law Medical Officers Association, inveighed with all the rhetoric of nineteenth century fundamentalism:

It has often been asserted that the inmates of a workhouse are generally worthless people, but I demur to that conclusion entirely. Of this I am certain, that many a person who has died in the infirmary of the sick ward of a workhouse has gone straight to Abraham's bosom as has ever passed from a bishop's palace or the death chamber of a king or a queen . . .[2]

Rogers was only one of many. Looking a little more closely at the climate of public opinion which existed in the England of the sixties and seventies, there is discernible a developing spirit of public responsibility towards the poor and the sick poor, reflected in periodical writings. Thomas Wakley, founder of the reforming medical journal the *Lancet*, headed the crusade, and newspaper articles began to follow his lead.[3]

[2] Joseph Rogers, *Reminiscences of A Workhouse Medical Officer* (London: T. Fisher Unwin, 1889), p. 244. Rogers, the descendant of three generations of medical men, devoted his life to the reform of medical relief to the indigent poor. He was one of the agitators for the prohibition of intramural interment in London and the repeal of the window tax.

[3] Thomas Wakley (1795-1862) founded the *Lancet* in 1823, after a number of years in medical practice, to expose abuses in hospital administration and to report medical lectures. A close friend of William Cobbett, Wakley was one of the leaders in the medical reform movement of the first half of the century. He became a medical authority in Parliament, where he represented Finsbury from 1835-1852. Wakley speared the

When she described the time-spirit of the mid-Victorian age, Beatrice Webb, that charming and spiritual pragmatist, suggested that it was a period when " the impulse of self-subordinating service was transferred consciously and overtly, from God to man." [4] Certainly public attention to the sick poor was only one part of the new humanitarianism driving members of the English middle class to look outside themselves for a greater personal fulfillment. Organizations like the Society for the Relief of Distress and the London Society for Organizing Charitable Relief and Repressing Mendacity selected their memberships from a charitable and religious middle class group, anxious of ridding themselves of the fundamental conflict between the Christian ethic and the struggle for survival. Despite this, the spirit of the greatest of utilitarians, Jeremy Bentham, was still strong, and Joseph Rogers wisely used utilitarian as well as humanitarian arguments to urge the advantages of a more generous view toward the sick poor saying:

... that a more liberal administration of poor relief meant true economy to the rate-payers, because if they cut short the sickness of the poor, and if they diminished the amount of deaths that took place among the breadwinners, they would, as the ultimate result, economize expenditure and out-relief.[5]

The late sixties had continued to be a period of depressed trade conditions, and an average of 4.6 per cent of the total population of England and Wales, slightly over one million persons, was forced to apply for poor relief during the years 1866-1871.[6] Economic recovery was slow especially in London. The national expenditure for poor relief, as recorded by the Local Government Board, advanced steadily from £6,439,517 in 1865-1866, to £7,673,100 in 1868-1869 and rose to £8,007,403 in 1871-1872.[7]

It was in this *Zeitgeist*, whose philosophic and economic threads can only be traced briefly here, that some four thousand poor law medical officers carried out their duties in hundreds of parishes throughout Eng-

Lancet campaign to eradicate the common practice of adulteration of foods and drugs, and took part in the movement to improve poor law medical service, shortly before his death. See Samuel Squire Sprigge, *The Life and Times of Thomas Wakley* (London: Longmans, Green and Co., 1897), *passim.*

[4] Beatrice Webb, *My Apprenticeship* (London, New York, etc.: Longmans, Green and Co., 1926), p. 138.

[5] Rogers, *op. cit.*, p. 239.

[6] J. H. Clapham, *The Economic History of Modern Britain: Free Trade and Steel, 1850-1868* (Cambridge: Cambridge University Press, 1952), p. 432.

[7] *Annual Report of the Local Government Board for 1876-1877*, p. xv. The total population at this time was recorded as between 21,000,000 and 22,000,000.

126

land and Wales.[8] The period 1871-1900 is an interesting one in which to examine some of the facets of poor law medical care and the role of the poor law medical officer in advancing that care. It was a period marked by the establishment of a new central authority for public health; a span of years of great importance in scientific advancements, both in preventive and curative medicine; a period of changing public attitudes towards the functions of the central government in caring for the health of the people of England and Wales.

Qualifications of the Parish Doctor

By 1870 poor law medical officers, who earlier in the century had been chosen "without regard to merit or qualification, and mainly for their willingness to accept the lowest rate of pay,"[9] were appointed more selectively. Following passage of the Medical Qualification Act of 1858, the Poor Law Board demanded that all poor law medical officers should be registered and should possess a legal qualification to practice both medicine and surgery in England and Wales.[10] This double qualification required that the poor law medical officer have obtained better professional training than many of his medical colleagues in private practice. This is not to say, of course, that all parish doctors ranked with Harley Street men. But their status within their profession and in the eyes of the public, had increased remarkably.[11] For the most part they were engaged on a fairly permanent basis, and in many large cities employed full-time as medical officers for the workhouses. Salaries were set by local Boards of Guardians, varied greatly, and were the cause for frequent complaint. Despite this, at the close of the nineteenth century, the posts were sought

[8] The annual reports of the Local Government Board during the period 1871 to 1900 irregularly cite numbers of poor law medical officers. For example, the 1874-75 report lists 4,212; the 1876-77 report, 4,233; the 1886-87 report, 4,293 medical officers. Hereafter, the annual reports of the Local Government Board and of the Poor Law Board are cited respectively as *Ann. Rep. L.G.B.* or *Ann. Rep. P.L.B.*

[9] B. L. Hutchins, *The Public Health Agitation. 1833-1848* (London: A. C. Fifield, 1909), p. 127.

[10] Ruth G. Hodgkinson, "The Medical Services of the New Poor Law, 1834-1871," Ph. D. dissertation, University of London, 2 vols., 1950, vol. 2, p. 588. A summary of this dissertation was published under the title "Poor law medical officers of England, 1834-1871," *J. Hist. Med. & Allied Sc.*, 1956, *11*: 299-338. As early as 1842 the Poor Law Commissioners in their General Medical Order Number 5 had set up four alternative licensing requirements for poor law medical officers, not all of which, however, required a double qualification in medicine and surgery. See *Ann. Rep. Poor Law Commissioners, 1842*, p. 130.

[11] Hodgkinson, "Poor law medical officers of England, 1834-1871," pp. 332-333.

after competitively, as they carried many advantages—often providing the holders with a " publicly guaranteed introduction to the neighborhood." [12]

As early as 1868 the Poor Law Board had also expressed themselves firmly on the use of unqualified assistants to poor law medical officers, saying: " The Board feel it necessary to request the cooperation of Boards of Guardians in discouraging the employment of unqualified assistants." [13] Poor law medical scandals, frequent in the forties, showed a marked reduction by the eighteen sixties. When, in 1869, the Poor Law Board began to include in its annual reports the number of dismissals of medical officers, the number was negligible.[14] The Poor Law Medical Officers Association had worked industriously to raise the professional standards of its members throughout the country. Nevertheless, much remained to be done in the years after 1870 before the higher standards of professional competence were uniformly applied by Boards of Guardians throughout the country.

Poor Law Medical Officers and Central Supervision

As is often the case, the relationship between the Local Government Board and the poor law medical officer was more centralized and authoritarian on paper than in practice. Geographical distance from authority often provides a comfortable excuse for ignoring rules and regulations; in many instances this was the case with poor law medical care.

The new Local Government Board, set up in 1871 and largely dominated by administrative personnel of the defunct Poor Law Board, controlled the administration of grants to local authorities and sent out directives and circulars regarding administrative procedures and the medical treatment of the poor. The Local Government Board also maintained a central inspectorate for poor law purposes.

Central Inspection. One of the greatest difficulties in the central poor law inspection service in this period was the lack of adequate medical supervisory staff. Local Government Board inspectors (like the old Poor Law Board inspectors) were laymen, not physicians, and yet they were empowered to survey and report regularly upon the quality of medical treatment to the sick poor.

The lack of medical supervision had earlier in the century been brought to the attention of an investigating committee in 1854, when a majority

[12] Samuel S. Sprigge, *Medicine and the Public* (London: William Heinemann, 1905), p. 146.
[13] *Ann. Rep. P. L. B. for 1868-69*, p. 32.
[14] Hodgkinson, *op. cit.*, vol. 2, p. 712.

of the doctors giving evidence advocated a medical supervisory staff in the Poor Law Board. Dr. Henry Rumsey had noted in his *Essays on State Medicine* of 1856 that the lay inspectors of the Poor Law Board although they:

... unanimously deprecated the appointment of *medical* authorities, they nevertheless admitted that there were no securities for the proper treatment of the sick beyond the legal or nominal standard of qualification possessed by the medical officers and ... that there was no supervision of practice, except a cursory perusal by the Board of Guardians of the weekly sick lists presented to them ...[15]

Some small attempt at central medical inspection had been made by the appointment of Dr. Edward Smith as a poor law inspector in 1865, with special reference to medical relief. Dr. Smith was in no sense, however, a general or administrative supervisor of the local poor law medical officers. His early duties dealt with an investigation into workhouse hospitals in the " metropolis and provinces " and with the improvement of poor law dietaries. In March of 1872 Dr. Smith's office was abolished.[16]

There were later added to the Local Government Board two medical inspectors, Dr. Fuller for provincial England and Dr. (later Sir) Arthur Downes for the London area. The number was far too limited to provide any real medical supervision.[17] Dr. Fuller's visits in the provinces were customarily only made upon the general request of the district lay inspector. Sir Arthur Downes, who served as Medical Inspector of the Board from 1889 to 1918, was to be instrumental in improving London poor law hospital treatment of pulmonary tuberculosis.[18] During the period 1871-

[15] Henry Rumsey, *Essays on State Medicine* (London: John Churchill, 1856), p. 274.
[16] Local Government Board, Government Office Correspondence, Nos. 17557/72 and 17558/72, of March 25, 1872.

Dr. John Simon, the Medical Officer of the Local Government Board who was finally defeated in his reforming efforts by the officialdom of the Board, commented on Dr. Smith's duties as follows: ". . . according to all I have heard in after years from Dr. Smith on the subject of his work in the office, the old secretarial belief as to the best way of dealing with matters of medical administration, had vigorously survived the fact of his appointment as Medical Officer of the Board; and I understand that he, in relation to such matters, was not expected to advise in any general, or any initiative sense, but only to answer in particular cases on such particular points as might be referred to him." Simon, *English Sanitary Institutions*, 2nd ed. (London: John Murray, 1897), p. 352.

[17] Sir Arthur Newsholme, *The Last Thirty Years in Public Health, Recollections and Reflections on My Official and Post-Official Life* (London: G. Allen Unwin, 1936), pp. 92-93.

[18] Sir Arthur MacNalty, *The History of State Medicine in England, Being the Fitzpatrick Lectures of the Royal College of Physicians of London for 1946-1947* (London: The Royal Institute of Public Health and Hygiene, 1948), p. 65.

1900, however, these two medical inspectors had relatively little effect on the over-all pattern of poor law medical care.

The staff of general inspectors who supervised the work of poor law medical officers from 1871-1900 was well imbued with poor law principles. Only a dozen in number for many years (covering all of England and Wales), by 1888 the small group had been strengthened to 15 and by 1894 totalled 18. Inspectors were charged with interpreting the policy established by the Board to local Guardians, and with supervising the administration of central policy in the local districts. Implementing these charges included an inspector's attending meetings of each Board of Guardians within the district at least once or twice a year, making semi-annual visitations to all poor law establishments in the district and preparing annual reports upon conditions.

A German investigator of the eighties, Paul Aschrott, commented that " the social position of the inspector is such that there can be no suspicion of personal interest in the advice which he gives as to local administration." [19] Indeed, when he queried the qualifications of the inspectors, Aschrott was told by the Local Government Board: ". . . they must, above all, be gentlemen, who, on account of their previous occupation and their position in life, enjoy consideration and are accustomed to exercise authority. Stress is laid upon a certain talent for organization, and they must already have shown some interest in the welfare of the poor." [20]

From the quality of their reports, it is clear that at least a good proportion of the general inspectors were able and well-motivated men. But there was little in either the inspector's duties or social position which qualified him to judge the professional adequacy of the poor law medical officer.

Central Directives. The central control which operated on the parish doctor other than in the figure of the district inspector lay in the General Orders and circular policy statements which the Local Government Board issued from time to time. An examination of these sporadic directives together with ancillary material in the otherwise invaluable correspondence files of the Local Government Board gives a very limited picture of the

[19] Paul Felix Aschrott, *The English Poor Law System, Past and Present*, 2nd ed. (London: Knight, 1902), p. 207. Dr. Aschrott, a Berlin judge, was a thorough, highly skilled analyst, whose study was recognized by contemporary officials of the English poor law system as an excellent survey. The book was translated from the German by Herbert Preston-Thomas, one of the most able of the poor law inspectors, and issued in two editions (1888 and 1902).

[20] *Ibid.*, p. 208.

relationship between central policy and the extension of the poor law medical service.[21]

Critics of the poor law system claimed that such regulations as existed were of too permissive or suggestive a nature to be used to compel local Boards of Guardians to provide adequate medical care for their poor. Even when certain directives were called to the attention of local Boards, they might be ignored.[22] In the main, the over-all outline of duties seems not substantially to have changed during the period 1871-1900. New orders for District Medical Officers had been issued in April, 1871, revising the orders of 1847, to make provision for the new establishment of infirmaries. The 1871 orders instructed District Medical Officers to attend the workhouse dispensary every day except Sundays for a minimum of an hour, or for a longer period as directed by the Guardians. Provision was also made in the same orders for attendance:

. . . at the home of the poor person on whose behalf application is made, or else-

---

[21] At the time the correspondence files of the Local Government Board were used for this research, and for study of other medical activities of the Board, the files were under the administrative jurisdiction of the Ministry of Housing and Local Government. The volume of records preserved by the Ministry is considerable. Over 9,000 bound volumes of manuscript and typescript materials of the Poor Law Unions are in existence, in battered but legible condition. The most valuable material for locating central policy of the Local Government Board during the years 1871-1900 is contained in two categories of papers: 1. Local Government Board "Government Office Correspondence" (75 volumes, 1872-1896), and Local Government Board "Miscellaneous Correspondence" (160 volumes, 1872-1900). The "Government Office Correspondence" is particularly valuable, containing detailed material on the Board's administrative procedures, drafting of Government Bills, correspondence with other Government offices, internal administrative memoranda and draft LGB orders. The Board, at its inception, adopted the useful system of mounting correspondence and memoranda on large paper, and circulating these papers within the Board for official comment. This material, as preserved in the bound files, enables the observer to trace much of the development of the Board's policy. The large file of "Miscellaneous Correspondence" is also useful for interpretations of policy to the public, for origins of policy within the Board, for reports of inspectors, and correspondence with local authorities.

All of these unpublished materials are an invaluable supplement to the published annual reports of the Local Government Board, which appear in the *Parliamentary Papers*.

[22] The *Lancet* reported several interesting instances where the Brentford Guardians informed the Local Government Board that they would do nothing to remedy the sanitary situation in their workhouse. The *Lancet* commented on a similar case of open defiance by the local authority, and noted that the Board seemed to be "utterly impotent to enforce commands given out with an air of apparent authority." (The *Lancet*, 1875, *1*: 100). Open defiance was probably the exception, but by an easy sliding over the central orders, local Guardians managed to pursue policies very different than were actually laid down by the Local Government Board.

where as the case may require, and supply all requisite medical or surgical advice and assistance to every pauper in the District placed under his charge . . .[23]

Addditional regulations provided for the maintenance of a medical relief register, notification to the Boards of Guardians of paupers named semi-annually to a permanent medical relief list, and attendance at meetings of the Dispensary Visiting Committee when required.

Duties prescribed in 1896 for medical officers attached to the work-house were very similar: personal attendance upon " as far as may be practicable the poor persons entrusted to his care," reporting to the Guardians as required upon the conditions of paupers, attendance at the workhouse at fixed periods, examining the state of paupers on their ad-mission, maintenance of records, giving directions for the classification and treatment of sick paupers, children, and nursing mothers.[24]

With a more adequate professional inspection service the quality of medical care provided to the poor under these over-all regulations might have been better. Without the presence, either of adequate enforcing authority or of any national standard of performance, such general and permissive regulation made for not only considerable variation in per-formance but outright abuse.

Indigenous Limitations in Poor Law Medical Care

More than general regulations and ineffective inspection severely limited the actual and potential role of medical officers treating the poor. The basic dichotomy of poor law medical service was as present in 1871 as when it was expressed by Beatrice Webb in 1909:

What many members of the Poor Law Medical Service feel most is not the miserable pay they get, not the lack of official appreciation, or encouragement nor even the absence of honours and dignity, but the *extraordinarily narrow scope* that, under the necessary limitations of the Poor Law they find for useful work. It is not encouraging, for instance, to have pass through one's hands (as the Poor Law Medical Officer does) one third of all the deaths from phthisis; and yet, as several Poor Law doctors told us, never to have seen among them a single curable case. It breaks the spirit of a man who cares anything at all about his professional work to have to go on year after year merely pretending to deal with cases, which have come to him only when destitution has set in, and therefore usually too late for any permanently remedial treatment under structural and other conditions

[23] *Annual Report L. G. B. for 1871-1872*, Appendix A, p. 9.

[24] Unnumbered circular, Local Government Board, Government Office Correspondence for 1898, "Extracts from the General Orders of the Poor Law Commissioners, the Poor Law Board and the Local Government Board Relating to the Duties of Workhouse Medical Officers."

which he knows will prevent cure, but which he, as a mere Poor Law Doctor, has no power to prevent.[25]

Measured against the curative potential of medicine today, late nineteenth century medical and surgical care was obviously very limited, and poor law treatment even more constricted. At its best poor law care was palliative treatment, most often with limited resources, and without chance of prevention.

One aspect of this fundamental problem was reflected in the provision of " medical extras." The significance of strengthening foods, often a high protein diet for the recovery of the sick, was well recognized by 1871. Yet the final decision as to whether a seriously ill workhouse patient was entitled to such " medical extras " as meat broth or stimulants rested not with the poor law medical officer, but with the Boards of Guardians. In February, 1871, the *British Medical Journal* reported the case of a Shropshire medical officer, Dr. W. P. Brooks, who complained to the Poor Law Board when an Assistant Overseer of the workhouse counteracted his order for two pounds of meat to make broth for a patient suffering from inflammation of the womb. The Poor Law Board, however, replied that they " consider that a certificate given by a Medical Officer for the allowance of nourishment or stimulants to any of his pauper patients can only be regarded as a recommendation or expression of his opinion as to what is required for such patient," and that the final decision rested with the relieving officer or Guardians. The *British Medical Journal* commented gravely: ". . . we think that the discretion of the medical officer to order nourishment necessary on medical grounds should be so far absolute as not to be interfered with by subordinate officers, whose means of judgement must be inferior to his own." [26]

The objective of the Poor Law Board, and later the Local Government Board, in leaving the final decision to the lay authorities was, of course, the pursuit of " less eligibility," and the fear that the poor law medical officer, given free reign over medical extras, would send the costs of medical relief soaring. The problem of medical extras arose repeatedly in the period 1871-1900, and the Poor Law Medical Officers Association discussed it on a number of occasions.

As the years passed after 1871, concomitant with the gradual evolution

[25] Beatrice Webb, *The Poor Law Medical Officer and His Future* [Papers Used at the Conference of the Association of Poor Law Medical Officers, 6 July 1909] (London: National Committee for the Break-up of the Poor Law, 1909), p. 4.
[26] *Brit. M. J.*, 1871, *1*: 135.

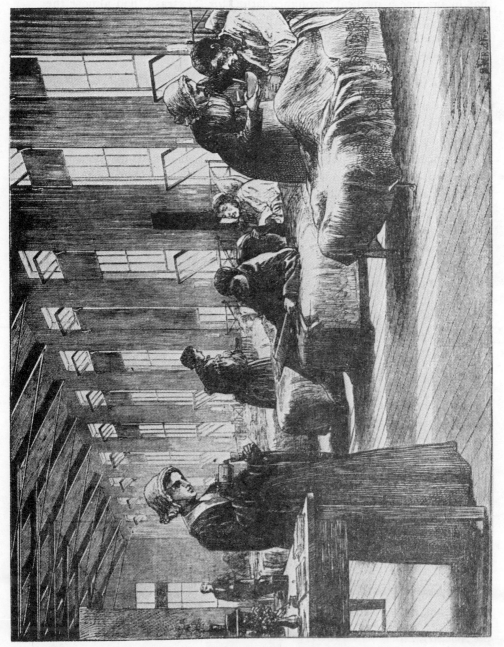

FIG. 2. A WARD IN THE HAMPSTEAD SMALLPOX HOSPITAL. From *The Illustrated London News*, October 7, 1871, p. 345.

133

in the concept of public responsibility for curative treatment, there developed a gradual relaxation in the application of " less eligibility," particularly in the larger cities. Aschrott was to note in the late eighties that in practice a medical recommendation for " extras " had almost the same effect as a direct order. Nevertheless the situation made for tension between medical officers and guardians or relieving officers, and continued to be resented by poor law medical officers.[27]

Extension of and Improvement in Poor Law Medical Facilities

One area of treatment for the sick poor underwent a marked change from 1871-1890—namely, the improvement of hospital and dispensary facilities. Early efforts of the Poor Law Medical Officers Association, in conjunction with the vigorous campaign carried out by the *Lancet* in 1864-1865, successfully aroused public opinion to the need for a reform of poor law hospital and infirmary conditions. Even before the establishment of the Local Government Board, the Poor Law Board had fully accepted the need for an improved infirmary service, and in the late sixties new institutions for the care of the sick poor began to be constructed in populous areas throughout England and Wales. Outbreaks of smallpox and the building of public infectious disease hospitals in the seventies stimulated the building of separate poor law infirmaries to replace the old sick wards in workhouses.

The greatest improvements in furnishing hospital service to the poor took place in London, where the existence of the Metropolitan Common Poor Fund facilitated the erection of the new buildings. The Metropolitan Poor Act of 1867 had been beneficial to London poor law districts in standardizing poor law medical facilities and, for the first time, bringing to the poorer districts measures of assistance which would not have been possible for them alone. In the first nine years of the operation of the Act in London, twenty-two separate infirmaries for the sick poor were opened. By 1877, only six London parishes still housed their sick poor in mixed workhouses.[28]

Extension of hospitalization for the destitute poor was accompanied by a similar provision for the class just above the destitute. Under the stimulus of the humanitarian reform pressures of the sixties and seventies, the Local Government Board moved to a position which encouraged hospital care for the poor who could not be technically classified as desti-

[27] Aschrott, *op. cit.*, pp. 237-238.
[28] Bethnel Green, Fulham, Lewisham, Paddington, Hampstead, and Mile End Old Town. See *Ann. Rep. L. G. B. for 1876-1877*, p. xxvi.

tute.[29] This new approach was originally justified on grounds of protecting the public against persons suffering with infectious diseases, whose homes did not offer adequate isolation facilities.

From 1875 it became the official policy of the Local Government Board to admit to poor law hospitals, without an order, anyone afflicted with fever or smallpox, if refusal to admit such patients involved danger. Under the Poor Law Act of 1889, the managers of the Metropolitan District Asylums were legally empowered to admit patients suffering from fever who were other than paupers.[30] The Public Health of London Act of 1891 permanently removed the possible disqualification by admittance to a pauper hospital.

It is both curious and significant that the whole process of extending poor law medical treatment to other than the destitute or to those suffering from infectious disease evolved through central administrative encouragement, from an administration still heavily scented with deterrence in other respects.

Improvements in staffing and equipment of poor law infirmaries also developed in the seventies and eighties, most notably in London and gradually in other large cities. By 1879 the Local Government Board related with satisfaction the disappearance from London inspectors' reports of such criticisms as: " no day rooms for the sick or separate kitchen, bad ventilation, inadequate lavatories, no paid nurses or nurses for sick children, no hot water supply, no infectious wards, poorly constructed sick wards." [31] The amount of space per patient, which in 1866 had been 500 to 600 cubic feet (exclusive of day room), had been improved by 1883 to 850 cubic feet. This did not equal the usual allotment of a general hospital, but was " regarded as sufficient for diseases of the chronic class treated in poor law infirmaries." [32] The ratio of poor law

[29] Beatrice and Sidney Webb, *English Poor Law Policy* (London, New York, etc.: Longmans, Green and Co., 1910), pp. 211-212.

[30] Temporary legalization had been granted under the Diseases Prevention Act of 1883, which was renewed annually. This temporary Act ensured that admission under such conditions did not carry with it the stigma of disqualification. An earlier attempt in Section 15 of the Poor Law Act of 1879 had given Managers of hospitals optional power to make contracts with vestries for the admission of non-paupers, but this had not been much applied. By 1900 the Annual Report of the Metropolitan Asylums Board stated they " possessed today hospital accommodation to the extent of upward of 6,000 beds, open to any person of whatever social position who may suffer from certain classes of infectious disease."

[31] *Ann. Rep. L. G. B. for 1878-1879*, pp. xxxii ff.

[32] *Ann. Rep. L. G. B. for 1883-1884*, p. xxxiv. Most persons admitted to poor law

medical officers to patients had not been increased by 1883, but in London a majority of the medical officers served full time, and were no longer engaged in private practice.

The new standards of treatment which stemmed from scientific advancement also gradually found their way into poor law treatment, despite an undoubted time lag. Asepsis, anaesthesia, better technical equipment and the new emphasis upon skilled nursing which arose from the Nightingale tradition were all gradually adopted as the official policy of the Local Government Board, usually some time later than their general use in the large London hospitals. From time to time the lay inspectorate of the Board drew the attention of Boards of Guardians to advances in medical and hospital care, commenting on the presence or absence of the new facilities. By 1893, Robert Hedley, poor law inspector in London stated (albeit somewhat complacently) before the Royal Commission on the Aged Poor:

The infirmaries of the metropolis are equal, I think, in their treatment of the poor to anything the poor will get in what are called the large hospitals of the metropolis . . . They are all built on the best principles of ventilation and they are all provided with medical officers . . . The Poor Law infirmaries of the metropolis now furnish between 12,000 and 13,000 beds, whereas what are called the hospitals of the metropolis, the large hospitals, St. Thomas', Bartholomews, and Guy's, I believe only provide about 5,000.[33]

The improvements in some large cities did not extend to rural areas, where poor law infirmaries were considerably less than satisfactory at the end of the century. And even in some large cities, local Boards of Guardians kept up resistance to the central policy of lessening deterrence and expanding the curative principle.[34] Outside of the big cities the lag was marked. Poor law reformers in 1909 were to comment dismally that apart from the populous cities:

. . . the sick are still in General Mixed Workhouses—the maternity cases, the cancerous, the venereal, the chronically infirm, and even the infectious, all together in one building, often in the same ward where they cannot be treated. For the

infirmaries suffered from such chronic diseases as bronchitis, cancer, renal disease, " senile decay," paralysis. *Ibid.*, p. xxxv.

[33] Questions 1154 and 1247, *Minutes of Evidence, Report of the Royal Commission on the Aged Poor*, 15 February 1893. See also comments on improved care in the *Ann. Rep. L.G.B. for 1898-99*, p. 85.

[34] The Manchester Guardians, for example, in an effort to exclude all but the destitute poor, forced all who applied to the poor law hospital facilities to enter through the workhouse gate. *Report of the Select Committee of the House of Lords on Poor Relief*, p. viii.

phthisical, for instance, there is (except in a few unions) no proper provision at all . . .[85]

Local Government Board officials were well aware of this lag and of the financial problem of providing separate infirmaries throughout England and Wales. In the 1894-95 annual report the following statement appears:

It must . . . be borne in mind that the workhouses in the country districts of Wales are for the most part very small, the inmates very few, accustomed to an exceedingly simple and primitive style of life; and it takes a long time to convince the Guardians of such unions of any necessity for marching with the times so far as providing trained nurses and modern hospital appliances. Still, matters are improving steadily, if slowly.[86]

Poor Law Nursing Service

A word must be included on the gradual improvement in poor law nursing service. By the late sixties and early seventies abuses in pauper nursing care began to receive considerable publicity. Dickens' Sairey Gamp caricatured an uncomfortable reality. The foundation of the Workhouse Nurses' Association in 1879 to develop a program of trained nurses for the care of the sick poor was to be a watershed in the improvement of poor law nursing. Louisa Twining and her associates also helped to set standards and recommended accredited nurses to Boards of Guardians. By 1899 the Association, while still lamenting degrees of imperfection in nurses' training, reported to the Local Government Board on the " neat and becomingly dressed young women in suitable uniform, in place of the wretched old creatures who, in pauper dress and black caps, prowled about the beds of our sick poor." [37]

Dr. Arthur Downes, in 1865, had been successful in persuading the Poor Law Board to recommend to local Guardians that they " as far as possible discontinue the practice of appointing pauper inmates of the work-

[85] *The Failure of the Poor Law*, Pamphlet issued by the National Committee to Promote the Break-up of the Poor Laws (no place of publication, 1909), p. 7.

There were, however, very few questions raised in Parliament on the subject of Poor Law medical treatment in the eighties and nineties. Only very occasionally, as in the instance of the management of the Eastern Hospital at Homerton (See *Hansard*, January 23, 1891), was the Local Government Board asked for any public accounting of poor law medical policy.

[86] *Ann. Rep. L. G. B. for 1894-1895*, Appendix B, p. 63. See also the statement of Inspector Preston-Thomas in the *Ann. Rep. L. G. B. for 1898-99*, Appendix B, p. 133.

[37] L. G. B. Misc. Corres., No. 42722/89, Paper of the Workhouse Nurses' Association sent to the Local Government Board, April 1889.

138

house to act as Assistant nurses in the infirmary and sick wards." [38]
Considerable improvements were made from 1865-1895 in the introduction
and extension of a paid nursing service. But the Local Government
Board's policy still gave excuse for many Guardians to continue with
the employment of paupers as attendants to the sick.

By the end of the century it was officially recognized that the nursing
of sick paupers left much to be desired. Although Guardians might be
forbidden to employ paupers as nurses, it was still very difficult to find
qualified women willing to serve in workhouse infirmaries.[39] Even in
London, George Lansbury's testimony before the Royal Commission on
the Aged Poor stated:

The wards in the workhouse [of the Poplar Union] are very much understaffed;
there are not enough nurses, and we have to rely a very great deal—very considerably—on the inmates to assist in the work of nursing and attending to the
aged, infirm and sick.[40]

More especially in rural areas, Guardians were reluctant to provide
in infirmaries and workhouses a degree of trained nursing service which,
in time of sickness, "neither they themselves, or their families or the
independent labouring classes could afford . . ." [41]

Outdoor Medical Care

The care of the sick in poor law infirmaries was only a part of the
program. "Outdoor" medical care for the poor not confined to hospitals
or infirmaries also underwent several changes from 1871 to 1900, including the building of dispensary facilities and a restriction of the extent
of outdoor relief (in favor of indoor treatment).

During the period 1847-1871, outdoor medical attendance had been
encouraged by the Poor Law Board, with no attempt to force the sick
into workhouses. During the middle sixties central inspectors, together

[38] L. G. B. Gov't. Office Corres., unnumbered memorandum dated 1 April 1892 (in
Vol. 150 of 1895).
[39] *Ann. Rep. L. G. B. for 1895-1896*, Appendix A, p. 112; *Ann. Rep. L. G. B. for 1897*,
Appendix B, p. 27; "Workhouse Infirmaries," *Macmillan's Magazine*, July 1881, p. 225;
Ann. Rep. L. G. B. for 1893-1894, Appendix B, p. 133.
[40] *Minutes of Evidence, Report of the Royal Commission on the Aged Poor*, 13 February
1894, Questions 13852 and 13856. Lansbury at that time was a Guardian of the Poplar
Union. A return to the House of Commons from the L. G. B. dated 12 August 1896
showed as of 1 June 1896 there were 13,428 sick and bedridden in London infirmaries,
with a total of 1,514 nurses for their care.
[41] *Ann. Rep. L. G. B. for 1894-1895*, Appendix B, p. 20. See also the Report of Mr.
J. S. Davy in the same annual report.

with the Poor Law Medical Officers Association, began to urge the building of dispensaries at which the swelling numbers of pauper sick could regularly be treated by poor law medical officers.

The Poor Law Board in 1867 called the attention of all Boards of Guardians in London to sections of the Metropolitan Poor Act of that year which related to the provision of dispensaries in London.[42] By 1871 six poor law dispensaries had been started in London; the following year nine appeared in the provinces, and inspectors urged the use of the dispensary system in other urban and rural districts of England and Wales. Outside London, however, building of dispensaries proceeded slowly in the following years.

In part the lag was associated with a new policy initiated in 1871 by poor law-Local Government Board authorities aimed at reducing outdoor relief and forcing the sick poor into the newly erected infirmaries. This policy, so close to a reversion to the principles of 1834, was carried out during the period when admission of other than the purely destitute to poor law infirmaries was being extended. The policy of restricting outdoor relief was enforced through the Board's inspectorate rather than by any specific circulars of the Local Government Board.[43] In actuality, infirmary treatment was often a considerable improvement on the normal housing conditions of the poorer classes.

Gradually, however, more and more dispensaries began to make their appearance. By 1886 forty-four serviced the London poor, and the Local Government Board noted that the original objections of some London guardians to establishing dispensaries on the grounds of expense had disappeared by 1888. However, there was no significant change in the numbers of paupers treated in outdoor medical care from the mid-eighties until the end of the century,[44] and testimony before the Royal Commission on the Aged Poor in 1895 confirmed the prevalence of a policy which still restricted outdoor care in favor of indoor treatment.[45]

[42] Ann. Rep. P. L. B. for 1868-1869, p. 18.
[43] Beatrice and Sidney Webb, op. cit., pp. 208-209.
[44] The annual reports of the L. G. B. show the following numbers of paupers attended in outdoor relief (including those both on the permanent medical list, and those for whom orders for attendance were issued):

    1887 (116,267);   1888 (116,218);   1889 (113,072);   1890 (119,041);
    1891 (115,961);   1892 (118,610);   1893 (131,440);   1894 (118,527);
    1895 (132,645);   1896 (116,893);   1897 (112,956);   1898 (110,419).

[45] Minutes of Evidence, Report of the Royal Commission on the Aged Poor, 1895, Questions 2633, 2638, 17456 ff.

The Poor Law Medical Officers Association and Reform

It was among these changing trends in poor law administration that the parish doctor carried out his daily routine. Shifts in policy affected individual poor law medical officers at different times, depending on the attitudes of local Boards of Guardians. The poor law medical officer, of course, was not merely the passive instrument of authority in all this, but was also a participant in the evolution of a broader, more humanitarian administration of the service.

The relation of the parish doctor to the widening of society's obligation to the sick poor cannot be evaluated by any precise scientific measurement. Like all pressures in the complexities of industrialized society it was only a part of the kaleidoscope pattern of a rapidly changing world. It is impossible under traditional methods of historical research to utilize the individual annual reports of over 4,000 poor law medical men serving in England and Wales for this thirty year period. Many, indeed, have been destroyed, or exist only in local files. Nor is there any evidence which (if such task could be performed with the relentless efficiency of IBM methods) could determine the reactions of the Guardians to these reports. We thus must view the poor law medical officer primarily through reported activities of his group association.

The Association. By 1871, there was in existence an articulate professional organization, headed by the redoubtable Dr. Joseph Rogers, which represented the poor law medical officers of England and Wales. Stemming originally from the membership of the Poor Law Committee of the Provincial Medical and Surgical Association, the group had passed through several stages. In 1868 the organization known as the Metropolitan Association of Poor Law Medical Officers re-constituted itself as the Poor Law Medical Officers Association, and its Council was revised to include an equal representation of metropolitan and provincial members.[46] The Association had attracted considerable support as well as publicity by efforts in the late sixties to bring about reforms in poor law care. Together with the *Lancet* and the Association for the Improvement of Workhouse Infirmaries, the Poor Law Medical Officers Association had been instrumental in securing passage of the Metropolitan Poor Relief Act of 1867.

Joseph Rogers, following a bitter personal struggle with the Guardians of the Strand Union, embarked upon a new program of strengthening the

[46] *Medical Press and Circular*, August 5, 1868, p. 125.

Association at the close of the sixties. Touring Ireland, he observed that the all-embracing program of medical relief there seemed to offer considerable improvement on the English system. Rogers also visited the principal cities of England and induced a number of cities to adopt legislation similar to the Metropolitan Act.[47]

Meanwhile, other supporters of reform of relief to the sick poor had joined in the fray. Dr. J. H. Stallard (M. D. Lond.) published a study of London pauperism, offering plans to revise the structure of poor law administration towards more efficient, central control. Dr. Thomas Hawkesley, Physician to the Infirmary for Consumption and Diseases of the Chest, spoke to the Association for the Prevention of Pauperism and Crime in London on the plague " constantly raging in our midst . . . more dangerous because overlooked in forms of poverty that from familiarity with them we come to view as inevitable . . ." [48] The medical journals maintained a repeated clamor in support of the poor law medical officers [49] and reports of poor law inspectors provided grist for reformers' mills.[50]

Demands in the Seventies for Reform. During this decade the Poor Law Medical Officers Association was to reach a new high in their calls both for improved working conditions for themselves as well as improvements in the quality of medical care for the poor.

By February of 1871 the Association had drawn up a nine-point reform program which was circulated in the leading medical journals.[51] Six of

[47] Rogers, *op. cit.*, p. xxi.

[48] Thomas Hawkesley, *Charities of London and Some Errors of Their Administration* (London: John Churchill & Sons, 1869), p. 19.

[49] See, in part, *M. Press and Circular*, 1868, *1*: 123-124, 378, 444, 249. Also *Lancet*, 1871, *1*: 60 and *Brit. M. J.*, 1869, *1*: 380; 1869, *2*: 539-540.

[50] See especially the *Ann. Rep. P. L. B. for 1870-1871*, Appendix, p. 188.

[51] 1. Permanency of poor law medical officer appointments and the entire payment of salaries out of the consolidated fund. 2. Adequate and uniform remuneration. 3. Increased salaries for length of service, and promotion to higher inspectorial appointments. 4. Consolidation of the various offices of registrar, vaccinator, medical officer, and medical officer of health, with fitting remuneration. 5. Drugs and surgical instruments to be provided by the Guardians, and dispensers and dispensaries to be established wherever practicable. 6. To obtain for the medical officers the responsible control of all midwifery cases. 7. The provision of a basis for consultation and united action in cases of difficulty. 8. Payment for surgery and midwifery in the workhouses as provided for in District work, and an extension of the list of operations for which extra fees were paid. 9. To raise the status of the poor law medical officer, to increase their influence and usefulness, and consequently their remuneration, and to provide a channel through which all the defects of the poor law medical service may be brought to light and " discussed with a view to their removal or amelioration." See *Brit. M. J.*, 1871, *1*: 134 and the *Lancet*, 1871, *1*: 175.

the points were aimed at improving the status of the poor law medical men, but three called for reform in medical care—namely establishment of additional dispensers and dispensaries, provision for consultation service and placing midwifery cases under the authority of the medical officers. Commenting on these demands with sound utilitarian sentiments, the *British Medical Journal* observed:

All of us who have considered the question and the medical officers of the Poor-law service especially, have long since aimed at the conclusion that a very large amount of pauperism which weighs upon the resources of the nation, arises from sickness of preventable character; and that under a better organized system of Poor-law relief, and especially by attributing to the medical officers of the Poor-law preventive as well as curative functions, much of this pauperizing sickness would be prevented, and where it is unavoidable, it might be more promptly and effectively cured.[52]

The following February (1872), a deputation called hopefully upon James Stansfeld, the new President of the Local Government Board. The deputation was headed by Corrance and Rogers (representing the Association) and was also accompanied by Dr. Ernest Hart, voluble editor of the *British Medical Journal* and Chairman of the Poor Law Committee of the British Medical Association. They asked Stansfeld for a thorough overhauling and reorganization of the poor law medical service, appointment of more medical officers, payment of drugs from the rates instead of by poor law medical officers, a greater degree of independence for medical officers in their relations with Boards of Guardians, and, further, they urged that medical officers of health strengthen their enforcement of sanitary measures.[53] These were, on the whole, less self-interested demands —aimed at a more general reform than were the previous year's list. Stansfeld, following an old pattern, promised consideration of the matter, but no sweeping administrative changes followed.

Two years later, in 1874, the Association made another attempt, this time through passage of a resolution with only one aim—extension of dispensary facilities:

That seeing that the greater portion of our annual outlay of £8,000,000 for poor relief is expended on the maintenance of the sick and on those dependent on them, and that the administration of medical relief in the provincial towns and rural districts of England and Wales is chaotic and based on no recognized principles, this meeting is of opinion that the system is most unsatisfactory and wholly and palpably inadequate to meet the necessities of the poorer classes. The Association trusts therefore that her Majesty's Government may see fit to introduce a measure

[52] *Brit. M. J.*, 1871, *1*: 509.
[53] *Brit. M. J.*, 1872, *1*: 187-188.

in the present session of Parliament or as soon after as may be practicable, having for its object the reform of such system by the establishment of district dispensaries, as recommended in the Report of the Royal Sanitary Commission by those Poor-law inspectors who were specially deputed to institute inquiries, and which dispensaries have been found in Ireland to work so beneficially in diminishing sickness and mortality, and in curtailing poor relief expenditure.[54]

When this memorial was presented to the Local Government Board, a supplementary paragraph was appended, again requesting superannuation rights for poor law medical officers through compulsory Parliamentary legislation. But the response was slow. Dispensary building was underway in the metropolis, but rural Boards of Guardians needed more than a resolution to solve the problem.

Another mammoth push for reform came in February 1878 when, acting together with the *Lancet*, the Poor Law Medical Officers Association rounded up eight thousand signatures to a new, comprehensive memorial addressed to the Local Government Board. In good Benthamite language this document emphasized that the petitioners' "claim to a hearing must be understood to be based upon the strictly utilitarian and economizing view of the subject on which we speak." [55] Once again some of the old complaints were put forward: local poor law medical officers should be responsible to the Local Government Board [not the Guardians], better pay was needed, medical officers should not be responsible for the supply and dispensing of drugs. The " memorial " also urged that medical treatment of the poor should be separate from the workhouse, that medical officers should have direct control over the supply of "necessaries" ["medical extras"] for the sick poor, that paid nurses be available for home nursing, and that a departmental or legislative commission be appointed to investigate these matters.

The Local Government Board took a leisurely approach to the memorial. Six months after it had been received, John Lambert, the Board's Permanent Secretary, responded casually stating that the pressure of business had heretofore prevented consideration and he hoped, shortly, to be able to communicate the Board's views on this subject.[56] On November 13, 1878, the Board finally dispatched a formal reply to the memorial, stating coolly:

1. The proposal for greater responsibility of the Poor Law Medical Officer to

[54] *Lancet*, 1874, *1*: 528.
[55] L. G. B. Misc. Corres., No. 15574/78 of 1878, "*Lancet* Memorial."
[56] L. G. B. Misc. Corres., No. 52410/78, 20 August 1878. See also *Ann. Rep. L. G. B. for 1878-1879*, p. xliv.

the Local Government Board is at variance with the policy of Poor Law Amendment Act, 4 & 5 William IV, which left the main control in the hands of the Guardians.

2. From time to time, the Board attempts to improve the salaries of the Poor Law Medical Officer.

3. The Board cannot agree, especially in rural districts, to a separation of drugs and provision of dispensers.

4. The Board cannot see anything in the nature of medical relief which requires it to be regarded as a matter distinct from the Workhouse.

5. The Board feels that leaving the supply of necessaries to the Medical Officer instead of the Relieving Officer would 'unquestionably increase the expenditure for the relief of the sick poor and diminish the control of the Guardians.'

6. With reference to paid nurses, there was nothing to prevent the Guardians from providing such assistance.[57]

The reply concluded that the Board saw no grounds which necessitated further investigation.

Such a reply might have dashed the hopes of any reformers. Part of the Board's rigidity was undoubtedly due to the authoritarian personality of John Lambert, a man who tended to regard all change as suspect. But a deeper factor than Lambert's reactions, or the central acceptance of recalcitrance of Boards of Guardians motivated the reply: namely central assumption that final procedural responsibility rested with the local authorities.

Following this 1878 set-back an extended lull fell over efforts of the poor law medical officers to change central policy. Much of the Association's energies during the eighties and the early nineties were concentrated upon the defense of particular medical officers who fell afoul of their Boards of Guardians, as well as in efforts to obtain superannuation, the payment of medical witnesses, and improvements in salary scales.[58] The medical journals and files of the Board's correspondence do not record major petitions again being placed before the Board for a number of years. The annual meetings of the Association continued to discuss the familiar poor law medical problems, as did poor law district conferences which had been held annually since 1868. The district conferences, which had been founded by Mr. Barwick Baker in the West Midlands, aimed at an exchange of views of "men of practical experience in poor law

[57] L. G. B. Misc. Corres., No. 77841/78, 13 November 1878.
[58] The fight for superannuation was bitter. Permissive legislation in 1864 and 1867 had given Boards of Guardians the right to provide for superannuation of union officers. This discretional right had been rarely exercised by local Guardians and, after a lifetime of public service in the community, the parish doctor was usually retired without remuneration.

administration with regard to the measures adopted in particular districts and their results." [59] Discussions at both the district conferences and at annual central conferences of poor law authorities, which were convened from 1871 on, kept alive the many problems in treatment of the sick poor.

Poor Law Medical Reform in the Nineties

By the early nineties a variety of new agents were at work unearthing fresh evidence of drawbacks in the whole poor law system. Charles Booth's studies on *The Life and Labour of the People in London*, carried out with a team of early " research investigators," began to appear in 1892; Booth's *Aged Poor in England and Wales* emerged in 1894. Fabian researchers were active on the subject. The growth of the trade union movement had also brought into articulate being united forces living close to the lives of the destitute and acutely aware of their needs.

In 1888 a select committee of the House of Lords was appointed to investigate the powers held by the Guardians and their adequacy to cope with distress which might occur in London or other heavily populated cities. The Lords' investigation was not an exhaustive one, and it did not take testimony from local poor law medical officers or from the Association. Some of the gains in poor law medical care were pointed out by Sir Hugh Owen, Lambert's successor as Permanent Secretary to the Board—particularly the increase in numbers of whole-time medical superintendents of poor law infirmaries and the improved dispensary system in London. It was officially admitted, however, that the medical staff serving under the poor law had not been sufficiently increased to cope adequately with the medical needs of the poor.[60]

The report of the 1888 select committee, insofar as it related to medical relief of the poor, was quite favorable. It observed that because of the excellence of treatment in London poor law infirmaries there was even a tendency to " regard them as a kind of state hospital, entrance into which does not imply that the patient is a pauper." [61]

By the early nineties, the public and central government's attitude towards medical care to the poor had altered considerably, and in 1893 the Poor Law Medical Officers Association decided on another major push for further reforms. In March a deputation headed by the Association's

[59] Aschrott, *op. cit.*, p. 86.
[60] *Report of the Select Committee of the House of Lords on Poor Relief, 1888, Minutes of Evidence*, pp. 7 and 604.
[61] *Ibid.*, p. viii. The report also suggested increased reliance on provident dispensaries and medical benefit funds to cut down on the use of poor law medical facilities.

Council members called upon the president of the Local Government Board, Sir Walter Foster, and presented a list of reforms on which the Council felt the time had arrived for legislation. Five points were stressed: first, the advisability of extending the successful London dispensary system to all large towns throughout England and Wales. Second, the parish doctors urged again that the practice of forcing them to pay for medicines should be eliminated. Next came the old question of superannuation; fourth, a reminder of the insufficiency of pauper nursing, and finally the Board was reminded that no official provision had been made for the use of anesthetics in poor law work.[62] Although for the past thirty-five years anesthetics had been in general use in medical practice, the Association's delegates stated that in many unions " operations were performed where private patients would undoubtedly have anaesthetics, whereas the pauper had to suffer without them." [63]

The Association delegates were accorded a far more favorable reception in 1893 than they had had from John Lambert in 1878. Sir Walter Foster assured the group of his " strong sympathy " with respect to the extension of the infirmary system throughout the country, as far as it might be feasible. The encouragement of infirmary building was, he emphasized, the official policy of the Board. The Board had discouraged the system of making medical men buy drugs and would continue to do so. With respect to anesthetics, Sir Walter assured the delegation of his entire willingness to support the provision of anesthetics. The Board had already sent out a circular on the provision of trained nurses, and had discouraged pauper nursing insofar as possible. Sir Walter recommended further, with respect to superannuation, that the Association draw up a workable scheme.[64] Shortly after the March deputation, the Local Government Board issued an order for the provision of anesthetics in pauper treatment.

This was heartening news for the Association. The changed, cooperative attitude of the Board and the widened public humanitarianism to the poor were also evident in central orders permitting a weekly screw of tobacco for paupers in 1892 and later considerable improvements in the diet under a General Order of 1900.[65]

[62] The deputation told Sir Walter that paupers were entirely dependent upon "the goodwill and charity of their medical attendants for the administration of anaesthetics. If they had not anaesthetics in any case it was because it was out of the power of the medical man to provide them." *Lancet*, 1893, *1*: 489.

[63] L. G. B. Govt. Office Corres., 1893 (Vol. 127), No. 40904/93.

[64] *Lancet*, 1893, *1*: 490.

[65] Newsholme, *op. cit.*, p. 78.

The same humanitarian outlook was to inspire the appointment of a royal commission in 1895 to investigate the condition of the aged poor. At this time almost a third of the old people in England and Wales received poor relief. Neither the Royal Commission of 1895 nor a Select Committee on the Aging Deserving Poor three years later, however, made any major recommendations for improvement in the care of the aged sick poor. The Poor Law Medical Officers Association, however, in 1896 passed a resolution stating that ". . . the time has arrived when Boards of Guardians should take into their serious and earnest consideration the necessity of providing for the aged and infirm inmates of workhouses accommodation which will be more suitable to their infirmities and other requirements than now exists." [66]

This resolution had little or no effect within the next few years, however. An important step in improving the position of the poor law medical officer occurred in 1895, when Walter Long, former Parliamentary Secretary to the Local Government Board, introduced an Association-supported bill to provide superannuation allowance for poor law medical men. The bill was successful and the cause of many years of strife finally resolved. Although superannuation had been one of the major planks in the formation of the Association, the Council meeting in March 1897 unanimously resolved that the passing of the Poor Law Officers Superannuation Act " had by no means rendered the further existence of this society unnecessary." [67]

The Position by 1900

The years between 1870 and 1900 unquestionably had brought improvements in public care for the sick poor. New infirmaries, particularly in the large cities, stood as sizable evidence of loosened purse strings of formerly unwilling Guardians. Society had quite fully accepted Dr. Henry Rumsey's mid-century statement that " the simple refusal of medical relief, will neither cure their destitution nor prevent their improvidence." [68]

As the great Poor Law Commission of 1909 was to reveal a few years later, however, the defects of medical service to the poor were still manifold in 1900 and the Poor Law Medical Officers Association had been unable to bring about a major material betterment. Public opinion continued for many years to be tolerant of abuses in treatment. While some

[66] *Lancet,* 1896, *1*: 860.
[67] *Lancet,* 1897, *1*: 661.
[68] Rumsey, *op. cit.,* p. 255.

148

large cities by 1900 had established fairly advanced programs,[69] other
areas were slack, even callous, in their administration of the program.
Not all parish doctors were men of the stamp of Joseph Rogers. George
Lansbury, indeed, in discussing the London poor law medical service had
claimed that " workhouse doctors do neglect their duty." [70] The actual
efficiency or inefficiency of the poor law medical officers is immeasurable.
Those in the best position to testify, the sick poor, were historically
voiceless.

Out of this changing pattern, however, there had clearly emerged a
greater affirmation of the principle of curative treatment for all. Clearly
recognizable were the stirrings of a new public attitude, characterized
by Thomas Mackay: " The subject is now approaching a critical stage.
There is a strong momentum bearing down on all opposition and leading
to an almost gratuitous treatment of sickness." [71] Legislation in the first
decade of the twentieth century was to make these words prophetic.

Insofar as he was able, the poor law medical officer had testified to
the abuses of the system in which he worked, had at times been baffled
by the spectacle of central acceptance but local deviation in the application
of reforms, and had been supported by the new forces of social reform in
the community. By 1900 he was still awaiting that sweeping investigation
of the massive problem of poor relief—to come nine years hence—as a
result of which England was to enter into a new age of social responsibility.

[69] The city of Liverpool, for example, at the end of the century had commenced the
erection of a tuberculosis sanitorium for the poor.
[70] *Minutes of Evidence, Royal Commission on the Aged Poor*, Questions 14022, 14023.
[71] Thomas Mackay, *Public Relief of the Poor* (London: John Murray, 1901), p. 171.

HEALTH AND POLITICS: THE BRITISH PHYSICAL DETERIORATION REPORT OF 1904 *

BENTLEY B. GILBERT **

The social reform legislation of the New Liberalism that culminated in David Lloyd George's famous scheme of national health insurance grew directly from the fears of national decline that disturbed Britons during the Boer War. The military disasters of December, 1899, at the hands of a few thousand unorganized Dutch farmers and the clear incapacity of the War Office evoked questions very early in the conflict about whether English ways of doing things were any longer invariably the best. The advantages of amateurism in military affairs, of rule of thumb in commercial technology, of dependence on heroism rather than staff work, seemed less clear than they once had. Thus, for many months Englishmen had been engaged in a serious and rather frightened reappraisal of the old assumptions about their civilization, when, early in 1902, all their doubts and fears were reinforced by alarming revelations about wide-spread weakness and positive physical disability of men volunteering for military service.

The result was the search for what came to be termed "national efficiency." Usually, national efficiency meant, above all, physical efficiency. A great empire needed a martial and vigorous race. Instead, there was a declining birth rate and, apparently, a deteriorating, incapacitated manhood. Because the Boer War was the first time since the struggle in the Crimea that large numbers of English males had been weighed, measured, and tested for physical weakness, no one could be sure whether the conditions reported were the result of progressive racial degeneracy or of an unhealthy urban environment.[1] But for most people, in any case, the distinctions were unclear.

* Read at the thirty-seventh annual meeting of the American Association for the History of Medicine, Bethesda and Washington, May 1, 1964.

** Supported by the National Institutes of Health, grant no. GM1140-01, and by the American Philosophical Society and the Colorado College Faculty Research Committee.

[1] Enough comparative statistics were available to suggest, alarmingly, that the average English physique was indeed weaker than it had been fifty-five years before. In 1845, for instance, 105 men per thousand recruited for the army had been under the standard height of 5' 6". In 1900, 565 per thousand were under this height. In 1901, the army had finally obtained permission to enlist men down to a minimum height of 5 feet. George F. Shee, "The deterioration in the national physique," *The Nineteenth Century*, (May) 1903, *52*: 798.

To allay public fears on the subject the Balfour government reluctantly appointed, in the fall of 1903, the Interdepartmental Committee on Physical Deterioration. The Unionists, already disturbed by the war, wanted no new alarms about physical deterioration. They attempted to assure that none would be raised by appointing a relatively low-ranking committee made up exclusively of civil servants, who could usually be trusted to support their political masters. But contrary to expectations, the interdepartmental committee published in 1904 an altogether full, honest, and frightening report revealing widespread physical weakness among the working class. The committee found, to be sure, no clear evidence of inherited physical degeneracy, but it found much evidence of physical unfitness caused by dirt, neglect, and ignorance—conditions well within the power of the government to correct. The committee's report contained nothing new to anyone who had read the accounts compiled by innumerable investigators of East London in the last two decades of the nineteenth century. Moreover, its recommendations only repeated the proposals for improving the conditions of the people that social reformers had been urging upon the nation for twenty years. But the Physical Deterioration Committee report made for the first time the connection between evil environmental conditions in the slums and national security. An unhealthy citizenry meant declining national power. Physical weakness meant military weakness. As a result, what philanthropy had been unable to accomplish in the nineteenth century, national interest made necessary in the twentieth. National efficiency became the topic of the day. The search for national efficiency gave social reform the status of a respectable political question, while Unionist neglect of the problem insured that welfare legislation would be a major parliamentary goal of the New Liberalism. In the name of national physical efficiency the state assumed responsibility for feeding children in state schools—regarded as an alarming invasion of parental responsibility at the time—and later for the physical inspection of school children. A longer delayed, but only slightly less direct, result was the great National Insurance Act of 1911, which provided the foundation for Britain's present welfare state.

The first unheeded warnings about the physical condition of the industrial worker attempting to enlist in the army came in 1901. Arnold White, a sensationalist writer on imperial topics, charged that among men volunteering for service in the army in 1899 at the Manchester recruiting depot, three of every five had been rejected as physically unfit.[2]

[2] Arnold White, *Efficiency and Empire* (London: Methuen, 1901), pp. 101-102.

A few months later, a much more sober and scientific writer, B. Seebohm Rowntree, confirmed White's finding. Rowntree discovered that among 33,600 potential recruits applying at the York, Leeds, and Sheffield depots between the years 1897 and 1900, the army had summarily rejected 26½% as unfit and had accepted a further 29% as "specials." If the physical condition of men in the rest of the country were no better, Rowntree concluded, at least one-half of the manpower of England was unfit for military duty.

Even if we set aside considerations of physical and mental suffering, and regard the question only in its strictly economical and national aspects, there can be no doubt that the facts . . . indicate a condition of things the serious import of which can hardly be overestimated.[3]

Perhaps because serious thinkers tended to disregard White, and because Rowntree's study, conversely, had so much other material in it that was new, the general public appears to have missed these two well-known writers' remarks on the physical condition of army recruits. General apprehension of the matter came only in January, 1902, with the publication in the *Contemporary Review* of an article by Major General Sir John Frederick Maurice, entitled "Where to Get Men."[4] Maurice's article essentially restated the conclusions of White and Rowntree. The environmental conditions of English working class life, he argued, were dangerously reducing the reserve of physically qualified men from which soldiers had to be recruited.

What I want to insist upon is that a state of things in which no more than two out of five of the population below a certain standard of life are fit to bear arms, is a national danger which cannot be met by any mere schemes of enlistment, and that true patriotism requires the danger be recognized.[5]

With Maurice's article the national debate on physical deterioration began. The state of the nation, it was argued, was a reflection of the state of the race.[6] The state of the race had to be determined, on the

[3] B. Seebohm Rowntree, *Poverty, A Study of Town Life* (London: Macmillan, 1901), pp. 216-221.
[4] "Miles" (Major General Sir John Frederick Maurice), "Where to get men," *Contemporary Rev.*, (January) 1902, *81*: 78-86.
[5] *Ibid.*, p. 81.
[6] Maurice followed his first article with a second, under his own name, in January, 1903. Referring to the controversy which had arisen since his first article, Maurice emphasized now that the physical condition of recruits was perhaps even worse than statistics indicated because patriotism was bringing forward a better class of men. At the same time, he charged, physical requirements had been relaxed, while recruiting

average, by the condition of the working class. If three-fifths of the English working class were unfit for military service, Great Britain would soon disappear from the ranks of first-class nations. Behind these unhappy reflections lay the menace of an armed, vigorous, populous German Empire.

Early in the spring of 1903, the Inspector General of Recruiting, in response to many demands, laid before Parliament a special report on the manpower problem. Referring specifically to Maurice's writings, the report agreed that his charges on the physical condition of recruits were substantially true. The army felt that the class from which it drew soldiers was, indeed, suffering progressive physical deterioration, and this was a matter of concern to the military authorities.[7]

Official confirmation of Maurice's assertion convinced even the stoutest skeptics of the dangers of physical unfitness. In a lead article on July 25, 1903, the *British Medical Journal,* which hitherto had taken no position on this subject, noted that among the 2,673,676 children reported by the 1901 census of England and Wales to be between the ages of ten and fourteen, 138,130 boys and 7,262 girls were at work.[8] (There were, in fact, 142 ten-year old charwomen.) If, said the *Journal,* the stunting effect of work on children were combined with lack of sunshine, outdoor exercise, and fresh air, and if the parents' earnings were insufficient to provide an adequate diet, it was easily conceivable that the British race would deteriorate. This was not a matter for the future, but a present crisis:

Now, more than at any time in the history of the British people do we require stalwart sons to people the colonies and to uphold the prestige of the nation, and we trust that the searching inquiry which the Duke of Devonshire's speech seems to foreshadow, if it does not dispel the fears engendered by the memorandum of the Director-General [sic. Inspector-General] may, at any rate, be a means of arresting the physical decline of the nation.[9]

The "searching inquiry" promised by the Duke of Devonshire, the Lord President of Council, would become six weeks later the Interdepartmental Committee on Physical Deterioration, which was finally appointed on September 3, 1903. The delay in naming a commission of investigation

sergeants were under orders not to reject summarily any applicant who might conceivably pass the physical examination. Major General Sir John Frederick Maurice, "National health; a soldier's study," *Contemporary Rev.,* (January) 1903, *83*: 41-56.
   [7] *Cd. 1501,* "Report of the Inspector General of Recruiting," 1903.
   [8] National health and military service," *Brit. M. J.,* 1903, *2*: 207-208 (July 25).
   [9] *Ibid.,* p. 208.

exemplifies the extreme reluctance with which the Unionist administration approached the matter of social reform. In this particular case, their unwillingness to attack a complicated and possibly expensive problem of public welfare was reinforced by a normal diffidence that inevitably arose when an inquiry would involve criticism by members of a government department of activities of their own, or allied, departments.

The physical welfare of the working population involved wide areas within the competence of the Local Government Board and the Home Ministry. Neither department desired an investigation at all.[10] In the beginning the government had intended only to use the interdepartmental committee to investigate whether the " allegations concerning the deterioration of certain classes of the population " ought to be the subject for an investigation by a royal commission. But by the end of the parliamentary session of 1903, it had become clear that even an interdepartmental committee composed entirely of docile civil servants would be bound to find a royal commission necessary. A ministry that had no desire for an investigation at all wished still less to see its works, or the lack of them, criticized by a body of non-political, independent experts. The government's solution, therefore, was to enlarge the terms of reference and to permit the interdepartmental committee to make what was essentially a royal commission report.[11]

The Committee published its report on July 29, 1904.[12] The document told the same dreary tale of poverty, malnutrition, and disease made familiar by the investigations of Charles Booth and B. Seebohm Rowntree. An important exhibit was the Johanna Street School in South London, not ten minutes walk across Westminster Bridge from Parliament Square. Here, the Medical Officer of Health for the London School Board, Dr. Alfred Eicholz, reported that ninety percent of the students were hindered in their studies because of some physical defect.[13] Basically, the students

[10] Almeric Fitzroy, *Memoirs* (London: Hutchinson, 1925), vol. II, p. 259.

[11] Speculating on the reasons that a committee charged with inquiring into public health contained no Medical Officer of Health nor any representative of the Local Government Board's public health authority, Gilbert Slater remarked in 1930: " Dog does not eat dog, nor do civil servants in one department of the national service readily cast aspersions on those in other departments, or depreciate the value of their work." Gilbert Slater, *Poverty and the State* (London: Constable, 1930), pp. 170-171. The exclusively official character of the committee was also noted by Sir John Gorst, who would nevertheless become a champion of the report. *Hansard, Parliamentary Debates,* 4th ser., CXL (August 10, 1904), col. 48.

[12] *Cd. 1275,* " Report of the Interdepartmental Committee on Physical Deterioration," 1904.

[13] *Cd. 2175,* p. 19.

154

did not get enough to eat. They got bread and tea for breakfast, bread and margarine for lunch, and about a penny's worth of food, usually fish fried in cottonseed oil, for supper. Witnesses confirmed Arnold White's original charge about the physical condition of men attempting to enlist at the Manchester depot. Among 12,000 men examined in 1899, 8,000 had been rejected as virtual invalids and only 1,200 were found, after service in the army, to be fit in all respects.[14] Nevertheless, there was no proof that the race was deteriorating. There was, to be sure, much ill health due to environmental conditions and lack of nourishment, but the unfitness disappeared when the conditions were removed. On the other hand, there were no adequate anthropometrical surveys covering the whole population. A uniform and continuous system of physical inspection became one of the most important of the committee's recommendations.

In summary, the committee recommended the enforcement of existing sanitary regulations, teaching girls proper methods of child care and cookery, the encouragement of physical exercise in state schools, and, most important, the establishment of an adequate system of physical inspection of school children and of a state-sponsored program for the feeding of school children of poor parents in order to ensure the child's ability to take full advantage of the education offered by the state. The committee proposed generally that the nation turn its attention to the care of children. Whether anything could be done for those who had become weak, malformed adults was uncertain. But humanity and national interest alike dictated that reform should begin with those not yet grown.

While the Physical Deterioration Report left no doubt that unfitness among the British working class population was a pressing and serious problem, the report did little to clear up the causes of this condition. The debate among the experts on the physical deterioration report revolved around two not precisely contradictory points of view. First of all, some serious commentators remained unconvinced by the assurance that no evidence existed of inherited racial physical decline. If progressive evolution had become degeneration, they argued, nothing could be done. So long as medical science insisted on insuring the proliferation and survival of stunted and untalented children while fit and intelligent parents failed to reproduce themselves, no amount of social reform legislation would improve the general condition of the race. This, basically, was the problem as it appeared to Karl Pearson and to Sidney Webb.[15] For these

[14] *Cd. 2210,* "Minutes of Evidence, Report of the Interdepartmental Committee on Physical Deterioration," 1904, p. 123.
[15] See Pearson's letter to *The Times,* August 25, 1905, entitled "National deterioration,"

155

men, the only possible solution was state action, not in favor of the depressed classes, but in favor of the talented classes, to encourage larger families. Webb called for a " revolution in the economic incidence of child-bearing," and his campaign for the " endowment of motherhood," mothers' pensions, was the result.[16] A number of the more enthusiastic, perhaps less conscientious, Darwinists—Arnold White, H. G. Wells, and George Bernard Shaw—as well as writers in widely-read periodicals of fashion of the type of the *Queen*, found an easy answer to the problem in the " sterilization of failures." [17]

Opposed to the Darwinists was the medical profession. Generally, the doctors refused to admit that the race was deteriorating. In some cases, they were suspicious of the report of the Physical Deterioration Commission itself.[18] Nevertheless, the profession was well acquainted with the physical condition of the working classes, and doctors generally supported measures designed to extend knowledge of hygiene and domestic science among the poor. The British Medical Association, once its interest was aroused, gave much attention to the committee report and was particularly active in bringing pressure on the government to begin physical exercise and medical inspection among school children.[19]

In the political world the promotion of the report fell to Sir John E.

in which he speaks of the "approaching crisis" resulting from the decline in birth rate among the talented. Any schoolmaster, he argued, admitted that it was already showing up. "The dearth of ability today must indeed depress thoughtful Englishmen. . . ." For a fuller discussion of Pearson's writing, see Bernard Semmel, *Imperialism and Social Reform* (Cambridge: Harvard Univ. Press, 1960), pp. 35-52. See also *The Times*, October 11, 1906, a two-part article by Sidney Webb, "Physical degeneracy, or race suicide." Webb pointed out that between 1896 and 1905, although the population of London County had increased by 300,000, the total number of children in the three to five year age bracket scheduled for school fell from 179,426 in 1896 to 174,359 in 1905.

[16] See Sidney Webb, *The Decline in the Birthrate,* Fabian Tract 131, London: Fabian Society, 1907.

[17] On Wells' proposals in this area, see William J. Hyde, "The socialism of H. G. Wells in the early twentieth century," *J. Hist. Ideas,* (April) 1956, *17*: 217-234. George Bernard Shaw agreed with Wells on the need for eugenic protection of the race, although the two agreed on little else.

[18] See, for instance, "The report of the Privy Council upon physical deterioration," *Lancet,* 1904, *2*: 390-392 (August 6).

[19] Through November and December of 1903, and January of 1904, the *British Medical Journal* published a series of articles on the question of national physical deterioration. While unwilling to recommend direct state welfare activity, the *Journal* did propose a wide range of regulatory measures—reduction of licenses of public houses, physical training in schools, care of poor children's teeth by the Poor Law medical service, the use of charitable funds to supply meals for underfed school children, and physical inspection in schools.

Gorst, formerly a member of the Balfour ministry as Vice-President of the Privy Council Committee on Education. (This was, in fact, the chief executive office of British state education. It was renamed, less cumbersomely, Secretary to the Board of Education in 1902.) The Unionist cabinet had resolved before the interdepartmental committee had reported, in May, 1904, to permit no new expenditures on social welfare by local authorities. William Anson, Gorst's successor in charge of British education and a sincere reformer, had been told curtly by Balfour that in dealing with the findings of the interdepartmental committee he could "be as sympathetic as he liked, but there would be no increase in rates," (local taxes).[20] By the beginning of 1905, however, public discussion of the report, and Gorst's clamour in Parliament and the press, had begun to cause official nervousness. The government had no desire to convey the impression that the Unionist party was indifferent to the condition of school children.[21] There were fears that awkward questions might be asked during the debate on the King's speech in 1905. Among Unionist leaders the most energetic opponent of any government reform legislation was William Anson's own immediate chief, the president of the Board of Education, the Marquis of Londonderry, who appears to have determined cabinet policy towards the Physical Deterioration Report. Londonderry urged the cabinet on February 10, 1905, to avoid any parliamentary unpleasantness over the Physical Deterioration Report by the ancient device of the appointment of a second committee to investigate the findings of the first. Like its predecessor, the second committee should be made up exclusively of civil servants, said Londonderry. In this way, the government would

[20] R. L. Morant to A. J. Balfour, December 3, 1904, British Museum Add MSS, 49787, *Balfour Papers,* vol. CV, f 123. The above memorandum was the result of Anson's suggestion that the government should make some statement in reference to physical deterioration in the King's speech.

[21] Unionists affected to regard Gorst as a revolutionary whose presence in politics represented a danger to the British system of government. The proposal to throw upon the local authorities the duty of feeding as well as educating children at school, said *The Times* in a lead article anticipating state welfare provision from the cradle to the grave, should be stigmatized as a "dangerous and far-reaching change in our school system":

"Sir John Gorst presents a not unusual combination of cynicism and sentimentalism. He is very lacking in sympathy with other people's ideals, aspirations, and efforts, and he is very much wedded to his own notions. On this question he contentedly accepts all the exaggerations that may help to make out a case for sentimental legislation.

If instead of quickening parental sense of duty, we are going to weaken it, we shall have to begin with the newborn babe.

It is a race of fatherless and motherless foundlings to which Sir John Gorst's proposals point." (*The Times,* January 2, 1905).

. . . avoid the difficulty of having ["unsuitable" crossed out in original MS] persons pressed upon us who might approach the subject with preconceived conclusions, and this committee should meet as soon as possible, so in the event of any serious debate on the Address we may be aided in resisting premature or too far reaching proposals by referring to the lack of specific information and practical suggestions. . . .

It would always be possible, Londonderry reminded the cabinet, to propose waiting for the committee report.

The terms of reference were most important, Londonderry went on. The committee must " not be at liberty to make any far-reaching proposal that the Unionist party would be unwilling to support. . . ." Anything, for instance, that would require new legislation or new taxes should be resisted. On the other hand, he warned, the terms could not be too narrow or the government " would be accused of parking [?] discussion while taking no really effective steps to discover or bring about any practical remedies for the evils now generally admitted to exist." Londonderry said that he was personally opposed to any changes that would incur new taxes and suggested:

. . . that it would be politic to state this explicitly for the reassurance of many anxious members of the Unionist party. This would limit the researches of the committee, as would the decision to refuse the right to recommend new legislation, but no doubt there were many other points of great value that the committee could formulate suggestions about.[22]

About a month later, on March 14, 1905, spurred on by Gorst's daily attack, Londonderry appointed the Interdepartmental Committee on Medical Inspection and Feeding of Children Attending Public Elementary Schools. The committee was ordered in singularly unchallenging terms of reference: " to ascertain what is now being done in medical inspection and to inquire into methods employed, the sums expended, . . ." on feeding of school children, and to report whether it " could be better organized, without any charge upon public funds. . . ."[23] Bound by these terms of reference, the committee report, rendered in November, 1905, barely two weeks before the Unionist government left office, was as pallid and innocuous as Lord Londonderry could have wished.

Early in April, Gorst sought to force the hand of the government.[24] In

[22] Lord Londonderry to Cabinet, MS Memorandum, February 10, 1905 (subsequently printed with deletions), Ministry of Education. *Private Office Papers,* "Education (Provision of Meals) Bill, 1906, Papers Leading up to Bill," unsorted.

[23] *Cd. 2779,* " Report of the Interdepartmental Committee on Medical Inspection and Feeding of Children Attending the Public Elementary Schools," 1906.

[24] For a detailed study of Gorst's activity in behalf of children, see: Bentley B.

the company of Thomas J. McNamara, a radical Liberal M. P., who provided, with Will Thorne, most of Gorst's support in the Commons, the Countess of Warwick, and a physician, Dr. Robert Hutchison, Gorst visited the notorious Johanna Street School in Lambeth. There, among the students, Gorst found twenty boys whom Dr. Hutchison certified to be suffering from malnutrition so acute it made effective school work impossible. The group then made application for relief in the name of the boys to the Lambeth Board of Guardians. The guardians, suitably impressed by a visit from two members of Parliament and a peeress bearing one of the oldest names in England, immediately issued orders for the out-of-doors maintenance of all necessitous children within the Lambeth Union.[25] With the example of this concession, the reformers forced a debate in the House of Commons on April 18 on the resolution that " local authorities should be empowered . . . for ensuring that all children at any public elementary school . . . shall receive proper nourishment before being subjected to physical or mental instruction. . . ."[26]

Anson announced during the debate that the Local Government Board was about to issue a circular to all guardians permitting them to feed school children upon application from a school manager or teacher. A copy of the circular together with a letter from him would soon be sent to all schools.[27] Feeding, said Anson, could be accomplished as direct poor law relief or as a loan. The former, he admitted, would put the parent under the legal disabilities of pauperism. He was not sure whether the parent would be pauperized if the guardians undertook to recover the cost, in effect gave relief as a loan.

Before the division, Anson announced that the vote on the resolution would not be treated as a party question. As a result, the government was defeated and the resolution passed, 100 to 64.[28] Thus, over a year before formal sanction by legislation, the state undertook to feed necessitous school children and so gave effect to one of the first recommendations of the Physical Deterioration Report.

A resolution passed by a minority of an aging House of Commons advising, but not requiring, a reluctant government to permit local

---

Gilbert, "Sir John Eldon Gorst and the children of the nation," *Bull. Hist. Med.,* (May-June) 1954, *28*: 243-251.

[25] For Gorst's story of this excursion, see: Sir John Gorst, *The Children of the Nation* (New York: Dutton, 1907), pp. 86-87.

[26] *Hansard, Parliamentary Debates,* ser. 4, CVL (April 18, 1905), col. 531.

[27] *Ibid.,* cols. 526-563.

[28] *Ibid.,* cols. 567-568.

authorities to give food to hungry children hardly counts as an act of revolution. The resolution of April 18 is important only as the symbol of the movement, minute but clear, toward the assumption of state responsibility. A corner of the monument to the nineteenth century ideal of self-help had been chipped away.[29]

The principle ungraciously accepted by the Balfour administration in April, 1905, was to be confirmed by the Liberal government in the Education (Provision of Meals) Act of 1906. But by the time of the passage of this act, there was little new that opponents, or supporters, of the measure could say. State provision of meals had begun. The question only remained whether society should attempt to punish the parent for neglect of the child by casting the father into the legal category of a pauper, or by proceeding against him for the recovery of the cost of food provided for his child. Neither measure, in fact, would ever force a truly indifferent parent to care for the physical condition of his child. And no punishment could compel a parent without money to buy food. The alternatives, therefore, were not whether the state or the parent should feed the child, but whether the state should feed the child or permit him to go hungry. The same intractable logic would be applied in 1907 to medical care for school children and to state maintenance for the aged in the form of non-contributory old-age pensions in 1908. Finally, after providing for the helpless, British society through compulsory insurance established the principle that the physical welfare of the mature working man was also a matter of state concern. An efficient nation could not afford to permit its citizens to suffer the consequences of their own improvidence. So began the evolution of national insurance.

[29] A. V. Dicey designated the feeding of school children one of the first of the socialist measures that culminated in what was to him the deplorable National Insurance Act of 1911. Albert V. Dicey, *Lectures on the Relation Between Law and Public Opinion in England During the Nineteenth Century*, 2. ed. (London: Macmillan, 1930), pp. xlix-l.

SANITARY REFORM IN NEW YORK CITY:
STEPHEN SMITH AND THE PASSAGE OF
THE METROPOLITAN HEALTH BILL *

GERT H. BRIEGER **

" Frenzy in the South," proclaimed the bold headline of the *New York Times* on March 10, 1865. These were the last days of the long and bitter struggle, and New Yorkers welcomed the news. Each day they read about Grant and Sheridan in Virginia and of Sherman's impressive march up through the Carolinas. On March 16th, however, a different subject dominated the first two pages of the paper. Instead of the usual fare of war news, the *Times* provided its readers with the testimony of Dr. Stephen Smith presented before a joint committee of the New York State Legislature. He had given evidence about the sanitary conditions of New York City and on the urgent need for new health laws. Smith gave a stinging indictment of the municipal authorities responsible for the public health and described the miserable conditions of the city's streets and tenements. This testimony, based on a massive effort by a large group of reform-dedicated physicians, was the culmination of years of effort by numerous citizens of America's major metropolis.[1]

The horrible conditions which existed at the close of the Civil War were not peculiar to New York or to that period. As Ford has pointed out, the relationship between cellar-dwellings and disease production in New York had been discussed as early as the 1790's.[2] In 1820 David

* A portion of this paper was presented to The Johns Hopkins Medical History Club, March 14, 1966, and at the Hixon Hour, University of Kansas Medical Center, April 18, 1966. It is part of a larger project, a biographical study of Stephen Smith, in which I am presently engaged. See *Bull. Hist. Med.*, 1965, *39*: 85.

** This investigation was supported by U. S. Public Health Service Training Grant number 9T1-LM-105-06.

[1] Smith had presented the evidence to the legislative committee on 13 February, 1865. It was published in the *New York Times* a month later and was reprinted in Stephen Smith, *The City That Was,* New York: Allaben, 1911, ch. 4. The latter version contained only very minor changes.

[2] James Ford, *Slums and Housing*, with Special Reference to New York City, History, Conditions, Policy, 2 vols., Cambridge: Harvard, 1936, vol. 1, pp. 17-204. Ford describes many of the early health ordinances. The amount of space he has devoted to sanitary matters is an indication of the close relationship of health and housing. There are a number of other works that deal with health conditions and sanitary laws prior to 1866. A few examples are Susan Wade Peabody, " Historical study of legislation regarding

160

Hosack told the medical students of the College of Physicians and Surgeons that the filth in various parts of the city was marked and that amelioration could probably not be achieved without the aid of the State Legislature.[3] Benjamin W. McCready, in 1837, pointed to poor housing and insufficient space as a major source of ill-health among the workers.[4] In 1842, John H. Griscom, one of the truly important figures in the story of sanitary reform, appended to his annual report of the City Inspector's office a pamphlet entitled "A Brief View of the Sanitary Condition of the City," in which he described living conditions and the destitution and misery of cellar-dwellers. He urged upon the Common Council the necessity of better housing laws.[5]

In December, 1844, Griscom delivered a discourse at the American Institute which he published during the next year as *The Sanitary Condition of the Laboring Population of New York*. He reported the health problems which faced many tenement-dwelling New Yorkers, and he urged "SANITARY REFORM." He was anxious to profit from the experi-

public health in the states of New York and Massachusetts," *J. Infect. Dis.*, 1909, Suppl. no. 4, 156 pp.; Charles F. Bolduan, "Over a century of health administration in New York City," *Dept. of Health Monograph Series*, no. 13, 1916; John Blake, "Historical study of the development of the New York City Department of Health," typescript, *ca.* 1952, 128 pp.; Charles E. Rosenberg, *The Cholera Years*, The United States in 1832, 1849, and 1866, Chicago: Univ. of Chicago, 1962; George Rosen, "Public health problems in New York City during the nineteenth century," *N. Y. State J. Med.*, 1950, *50*: 73-78; and Howard D. Kramer, "Early municipal and state boards of health," *Bull. Hist. Med.*, 1950, *24*: 503-509.

I should also say at the outset that the city did have a health organization during the years prior to the Metropolitan Health Bill of 1866. A history of the department is in the process of being compiled by Professor John Duffy, who will give in great detail what I have perhaps too much simplified in this paper. It was the "felt reality" of the time, however, according to many physicians, that New York did not indeed have a health department worthy of that name. *Reports, Resolutions, and Proceedings of the Commissioners of Health of the City of New York For the Years 1856-1859*, New York: Clark, 1860, reveals that meetings were frequent, sometimes even daily, but that mostly they dealt with quarantine matters and occasionally with removal of nuisances.

[3] David Hosack, "Observations on the means of improving the medical police of the city of New York," in *Essays on Various Subjects of Medical Science*, 2 vols., New York: Seymour, 1824, vol. 2, pp. 9-86.

[4] Benjamin W. McCready, *On the Influence of Trades, Professions, and Occupations in the United States, in the Production of Disease*, Genevieve Miller, ed., Baltimore: Johns Hopkins Press, 1943, pp. 41-45.

[5] John H. Griscom, *Annual Report of the Interments in the City and County of New York for the Year 1842, with Remarks Therein, And a Brief View of The Sanitary Condition of the City*, New York, 1843. See also Lawrence Veiller, "Tenement house reform in New York City, 1834-1900," in Robert W. DeForest and Lawrence Veiller, eds., *The Tenement House Problem*, 2 vols., New York: Macmillan, 1903, vol. 1, pp. 71-75, in which Veiller has included long quotes from Griscom.

ence of English and French sanitarians, and their influence is evident in the text as well as the title.[6]

Griscom was one of the first to show that the system of subtenancy and the rental extortions of the sublandlord were among the principle causes of misery of so many of the city's poor. This system enabled the owner of one or several houses to rent them to a sublandlord, who in turn divided them into as many apartments as possible. He then extracted as much rent as he could, often from helpless immigrants. By making few repairs and providing little maintenance he realized a great profit. Often he owned the local store as well and fixed prices at relatively high levels. The working classes were virtually restricted to lower Manhattan because there was no means of inexpensive, rapid transportation which would have freed them from the packed tenement conditions.[7]

Griscom also clearly described the evils of cellar-dwellings, often soggy and lacking ventilation. Many of the cellar-apartments were below sea level. When high tides came, the rooms were submerged! During heavy rains, the streets drained into the cellars. The cellar-dwellers, or Troglodytes as they were often called, lived and slept on planks suspended well above the floors.

In contrast to McCready, who seems to have practiced and taught medicine in comparative quiet, Griscom continued active agitation for improved public health laws. He was one of the first to stress that the physicians in the public dispensaries of the city would be ideally suited for the jobs of health wardens or sanitary inspectors.[8] He was the first witness before the Select Committee of the New York Senate appointed in 1858 to

[6] Not only were New Yorkers influenced and inspired by the work of the Parisian and London sanitarians, but there were frequent allusions to the mortality rates in these cities, as compared to New York. New York usually fared second best. See also "Health. New York versus London," *Hunt's Merchant's Mag.*, 1863, *48*: 120-124; and "Health of New York, Philadelphia, and Baltimore, for 1860," *Am. M. Monthly*, 1861, *15*: 312-316. It was especially galling to New Yorkers that the over-all mortality rate of the United States was far lower than that of England (15 per 1000 *v.* 23 per 1000) yet in New York City it was much higher (36 per 1000). See *Report of the Committee on the Incorporation of Cities and Villages, on the bill entitled "An Act concerning the Public Health of the counties of New York, Kings, and Richmond,"* New York State Legislature, Assembly Doc. no. 129, 1860.

[7] The problem of tenements and housing reform has been fully dealt with by others. The role of housing in sanitary reform was a central one. See for instance, Ford, *Slums and Housing, op. cit.*; DeForest and Veiller, *The Tenement House Problem, op. cit.*; Gordon Atkins, *Health, Housing, and Poverty in New York City 1865-1898*, Ann Arbor: Edwards, 1947, which includes a good discussion of the sanitary reform of 1866. Roy Lubove, *The Progressives and the Slums*, Pittsburgh: Univ. of Pittsburgh, 1962, also deals with the formation of the Metropolitan Board of Health.

[8] John H. Griscom, "Improvements of the public health, and the establishment of a sanitary police in the city of New York," *Trans. M. Soc. State of N. Y.*, 1857, pp. 107-123.

investigate the health department of New York City. He then sat with the Committee during its interrogation of over twenty witnesses, often interjecting lively questions and barbed remarks.[9]

This Committee was appointed to investigate the " assertion that great defects exist, and great improvements are practicable in the health department and sanitary laws of the city of New York." [10] Three major questions were asked: 1. Whether the allegations were true that New York had a higher ratio of mortality than other large cities. 2. If true, what were the causes of this excess mortality. 3. What were the possible remedies.[11]

Almost unanimously the witnesses gave an affirmative answer to the first question. As to the causes, this report established what was to become a constantly recurring refrain. Almost all the witnesses ascribed the excessive mortality to over-crowded tenement houses, improper light, ventilation, and food, filthy streets, insufficient sewerage, and an almost total lack of a regularly constituted and effective department of health.

Contrary to the arguments put forward by the City Inspector, Mr. Morton, the committee stated that a properly constituted health department would require the talents of the best educated men, well versed in the recent advances of medical science. Not since 1844 had a physician been City Inspector. " A man when he wants his watch repaired," argued Dr. John McNulty, " does not take it to a shoemaker. . . ." [12]

The City Inspector and his men disagreed. Mr. Richard Downing, Superintendent of Sanitary Inspection, claimed that knowledge of the law, not medicine, was necessary. It did not require medical knowledge, he said, to smell an odor or to recognize a filthy street.[13] Mr. Morton added his feeling that physicians would not do the job; they would think it undignified to " go running through tenement houses and sticking their noses down privies, to see if they were healthy or not. . . ." [14]

For two years prior to the Senate Committee's investigation, the leading medical society, The New York Academy of Medicine, petitioned the legislature for modifications of the health laws. In 1856 the Academy sent a memorial to Albany which stated that " a large portion of the annual mortality of this city results from diseases, whose causes are more or less within our control, but which are totally unchecked by any public administration of proper sanitary precautions, and that from this

[9] *Report of the Select Committee Appointed to Investigate the Health Department of the City of New York,* New York State Legislature, Senate Doc. no. 49, 1859.
[10] *Ibid.,* p. 1.
[11] *Ibid.,* p. 3.
[12] *Ibid.,* p. 52.
[13] *Ibid.,* pp. 156-157.
[14] *Ibid.,* p. 174.

neglect, in addition to a very great and unnecessary loss of life, the city and State endure an incalculable detriment to their commercial and moral interests." [15] No bill was passed at the 1857 session.[16] Nor was a renewal of the petition successful the following year.

In the meantime, however, the legislature did pass the Metropolitan Police Bill, in 1857, an important model and precedent for future health legislation. By transferring to state control the city's police force, the Republican State Legislature created a new police district comprising the counties of New York, Kings, Richmond, and Westchester. The Board of Police was to consist of five commissioners, plus the mayors of New York and Brooklyn. New York's Mayor Fernando Wood resisted the new law and kept control of his original municipal force—most of whom had voted for him on the Democratic ticket. Only after rioting in the streets with the municipal faction, the arrest of Mayor Wood, and the use of the state militia, did the Metropolitan Police finally win their right to act as the city's legally constituted guardians of the peace.[17]

A recent historian of this episode pointed out how the situation was complicated by a growing political and social cleavage between New York City and the rest of the state.[18] Each mayor, in his annual messages of the succeeding years, used the argument that local problems, such as sanitation, should be kept under local control. Thus the sanitary reform measures, suggested repeatedly between 1856 and 1866 by the leading physicians of New York, took on increasingly complex political overtones. Health bill advocates found themselves fighting, not only for good health and efficient sanitary administration, but against political corruption and the control of Tammany Hall over the city.[19]

In the meantime, the New York Sanitary Association had been founded in January, 1859. The members immediately took up the fight for the health bill before the legislature, then in session. John Griscom and Elisha

[15] New York State Legislature, Assembly Doc. no. 129, *op. cit.*, p. 1.

[16] Not only was the bill refused, but, to add to the problems of sanitation, the City Inspector was at that time given supervision of street cleaning. As the New York Sanitary Association pointed out later, this was added to his already grossly neglected sanitary duties. *Reports of the Sanitary Association of the City of New York*, New York, 1859, p. 7.

[17] See Denis T. Lynch, "*Boss*" *Tweed*, the Story of a Grim Generation, New York: Boni and Liverwright, 1927, pp. 187-199; Samuel A. Pleasants, *Fernando Wood of New York*, New York: Columbia Univ. Studies in Hist., Econ. and Pub. Law, no. 536, 1948, ch. 5; James F. Richardson, "Mayor Fernando Wood and the New York Police force, 1855-1857," *N. Y. Hist. Soc. Quart.*, 1966, *50*: 5-40.

[18] Richardson, *op. cit.*, p. 6.

[19] Those interested in sanitary reform seem to have been well aware of their enemies. Stephen Smith frequently described corrupt practices such as the bribery to which the

Harris were officers of the group, and Stephen Smith, Joseph M. Smith, and Peter Cooper were among the members of the council.[20]

That winter the Association impressed upon the legislators the urgent need for a health bill. They used established arguments: New York's ratio of mortality was greater than that of most cities in the United States and Western Europe; those diseases which most contributed to this mortality were due to the absence of proper sanitary administrations and were just those diseases thought to be preventable; New York had three separate health authorities, none of which functioned properly. These were the Board of Health, composed of the Mayor, Aldermen, and Councilmen and rarely in session; the Commissioners of Health, including the Mayor, the Presidents of the Boards of Aldermen and Councilmen, the Resident Physician, and Health Officer of the Port; and the City Inspector's Department.[21] The sanitary association pointed out that there were about 112 individuals directly and indirectly supposedly concerned for the health of the people, but " that there is not one who feels it to be required of him to take note of, or to use any effort whatever to check the immense amount of disease. . . ."[22]

Once again the story was the same. Their bill failed to pass.

By the end of 1860, the Sanitary Association could say that its meetings had been well attended and that it considered itself a permanent organization. It continued to act as a lobby group in Albany. The membership increased to over two hundred and fifty, representing the professions of law, medicine, education, and divinity.[23]

As late as 1862 the group continued to hear interesting papers, but

Tammany-controlled City Inspector's Office allegedly resorted. The 1857 bill had been "effectually defeated by the paid agents of corrupt officials who succeeded, at a late period of the session, in sequestering or destroying all traces of the bill, both manuscript and printed." *Am. M. Times,* 1860, *1*: 423. It must also be noted that the friends of sanitary reform early realized that a health department with jurisdiction merely over New York, and not including Brooklyn or the other surrounding communities, would have been of little avail. The large interchange of people each day made the metropolitan concept a necessity. See "New York Health Bills," *Am. M. Times,* 1862, *4*: 70-71. For a brief, general description of New York City government see Seth Low, *New York in 1850 and in 1890,* New York: N. Y. Hist. Soc., 1892.

[20] N. Y. San. Assoc. *Report, op. cit.* Elisha Harris must have been everybody's favorite secretary. He held that job in the Sanitary Association, and later in the Council of Hygiene, the U. S. Sanitary Commission, and the American Public Health Association. See also, Wilson G. Smillie, *Public Health,* Its Promise for the Future, New York: Macmillan, 1955, pp. 289-290.

[21] N. Y. San. Assoc. *Report, op. cit.,* pp. 11-13.

[22] *Ibid.,* p. 13.

[23] *Second Annual Report of the N. Y. Sanitary Association* for the year ending Dec. 1860, New York, 1860, pp. 1-23.

166

the pressures of the war seem to have caused a cessation of its activities sometime in that year.[24]

While I have concerned myself primarily with matters of the public health, problems of personal health were not ignored. The sanitarians had the twin aims of improving the health laws and of educating the people, especially the poor, in the ways of proper hygiene. This, indeed, was also the aim of the numerous philanthropic organizations that flourished in New York at mid-century. The popular magazines and the newspapers often contained articles on health or advice on matters pertaining to diet or epidemics. One author, in 1856, thought that Americans should be the healthiest people in the world. If they were not, it was due to the hectic pace of life, with too much work and too little play.[25]

Medical teachers did not neglect the subject of hygiene, although often admitting that, in this area, ". . . the profession of medicine has hitherto grievously failed "[26]—this, even though the medical profession had expended an incredible amount of time and talent upon the subject of public and private hygiene in the quarter century before the Civil War.[27] And so, too, many doctors believed that hygiene and not quarantine was the true law of health.[28]

II

When the *New York Journal of Medicine* ceased publication in 1860, Stephen Smith shifted his editorial chair to the newly established *American Medical Times*, and he began four years of vigorous crusading in a large variety of areas. The older journal had contained few editorial comments in its bimonthly numbers, while its successor, a weekly, published lengthy editorials in every issue. In his writings he concerned himself with the

[24] Louis Elsberg's "The domain of medical police," *Am. M. Monthly*, 1862, *17*: 321-337, was delivered before the Association. This concept of medical police was a prominent idea in the writings of John Griscom too. See George Rosen, "The fate of the concept of medical police 1780-1890," *Centaurus*, 1957, *5*: 97-113. Actually the term "sanitary police" might be more applicable to the goals of the New York sanitarians. According to Shattuck, in the term "medical police," cure of disease is implied; while in the idea of "sanitary police" prevention is stressed. Lemuel Shattuck, *Report of the Sanitary Commission of Massachusetts 1850*, Cambridge: Harvard, 1948 (reprint).

[25] [Robert Tomes], "Why we get sick," *Harper's Monthly*, 1856, *13*: 642-647. The author noted that, "A host of diseases of the heart, the brain, nerves, and stomach, which exhaust the doctor's skill and fill his pockets, came in with modern civilization. To these diseases the Americans are far more subject than any other people . . . ," p. 642.

[26] Frank H. Hamilton, "Hygiene," *New York J. Med.*, 1859, *7*: 60-74, p. 60. Hamilton, a renowned surgeon, had been Stephen Smith's teacher and preceptor and remained a close friend in later years.

[27] *Ibid.*, p. 63.

[28] "Quarantine and Hygiene," *North Am. Rev.*, 1860, *91*: 438-491, p. 491.

role of medicine and the medical profession in society, including frequent expositions on wartime problems.[29]

Since Smith was a New Yorker, and because his journal was published in that city and presumably found most of its readers there, he usually devoted himself to local sanitary problems—primarily the need for legislative reform and the necessity for vigorous action on the part of the medical profession. In his first editorial in the new journal he set forth many of the precepts he planned to follow. He singled out the subject of hygiene to receive vigilant and faithful attention.[30] In the third number he elaborated on these ideas and stated his intention periodically to examine the more important questions relating to sanitary and quarantine systems of American cities and particularly the role and duty of the medical profession.[31] Despite the potential usefulness of his public health editorials nationally, he consistently focused on New York City.

During the summer of 1860 things looked bleak indeed. The country was threatened by division, political feelings ran high, and local sanitary problems continued to increase. More and more immigrants had to be fed and housed as each month passed. Smith shared the pessimistic mood of late summer when he noted that amidst legislative corruption it was not at all certain that improved health laws could be obtained: " And such are the necessities of the people, such the jeopardy of life and health as well as commercial interests, that our population cannot safely await the good time coming, when good laws and municipal reform shall effect the sanitary improvements now demanded. From various quarters the question comes up—What shall be done? "[32]

His answer was clear: he believed that more pressing than questions of quarantine were those relating to civic hygiene. More attention had

[29] Although Elisha Harris and George Shready were assistant editors, I have ascribed the editorials to Smith, throughout. Harris actually resigned in 1861 because of increasing work with the U. S. Sanitary Commission. Shrady apparently did most of the reports of medical society meetings. Furthermore, Smith published many of the editorials in his book *Doctor in Medicine* and Other Papers on Professional Subjects, New York: Wood, 1872, thereby claiming authorship for those included. In various letters to his wife, to be dealt with in a future study, Smith complained of the wearying task of his weekly editorials. In this paper I am concerned only with those editorials that dealt with sanitary reform.

[30] *Am. M. Times*, 1860, *1*: 15. Howard D. Kramer, " The beginnings of the public health movement in the United States," *Bull. Hist. Med.*, 1947, *21*: 352-376, gives Smith and the *American Medical Times* a great deal of credit for bringing about reform, p. 375. Also Kramer, " Early Municipal and State Boards," *op. cit.*

[31] " Our sanitary defences," *Am. M. Times*, 1860, *1*: 46-47.

[32] *Ibid.*, *1*: 100.

to be **devoted** to municipal sanitary arrangements, especially to those of New York.[33]

The cause of sanitary reform moved forward slowly during the Civil War. Although official population figures showed a slight decrease in the 1865 census as compared with 1860, the city's municipal problems became worse.[34] Stokes noted that the city's growth during the war had been checked, but not stopped entirely. Fewer buildings were erected and the misery of crowded tenements grew. The increase in production and the resultant higher wages probably did elevate the general standard of living, but often prices increased too so the poorest classes were left with a net loss.[35] The poor did not share in the profits of rising real estate values and the general business expansion—in fact these things operated to their disadvantage. The increase in luxury which " struck every observer " falls short of describing the condition of more than half of the population—the tenement dwellers.[36]

Although wages rose, prices rose faster. Eggs, fifteen cents in 1861, rose to twenty-five cents by the end of 1863; potatoes went from $1.50 to $2.25 per bushel during the same period. The increase in wages was generally about twenty-five percent, or less than half the increase of prices.[37]

Citizens interested in sanitary reform worked on through the war years. They helped introduce a bill into the state legislature each winter, but it failed to pass with each succeeding session. The daily papers and popular journals continued to clamor for both municipal and sanitary reform, building up to quite a pitch in the year prior to the success of 1866—the Metropolitan Health Bill.

The medical press was also active, especially the influential *American Medical Times*. Others, beside Stephen Smith, participated in the effort; but it is on Smith's role I wish to focus. I should note that his work in the early 1860's was of much broader scope than my emphasis on sanitation would indicate.

[33] *Ibid.*, 2: 47-48.

[34] For a general discussion see Emerson D. Fite, *Social and Industrial Conditions in the North During the Civil War*, New York: Macmillan, 1910, p. 229.

[35] I. N. Phelps Stokes, *The Iconography of Manhattan Island*, 6 vols., New York, 1895-1928, vol. 3, pp. 736-756; Milledge L. Bonham, Jr., " New York and the Civil War," in Alexander C. Flick, ed., *History of the State of New York*, 10 vols., New York: Columbia, 1933-1937, vol. 7, pp. 99-135.

[36] Allan Nevins, *The Evening Post*, A Century of Journalism, New York: Boni and Liverwright, 1922, p. 364.

[37] Fite, *op. cit.*, p. 184. Also Edgar W. Martin, *The Standard of Living in 1860*, Chicago: Univ. of Chicago, 1942, contains many useful data.

Prior to 1864, Smith's efforts in behalf of a Metropolitan Health Bill were confined chiefly to the numerous editorials praising each bill, exhorting his fellow physicians to exert influence upon the legislature, and bemoaning the lack of a properly constituted health department in the city.

In December, 1860, he asked: Will the next legislature provide a sanitary code for the city? [38] He pointed out that more than a fourth of the state's population resided in New York and Brooklyn. He noted that it was widely acknowledged that these million and a quarter people were " living under one of the most corrupt and corrupting municipal governments in the civilized world, and that reform without the interposition of State legislation is impractical." To call the existing Health Department by that name was a misnomer. " It does little for health, but much for disease and death." [39]

Early in 1861, Smith aimed his editorial guns in a violent attack on the City Inspector, who was to become a favorite target for the next five years.[40]

The City Inspector was really the only active health official in New York. It is true that there was a Physician of the Port and a Resident Physician, who, with the Mayor and Presidents of the Boards of Councilmen and Aldermen, constituted a Commission of Health. In fact, however, in matters other than quarantine, it was mainly the City Inspector and his 44 health wardens who looked after the sanitation of the city.[41]

In his report for 1860, the inspector, Mr. Daniel E. Delavan, a two year incumbent in the post, claimed a healthy condition for New York when compared to European cities.[42] What problems there were he attributed mainly to immigrants. His report admitted many of the sanitary

[38] " Health laws," *Am. M. Times*, 1860, *1*: 423-424.
[39] *Ibid.*
[40] " Health of New York in 1860," *Am. M. Times*, 1861, *2*: 63-64.
[41] See *Proceedings of a Select Committee of The Senate . . . Appointed to Investigate Various Departments of the City of New York*, New York State Legislature, Senate Doc. no. 38, February 9, 1865. In this 612 page report, which dealt only with the City Inspector's department, there is a wealth of information. Testimony revealed the buying and selling of jobs and the incompetence of the health wardens. The duties of the twenty-two wardens and an equal number of assistants was to report nuisances, inspect buildings, privies, and cesspools, report all diseases, and to prevent accumulation of garbage and offal on the streets and sidewalks, p. 345. Several health wardens admitted they did not go personally to see cases of disease. They generally admitted that some smallpox existed and " a few fevers," when in fact smallpox, typhus, typhoid, cholera infantum, and scarlatina were widespread, pp. 455-456. Several of the wardens also admitted that they " devoted " a month's pay—but usually claimed ignorance of the fact it was used to aid defeat of health bills in Albany, pp. 462, 467.
[42] *Annual Report of the City Inspector . . . for the Year Ending December 31, 1860*, New York: Board of Aldermen, Doc. no. 5, 1861, p. 10.

problems of New York and he gave some reasons for them. In the first place, he was very critical of the medical profession for their failure to cooperate in the proper registration of vital statistics. Thus he noted the paradox of " opposition among the very class whose leading spirits have been most active for some years past in this city in urging the cause of sanitary reform." [43] He admitted to the filthy condition of the streets, stating that the Common Council had removed $50,000 from his budget and that in November, 1860, money for street cleaning ran out; 300 miles of paved streets was a lot to sweep. [44] Mr. Delavan also was opposed to having the state legislature do for the citizens what they could best do for themselves. With a final thrust aimed at those working for reform, he said, " Nor is it necessary for the further efficiency of this department that it should become the nursery of students of medicine. . . ." [45]

Smith dealt harshly with this report. He noted that it contained ". . . its usual variety of loose and often absurd statements in regard to the public health, and deductions, the result of the most profound ignorance of sanitary science." [46] He objected mostly to the assertion that New York was a healthy city. The ratio of 1 death in 36 of its population made the mortality rate the highest of civilized cities.

Early in 1862, Smith bemoaned the singular indifference, which he felt was evident in the city, toward the fearful living conditions of most of its people. [47] The *Medical and Surgical Reporter* of Philadelphia agreed and said that the Augean stable had to be cleansed and a Hercules of sanitary science was needed to do the job. [48]

In February, 1862, Smith became more optimistic about the possibility of a health bill. There was good evidence at last that a reorganization of the health department was to take place. Perhaps he saw a turning point in the road to victory when he noted that, " the question which is presented this winter is not, Shall there be a reform, but, What shall be its character? " [49]

Optimism was short-lived. In early May he began an editorial plain- tively announcing the adjournment of the legislature without the enact- ment of a health bill. The metropolitan concept introduced into the pro- posed bill was distasteful to the mayor. Smith decided that Mayor Opdyke

[43] *Ibid.*, pp. 16-17.
[44] *Ibid.*, pp. 19-22.
[45] *Ibid.*, p. 60.
[46] *Am. M. Times*, 1861, 2: 63.
[47] " Sanitary legislation," *Am. M. Times*, 1862, 4: 28-29.
[48] *M. and S. Reporter*, 1862, 7: 349-351.
[49] " New York health bills," *Am. M. Times*, 1862, 4: 70.

had really joined the " Ring " and thereby had aided the defeat of "this most righteous measure." [50]

Others, too, " confessed to a very great disappointment " at the failure of the bill. The *Medical and Surgical Reporter* entitled its editorial, " Health Bills and a Diseased Body Politic." " Politicians, those curses of our country . . ." doubtless were to blame, said the *Reporter*.[51] And so again New York was left to its own sanitary devices, devices that were due to receive shocking public description and denunciation in the succeeding few years.

In what had become a cycle of editorial moods, Smith seemed most discouraged toward the end of 1862. It was an extremely busy year for him, personally. Besides the weekly editorial writing and editing of the *Medical Times*, he wrote a manual for military surgeons, used in the Civil War; he continued active teaching and practice at the Bellevue Hospital and its new Medical College, where he was the first Professor of the Principles of Surgery; and he served a stint in the military hospitals of Virginia as an acting assistant surgeon. But the sanitary reform of New York was still a pressing concern for him.

In November he wrote that prospects for a bill seemed discouraging, that many had been led to believe that subsequent efforts would lead nowhere and hence should be abandoned indefinitely. Smith disagreed. While thousands of New Yorkers were dying annually of what he firmly believed were preventable diseases, and while half the city's population lived in the cheerless, sunless, and airless tenements, it was unthinkable to yield in the struggle. Ceaseless agitation would be required. His feelings were perhaps neatly summed up when he noted in that November of 1862, " we should not, however, lose sight of the fact that we are striving to accomplish a reform which in importance and in magnitude rises superior to all civil, social, religious, or political questions of the time." [52] Allowing for the exaggeration and zeal of the reformer, this statement still, I believe, illustrates the extent of his commitment to sanitary reform, especially in view of the state of the nation's political and economic health.

He described the effects he envisioned from legislative enactments: First, they should protect the citizen, especially the impoverished one, from disease and thereby lengthen life; second, they would develop a strong and healthy generation of citizens; and third, all health reforms would add greatly to the sum of human happiness. So fully impressed

[50] " Failure of the health bill," *Ibid.*, pp. 250-251.
[51] *M. and S. Reporter*, 1862, *8*: 124-125.
[52] " The prospect of health-reform in New York," *Am. M. Times*, 1862, *5*: 276.

was he with the importance of sanitary reform that he felt, even though the prospect of success was not as great as it had been the year before, " we ought to put forth increased energy instead of relaxing our efforts." [53]

Public apathy was a major obstacle in the path of sanitary reform. This unconcern was as prevalent in much of the medical profession as it seems to have been in the general public. Numerous writers appealed to the educated, the rich, the influential, to raise their voices in protest. *Harper's Weekly* noted, for instance, " There is certainly no city in the world where intelligent and decent people surrender themselves to a band of knaves with such good humor as in New York." [54] The *Medical Times* noted that : " The country is horrified when a thousand fall victims in an ill-fought battle, but in this city 10,000 die annually of diseases which the city authorities have the power to remove, and no one is shocked." [55]

December 12, 1863, marked a turning point. On that day a group of the leading lawyers and merchants of the city, including Peter Cooper, John Jacob Astor, Jr., August Belmont, and Hamilton Fish, formed the Citizens' Association. They were organized " for purposes of public usefulness." [56]

At an Association meeting two months later, a committee was formed to solicit from the medical profession the " fullest and most reliable information relative to the public health." Shortly, twenty-four of the city's leading medical men received a letter from the Association—among them : Valentine Mott, Willard Parker, Stephen Smith, John H. Griscom, Elisha Harris, Austin Flint, Frank H. Hamilton, and Gurdon Buck.

Only a week later, on March 9th, the physicians answered the committee's request for information. The doctors pointed out that although New York with its many natural advantages ought to be one of the healthiest cities, the exact reverse was the case. They believed the high mortality rate was a reliable index of the city's miserable health conditions. They provided comparative statistics : mortality in New York was one in every 35.7 of the population, while in Philadelphia it was one in 43.6, in Boston one in 41.2, and in Hartford as low as one in 54.8. The city fared poorly in comparison to London and Liverpool as well. They pointed to Lyon Playfair's figures in Great Britain, which showed that for every death there were at least twenty-eight cases of illness.[57]

[53] *Ibid.*, p. 277.
[54] *Harper's Weekly*, 1863, 7: 786.
[55] " Sanitary interests in New York," *Am. M. Times*, 1863, 6: 21-22
[56] For a description of the founding of the Citizens' Association see Edward C. Mack, *Peter Cooper, Citizen of New York*, New York: Duell, Sloan, Pearce, 1949, ch. 19. See also the *New York Citizen*, Aug. 13, 1864.
[57] These two letters may be found in *Report of The Council of Hygiene and Public Health of the Citizens' Association of New York, Upon the Sanitary Condition of the City*, New York: Appleton, 1865, pp. ix-xiii.

In the meantime, the Citizens' Association busied itself with the task of lobbying for the health bill then being considered in Albany. Representatives appeared before the legislature on March 15 and 16, only to meet resistance from both Democratic and Republican members. The former regarded the sweeping measures proposed under a metropolitan, non-political health department as being aimed at their friends, which indeed it was. The Republicans were reluctant to interfere in city affairs, thereby hurting their chances in the upcoming presidential election that fall. The members of the Citizens' Association found, according to Stephen Smith, that to many members of the legislature, " the death of five thousand citizens was not so serious as the possibility of a presidential defeat." [58]

It must have been clear, at this point, to the Citizens' Association and the friends of sanitary reform, that what they really needed was a set of clear and extensive facts about the health conditions of the city—facts that would overcome the inertia of some legislators and facts which would once and for all clearly disprove the data which the City Inspector's Office had for so long been bringing to Albany to controvert any proposal for better laws.

A Council of Hygiene and Public Health was formed in April within the Citizens' Association. Its president was Joseph M. Smith, a prominent physician and writer who had made a monumental study of the epidemics of New York State.[59] Elisha Harris, a close friend and neighbor of Stephen Smith, was made secretary. The council consisted of sixteen physicians, many of whom had been recipients and signers of the letters noted above.[60]

To gather the necessary facts about the true health and sanitary conditions of New York and its three-quarters of a million residents, an extensive survey was planned. This survey was organized and directed primarily

[58] " Citizens' Association and health reform," *Am. M. Times*, 1864, *8*: 200. Also at the beginning of 1864 there was an investigation into the affairs of the City Inspector's department. Smith published excerpts from a letter written by Thomas N. Carr, who had been superintendent of street cleaning. Carr said that New York simply had no sanitary department worthy of the name. He felt that the only concern the City Inspector had was for the streets. Carr continued: "On an examination of the annual sanitary reports of England or France, the mind is astonished by the vastness of research, investigation, and scientific elaboration which these reports contain, and yet, strange to say, street cleaning, instead of being the all absorbing feature of these documents, is not even mentioned." *Am. M. Times*, 1864, *8*: 57.

[59] Joseph M. Smith, " Report on the medical topography and epidemics of New York," *Trans. A. M. A.*, 1860, *13*: 81-269.

[60] In 1865 Smith became the secretary. For the names of the members of the Council, see the first part of the introduction to the *Report, op. cit.*

by Stephen Smith.[61] It was to become, according to numerous commenters, the most complete sanitary survey ever made, and certainly an important landmark in the history of public health in America.

The survey began early in May, got under full swing by July, and was completed by mid-November.[62] The city was divided into thirty-one districts, each inspected thoroughly by a physician. It was intended, by means of the survey, to arrive at " positive knowledge of the amount of preventible disease existing in New York, the location of insalubrious quarters, the peculiar habitats of typhus, smallpox, . . . and the conditions on which the alarming prevalence of these diseases depend." [63] A month later, in late July, Smith noted, " It is nothing less than a full and accurate inquiry into the causes of disease in this city by competent medical men." [64] And thus it should also be credited as a landmark in the history of epidemiology.

Although there were numerous etiological theories current in 1864, in the sanitarians' view the environment played the most important part, especially the so-called localizing causes, or those which promoted the prevalence of disease in particular localities. Each of the thirty-one inspectors reported on his district and described his findings mainly in terms of cleanliness and filth.[65]

The inspectors were, for the most part, young physicians who were employed by one of the public (charity supported) dispensaries of the city. They were ideally qualified, for their patients mostly came from the poorer districts; moreover, they had had experience in visiting the tenements. They were given only token compensation ($40 per month)

[61] The evidence concerning Smith's role lies mostly within his own writings, especially *The City That Was, op. cit.* Charles F. Chandler, however, also gave Smith credit for organizing the survey. See *Stephen Smith, Addresses in Recognition of His Public Services on the Occasion of His Eighty Eighth Birthday,* New York: New York Academy of Medicine, 1911, p. 19, in which Chandler, then an old man himself, noted, " This work was organized and supervised to its completion by Dr. Stephen Smith." In 1864 Joseph M. Smith, the president of the Council, was seventy-five years old. Elisha Harris, the secretary, was mainly occupied by the U. S. Sanitary Commission.

[62] *N. Y. Times,* March 16, 1865, or *The City That Was, op. cit.,* p. 57.

[63] *Am. M. Times,* 1864, *8*: 307. The *N. Y. Tribune,* 3 June 1864, had great praise for the efforts of the Citizens' Association.

[64] *Am. M. Times,* 1866, *9*: 47.

[65] There is a long discussion of etiological factors in disease in the introductory portion of the *Report,* pp. xlvii-lxviii. See also Richard H. Shryock, " The origins and significance of the public health movement in the United States," *Ann. M. Hist.,* 1929, *1*: 645-665, especially pp. 650-652; Charles E. Rosenberg, " The cause of cholera: aspects of etiological thought in nineteenth century America," *Bull. Hist. Med.,* 1960, *34*: 331-354; and his *The Cholera Years, op. cit.*; and John Simon, *Filth Diseases and Their Prevention,* 1st Am. ed., Boston: Campbell, 1876.

for their labor. Their reports, charts, maps, and diagrams filled seventeen folio volumes. On his return from his work on behalf of the U. S. Sanitary Commission, Dr. Harris edited the 360 page report and added a 143 page introduction. The report was published in April 1865. The reviews of the book were uniformly laudatory, and many pointed out the great importance of the survey and the *Report* for the future of sanitary government in New York.[66]

The *Report* has been frequently cited in discussions of American public health and of housing problems. Indeed, it deserves to be ranked very high among primary documents, not only in the history of public health reform but in epidemiology as well. Furthermore, it affords an extremely detailed look at some aspects of the way of life in each of the wards of New York in 1864, and it should be of great interest in the study of urban history.

Epidemiology has been defined as "the study of the distribution and determinants of disease prevalence in man."[67] According to this concept, then, the *Report* belongs among the most important of nineteenth century epidemiological studies. It contains graphic, statistical, and descriptive information on population, number and size of tenement houses, prevailing diseases, schools, churches, stores, slaughter-houses, factories, brothels, drinking establishments, sewerage, streets, and topography.

Its impact was manifold. Certainly it did not "drop stillborn from the printer's hand," as had been the case with the Shattuck *Report* fifteen years earlier. Instead, as Kramer has pointed out for the Chadwick *Report*, it was a document that was alive; it aroused indignation and wonderment; it had emotional appeal beyond its intellectual content. And it led to effective legislation.[68]

[66] The *N. Y. Times* on July 7, 1865, said: "No volume of intenser interest has ever seen the light in this city. . . ." See also *Nation*, 1865, *1*: 250; *Am. J. M. Sc.*, 1865, *100*: 419-428.

[67] Brian MacMahon, Thomas F. Pugh, and Johannes Ipsen, *Epidemiologic Methods*, Boston: Little, Brown, 1960, p. 3.

[68] Kramer, "Beginnings," *op. cit.*, pp. 361-362. There were occasional descriptions of living conditions among the poor in the general press. See, for instance, Samuel B. Halliday, *The Lost and Found; or Life Among the Poor*, New York: Blakeman & Mason, 1859. Halliday was a member of the N. Y. Sanitary Association. Soon after the survey of the Citizens' Association was published there was a vivid article in the *Nation* by Bayard Taylor, entitled "A descent into the depths," 1866, *2*: 302-304. Although I have focused attention on the two societies in which Smith played a role, this is not to say that they were the only ones active in sanitary reform at this time. The A. I. C. P. and the various missions and tract societies were also active. The A. I. C. P. *Report* for 1853 contains a long discussion of sanitary needs. Its founder and leading spirit, Robert M. Hartley, was well known for his crusade against swill milk. See Roy Lubove,

Besides the descriptions of overflowing privies with their nauseous odors, garbage, offal, ashes, and generally dirty streets, the inspectors also wrote about slaughter-houses, fat and bone boiling establishments, and stables, all dispersed among the tenements. The streets were the main focus of complaint from the magazines and newspapers of the day as well. Youngsters, it is said, could easily earn nickels by standing along Broadway and sweeping a path through the muck for those who wanted to cross.[69] On Thirty-ninth Street, the inspector reported that blood and liquid animal remains flowed for two blocks from a slaughter-house to the river.[70] Another great source of nuisance was the wooden garbage box. These usually rotted, allowing liquid contents to flow out. It seems they also provided a ready source of wood for political bonfires.[71]

Occasionally the survey itself was responsible for immediate improvements. In parts of the third district the inspector noted progress with each succeeding visit he made.[72]

It was armed with the data from this comprehensive epidemiological study of New York City that Stephen Smith appeared before the legislature in Albany on February 13, 1865. The report had not yet been published, but Smith in his testimony, to which I alluded at the opening of this paper, quoted widely from it. He spoke before the joint committee of the Senate and Assembly, presided over by Andrew D. White. The committee had already heard testimony from Mr. Dorman B. Eaton on the legal aspects of the proposed bill.[73] Smith told them that he and the

"The New York Association for Improving the Condition of the Poor: the formative years," *N.Y. Hist. Soc. Quart.*, 1959, *43*: 307-327; and Atkins, *Health, Housing, and Poverty, op. cit.* Carroll S. Rosenberg's "Protestants and Five Pointers: The Five Pointers: The Five Points House of Industry, 1850-1870," *N.Y. Hist. Soc. Quart.*, 1964, *47*: 327-347, describes New York's most notorious slum and efforts toward amelioration. Also Allan Nevins has drawn attention to the reformers in his "The golden thread in the history of New York," *N.Y. Hist. Soc. Quart.*, 1955, *39*: 5-22.

[69] Israel Weinstein, "Eighty years of public health in New York City," *Bull. N.Y. Acad. Med.*, 1947, *23*: 221-237.

[70] *Citizens' Association Report, op. cit.*, pp. 261-262.

[71] *Ibid.*, p. 285; and *Annual Report of the City Inspector . . . for the Year Ending December 31, 1861*, New York: Board of Alderman, Doc. no. 4, 1862, pp. 21-23.

[72] *Citizens' Association Report, op. cit.*, p. 42.

[73] *City That Was, op. cit.*, p. 46; Andrew Dickson White, *Autobiography*, 2 vols., New York: Century, 1905, vol. 1, pp. 107-110. White reported the oft quoted testimony of one of the city's health wardens, who, when asked the meaning of the word hygiene, answered that it referred to bad smells arising from standing water. White also sat on a Senate committee during the investigation of the City Inspector's department early in 1865. Despite the pleas of the Citizens' Association, City Inspector Boole was not dismissed. See Stokes, *Iconography, op. cit.*, vol. 5, p. 1912; and Senate Doc. no. 38, 1865, *op. cit.*, p. 467. Eaton's testimony was given Feb. 2, 1865, and was published by

Citizens' Association had been inspired and aided by the work of similar organizations in Great Britain, notably the Health of Towns Association.

He further told the legislators that the best method of arriving at a complete understanding of the existing causes of disease was by a house-to-house inspection. Since it was disease that was the object of study, it could only have been carried out properly by sufficiently trained men, *viz.*, physicians.

He described conditions in general terms of cleanliness, stating that the degree of public health of a town was to be measured by its cleanliness and that in no way was the sanitary government of New York to be commended. He called the City Inspector's department a " gigantic imposture." The twenty-two health wardens and an equal number of assistants were grossly ignorant of sanitary matters, but that was to be expected in view of their backgrounds, since they were liquor store owners, local politicians, stonemasons, and carpenters. Not only were they ignorant of medical matters, but Smith also accused them of unwillingness to visit houses where known cases of disease existed. He told of one health warden who sent for an attendant of a smallpox patient in an upper room. Ordering the attendant not to approach too closely, he then advised: " Burn camphor on the stove, and hang bags of camphor about the necks of the children." Smith then asked the members of the Senate and Assembly:

To what depth of humiliation must that community have descended, which tolerates as its sanitary officers men who are not only utterly disqualified by education, business, and moral character, but who have not even the poor qualification of courage to perform their duties?

He ended his long testimony with the recommendation that New York heed the experience of other large cities in establishing a well-organized health board. That board, he opined, should be independent of politics and above partisan control. Furthermore the board must combine administrative ability with a knowledge of disease and its prevention. For this reason he felt that the composition of the board should include medical and non-medical members. His testimony, although well organized and at times forceful as well as eloquent, was not original. It represented the consensus of most of his co-workers. It is to his credit, however, that the problems of sanitary reform were continually held up before the medical profession through his editorials in the *American Medical Times*

"Friends of the Bill" later that year. Together with an appendix, his remarks take up 56 printed pages. *Remarks of D. B. Eaton, Esq., at a Joint Meeting of the Committees of the Senate and Assembly*, New York: Nesbitt, 1865.

and now were brought before the general public, with the aid of the *New York Times*. Equally to his credit was it that he had helped to write the medical portion of the proposed bill and, together with Dorman B. Eaton, a lawyer and a keen student of sanitary laws, had drafted the final version.

Why the *Times* hesitated for over a month before publishing his speech I cannot explain with certainty. It is entirely possible that when the testimony was given on February 13, the prospect of legislation was bright; but that by March 16, when the *Times* printed the speech, the bill was already in dire straits.[74] Henry Raymond and the *Times* were deeply committed to a health reform measure, as is attested by frequent editorials during the winter of 1865 and again during the next session in 1866. It may well be that the *Times* felt that publication of the facts would serve to bring pressure to bear upon the reluctant legislators.[75] That it did not achieve this result is a matter of record. But now the issues and the facts were clearly before the public. Because part of the Citizens' Association survey was published in the *Times* it achieved a wider public circulation for writing on the subject of sanitation than had ever been the case before. This was a milestone in New York history.

Unfortunately, Smith's testimony in February, its publication in March, and the subsequent appearance of the printed *Report* were not enough to sway the lawmakers in Albany. Frequent editorials in the *Times*, the *Tribune,* and the *Citizen,* a weekly paper founded by the Citizens' Association in 1864, did not seem to help either.

On January 16, 1865, the *Times* noted that typhus and smallpox were running rife. The " ignorant men called ' Health Wardens ' " were receiving annually an aggregate of nearly $50,000, but in the opinion of the newspaper, " The only persons who are doing anything for the public health are the agents of the Citizens' Association."

On March 3, the *Tribune* reported the continuing discussion in Albany and the testimony that had been given for the bill by the members of the

[74] On March 10 and 11, 1865, the *Times* noted that opposition was brewing from quarters formerly friendly to the bill. The paper warned that delay in passage of the bill was dangerous, so late in the session. Smith gave a great deal of credit to Henry J. Raymond, editor of the *Times*, calling him an ardent reformer. *City That Was, op. cit.,* p. 173.

[75] That some of the legislators were impressed by the testimony was attested to by at least one member of Smith's audience. After hearing the description of sweat-shop conditions in the tenements and of clothing, in the process of manufacture, draped over cribs of children with active smallpox, one of the committee supposedly said to Smith: " Why I bought underwear at one of those stores a few days ago, and I believe I have got smallpox, for I begin to itch all over." *City That Was, op. cit.,* p. 156. It should be stressed that this episode was forty-six years in the past when the book was published.

Citizens' Association and against it by Francis I. A. Boole the City Inspector, Lewis A. Sayre the resident physician, and Cyrus Ramsey the Registrar in the City Inspector's department. According to the *Tribune*, Ramsey attempted ineffectually to controvert the statements made by Smith, Eaton, and the friends of reform. The *Tribune*, somewhat incredulously, noted that Ramsey was driven to extremes in support of the existing corrupt system when he even went so far as to ridicule the idea that cleanliness was an important source of health.[76]

As March progressed, the *Times* pointed out that the Democratic members in the legislature hung together on every question, but not the Republicans. The health bill had, despite pleas from many sides, once again become a political and partisan issue.[77] The *Tribune* said, " To lose the rich *placer* of the City Inspector's department is to cut the winds of scores of active workers, whose only duty is to sign the payrolls and work for the party that gives them fat sinecures." [78]

On April 12, three days after Appomattox, the bill finally came out of committee into the House. Two days later, amid " perfect bedlam," it was defeated. Most New Yorkers, however, were probably much too dazed and saddened to read the account from Albany on the morning of April 15. The headline that day proclaimed " Awful Event." [79] It is not likely that in the days following the tragic and shocking death of Lincoln, those who had labored so hard that year for a health bill had any time for grief on its account.

In 1865 cholera threatened New York again, and the press of the city

[76] Ramsey was a physician but seems to have been completely under Tammany sway. Lewis A. Sayre was the Resident Physician of New York, as well as a leading teacher of orthopedic surgery. His difference of opinion with the members of the Citizens' Association seems, on the surface, to have been on intellectual grounds. Smith, who was a fellow faculty member of Sayre's at Bellevue, had once called the latter's job (as Resident Physician) a sinecure. *Am. M. Times*, 1862, *4*: 252. It is, of course, quite possible that Sayre's own vested interests prompted his belief in the status quo. His salary was about $5,000 per year.

[77] *N. Y. Times*, March 20, 1865.

[78] *N. Y. Tribune*, March 20, 1865.

[79] *N. Y. Times*, April 13, 15, 17; *N. Y. Tribune*, April 15. The *Times* on April 17 noted three reasons for the defeat of the bill: Several Union (Republican) members were absent owing to illness; several others were unwilling to create another commission for the Governor; and, City Inspector F. I. A. Boole had spent nearly the whole winter in Albany, armed with sufficient funds to kill the bill. This occurred in an Assembly in which the Republicans had a majority of twenty-four. For a discussion of Boole, see Gustavus Myers. *The History of Tammany Hall*, New York: Boni and Liverwright, 1917, pp. 205-208. An informative discussion of the state political situation at this time may be found in Homer A. Stebbins, " A political history of the State of New York 1865-1869," *Studies in Hist., Econ. & Pub. Law*, vol. 55, New York: Columbia University, 1913.

became increasingly alarmed over the prospects of another epidemic. The summer passed, however, and with a sigh of relief those concerned felt that with the approaching cold season the city would be safe, at least temporarily. But the need for legislative action became more acute.[80]

On November 9, the *Nation* claimed that New York was nearly as filthy as the Asiatic towns from which the cholera came.

It is awful yet comical to learn that the Board of Health, which at such a crisis ought to reign supreme, is such a disreputable body that, nobody having the power to adjourn it if once organized, the Mayor is afraid to call it together.[81]

The *Times*, a day later, noted that the Mayor considered the cholera the lesser of the two evils, and so left the Board alone.[82]

As 1866 opened, Mayor John T. Hoffman, a Tammany leader, stated in his first message to the Common Council that the Board of Commissioners of Health, would be " able to accomplish all that may be required of it." He was against a metropolitan bill, and he used the old argument that such a bill would be an interference with the municipal rights of New York.[83] The *Times* retorted that the only branches of the city government managed with honesty were Central Park, the Police Department, and the charities on Blackwell's Island—all created by the state legislature. As for the *Times*, it felt that, " We would prefer to live under a ' Legislative Commission ' to dying prematurely and painfully under the pure Democratic rule of a city constituency." [84]

All through January and February the *Times*, and occasionally the *Tribune*, continued to press for a bill. After a complicated fight between the Senate, which passed a bill including the names of four physicians who were to be commissioners, and the Assembly, which wanted to allow the Governor to name the members of the board, the whole thing was nearly scuttled once again.[85] Success was finally achieved on February 15th. The Assembly passed an amended bill allowing the Governor to name the commissioners. With the aid of an impassioned speech by Senator Andrew D. White, using some of the testimony Stephen Smith had presented the previous year, the Conference Committee of the two houses settled their differences and received assurances from Governor Fenton

[80] *New York Times*, Oct. 31, Nov. 9, 1865; *Nation*, 1865; *1*: 609.

[81] *Nation, ibid.*, p. 577.

[82] Quoted by Rosenberg, *Cholera Years, op. cit.*, p. 186. See also *City That Was, op. cit.*, p. 166.

[83] The speech is printed in the *N. Y. Times*, Jan. 3, 1866.

[84] *Ibid.*, Jan. 7, 1866.

[85] *Ibid.*, Feb. 7, 1866.

that none of his appointments would be on a political basis.[86] On **February 21**, 1866, the *Times* felt that the final victory for a health bill was not to be passed over without public notice. The dedicated physicians and philanthropists who, for ten years, had come each winter to Albany received due praise.

The official date of passage was February 26, and the title of the law was "An Act to Create A Metropolitan Sanitary District and Board of Health therein for the Preservation of Life and Health and to Prevent the Spread of Disease." [87]

The law, which in essence had been drafted by Stephen Smith and Dorman B. Eaton the year before, created a health department for the metropolitan area of New York. The new Metropolitan Board of Health, as it was called, was given extremely broad powers to make laws, to carry them out, and to sit in judgment of them, all at the same time. Questions of constitutionality would soon arise.[88]

The general implications of this bill of 1866 are several. It was undoubtedly a major triumph in the history of public health, as noted by Rosen.[89] Locally it served to give a great city the beginning of really effective sanitary government, carried out by professionals. Furthermore, as a major piece of reform legislation it may have been one of the beginning moves against a thread of corruption so strong that it was not broken until the Tweed "Ring" was finally deposed in the early 1870's. The Reverend Samuel Osgood may have had the health bill in mind when he said:

Careful legislation, with intelligent suffrage and a city government more on the plan of the national, and taking from the Common Council its temptations to base

---

[86] *Ibid.*, Feb. 16, 20, 1866.

[87] *Laws of New York, 1866*, ch. 74. Reprinted by Bergen & Tripp, Printers, 1866.

[88] Smith described Eaton's role and his activities in other spheres in chapter 6 of *The City That Was, op. cit.* This book, incidentally, was dedicated to the memory of Dorman B. Eaton. Eaton was perhaps best known for his work in civil service reform. See Ari Hoogenboom, *Outlawing The Spoils*: A history of the Civil Service Reform movement, 1865-1883, Urbana: Univ. of Illinois, 1961. Eaton was credited by Smith with having written the legal aspects of that bill. Eaton's views can be seen in his "The essential conditions of good sanitary administration," *Rep. and Papers*, Am. Pub. Health Assoc., 1874-1875, *2*: 498-514. He was a student of English sanitary law and patterned the New York bill on what he had learned in England. See Dorman B. Eaton, *Sanitary Regulations in England and New York*, New York: Amerman, 1872. See also Stephen Smith, "Development of American public health endeavor," *Am. J. Pub. Health.*, 1915, *5*: 1115-1119; Stephen Smith, "The origin and organization of the Department of Health of the City of New York," *M. Rec.*, 1918, *93*: 1115-1117; and his "The history of public health, 1871-1921," in *A Half Century of Public Health*, M. P. Ravenel, ed., New York: A. P. H. A., 1921, pp. 1-12; especially pp. 4-10 deal with the Metropolitan Health Bill.

[89] George Rosen, *A History of Public Health*, New York: MD, 1958, p. 247.

jobs, will set us right, and free us from being subject to the dynasty of dirt and sovereignty of sots.[90]

On a broader scale, the sanitary reform of New York City had several more specific results. In the first place it was the first comprehensive health legislation of its kind in the United States, and later it was to serve as a model for numerous local and state bills. In this respect too the reform movement seems to have united the sanitary interests of numerous physicians and laymen alike. Sanitary science was becoming a specialty in this country, as in Europe. The work in New York also led to the formation of the most important national health group, the American Public Health Association. Stephen Smith, who was one of the prime movers in its founding and its first president, gave credit to his work for the Metropolitan Health Bill and later as a Commissioner on the Board for providing the inception of the A. P. H. A. in 1872.[91]

Finally, the sanitary reform work in New York also played a role in the changing status or image of the physician and of medicine as a whole. Kramer has noted that before public health could be undertaken, medicine had to put its house in order.[92] But the reverse may have been even more the case: Effective sanitary legislation and the organization of competent health departments played a great part in helping medicine to re-establish the much needed order in the house.

[90] Samuel Osgood, *New York in the Nineteenth Century*, New York: N. Y. Hist. Soc., 1866, pp. 40-41. See also a review of numerous documents of the Citizens' Association, including the *Report of the Council of Hygiene*, by James Parton, " The government of the City of New York," *N. Am. Rev.*, 1866, *103*: 413-465. Deserving more work is an analysis of those who were involved in the health reform movement. What were their backgrounds, their motives, and how large a part did they actually play? Also, how was the health reform movement, if indeed one can call it a movement at all, related to other reforms and reformers of the time? Health legislation played an important role in the general amelioration of the urban environment and in the development of cities. This too is an aspect of nineteenth century public health that deserves much more study. See particularly Charles N. Glaab, *The American City*, A Documentary Study, Homewood: Dorsey, 1963. Also Arthur M. Schlesinger, " The city in American history," *Miss. Valley Hist. Rev.*, 1940, *27*: 43-66, and Blake McKelvey, *The Urbanization of America 1860-1915*, New Brunswick: Rutgers, 1963.

[91] Stephen Smith, " American public health endeavor," *op. cit.*, p. 1117. Eaton and Elisha Harris were also active in the early work of the A. P. H. A.

[92] Kramer, " Beginnings," *op. cit.*, p. 370.

GOVERNMENT'S ROLE IN AMERICAN MEDICINE—A BRIEF HISTORICAL SURVEY [1]

MILTON I. ROEMER [2]

The pattern of medical services in the United States has naturally followed the trend of the general social, political, and economic organization of the country. Probably one of the strongest heritages of the revolution that gave birth to the United States as an independent nation was a certain distrust of government—of strong centralized administration. This attitude, implementing as it did the interests of an expanding industrial economy, has been the most profound of influences on the pattern of medical services in our country.

The American Revolution may be epitomized as a social revolution of a rising young bourgeoisie, backed by farmers and intellectuals, against a powerful landed aristocracy of the mother nation. The political form taken by this economic conflict was expressed largely in the principles of states' rights and the sanctity of private property embodied in our federal Constitution. This victory of " Jeffersonian democracy " over Hamiltonian federalism was in its day a victory of the forces for social progress—a victory for the ascending class which had made and won a revolution. One of the most significant political facts of our era is the striking transposition of forces today in which the Jeffersonian principles of local sovereignty have become the slogans of the twentieth century Tories while Hamiltonian federalism has become the government instrument for enforcing the rights of the common man.

Medical Care and Colonial Poor Relief

These political developments of our nation have their precise counterparts in the field of medical service. The Colonial world naturally attempted to adopt the medical patterns known to the colonists in the mother country. With few physicians available, however, the colonists were at first thrown upon their own resources and folk practices were the rule. It is significant that the central figure in the early American conflict over inoculation was a clergyman, Cotton Mather, who promoted

[1] Presented originally before the New York Society for Medical History, March 4, 1943. Revised.

[2] Senior Assistant Surgeon (R), U. S. Public Health Service; assigned to the Office of the Chief Medical Officer, Farm Security Administration, Washington, D. C.

inoculation during the Boston smallpox epidemic of 1721. Insofar as physicians were to be found, however, the management of nearly all matters of health fell into their hands. This included not only general diagnosis and treatment, as we are accustomed to think of them today, but all matters of sanitation and communicable disease control, preparation of drugs, medical relief of the poor, and even medical care in the physician's home (as hospitalization) in some instances. The physician was often a powerful political figure in the Colonial community.

Even under the aegis of the rugged, independent Colonial practitioner, however, some medical service was supported directly by the government. This was the medical care of the poor relief group, assumed usually as charges of the local town government (or county government in the southern colonies) although sometimes provided by the church. In the seventeenth century, care of the sick poor was quite disorganized, being usually in the patient's home or in the home of a neighbor or friend with whom he was boarded. The physician was paid on an individual case basis. Gradually one physician would come to be utilized for nearly all the local cases and in the 1660's one begins to find physicians engaged for this work on the basis of an annual salary. These were the "town physicians."

As the population of the colonies increased it became necessary to provide some form of systematic shelter for the poor, particularly the sick poor. During the 1730's therefore, a number of the large colonial communities built almshouses at which a physician was customarily engaged for a stipulated annual salary. Since the assignment was usually given to the lowest bidder, the quality of services may well be imagined. Governmental support for these meager services was entirely on a local basis, although care for non-residents of a town was sometimes assumed by the colonial government. Since hospital facilities for those chronically ill with phthisis or lunacy or other diseases were not available, the poorhouse became also the haven for these sick persons. Thus, medical care was essentially an incidental feature of local poor relief, given after the pattern of the Elizabethan poor law of 1601.

In the ante-bellum South, under the slave economy a special system of "free" medical services by plantation doctors was developed for the slaves on some of the larger plantations. This service, the adequacy of which may be judged by available records of the high death and disease rates from typhoid, cholera, tetanus, and female pelvic disorders among the slaves, was not furnished by government, of course, but by plantation sires. Its past existence is worth recognizing, however, if only because it reflects the huge burden of health provision for the economically depressed Negro people which fell upon southern communities after the Civil War. Not that this burden has been adequately assumed, but its pressure accounts largely for the fact that the earliest development of full-time county public health departments took place in the southern states.

Hospitals

Hospital services for general illness were initiated on a voluntary basis but government played some part from the very outset. The Pennsylvania Hospital, usually claimed to be the first institution in the United States exclusively for the care of the sick (1751), was, for example, constructed and maintained by voluntary subscriptions supplemented by public funds. Continuing traditions of Christian charity, which in the Middle Ages gave rise to the first hospitals, the earliest institutions were intimately associated with almshouses and were intended primarily for the care of the sick poor. It was not until well into the nineteenth century that " self-respecting " citizens of means allowed themselves to be hospitalized for general illness and any appreciable support for hospitalization came from private patients, as distinguished from charity or government. In the twentieth century, as income from private patients has increased, proportionate income from philanthropy has declined and the part played by government has become greater.

It is enlightening to recall that among the earliest purely governmentally supported institutions in the United States were the asylums for the insane in the early nineteenth century, for here society's motive was to protect itself from the fury of maniacs. The first American hospital exclusively for the care of the mentally ill was established at Williamsburg, Virginia, in 1773 (now the Eastern State Hospital of Virginia), which accepted pay patients along with the insane poor. It was many years, however, before the influence of Pinel and the Tukes in Europe and Dorothea Dix in this country converted the jails and almshouses ordinarily used for this purpose into hospitals for mental disease. Increasingly, the care of the mentally ill has been recognized as a responsibility of State government. The number of mental hospital beds in the United States has grown at such a rapid rate, furthermore, that about 50% of all hospital beds in the country today are exclusively for mental patients—and over 95% of these are government supported.

The other chief disease early provided for on a governmental basis in the United States was tuberculosis. The menace of this disease as the nation's chief cause of death toward the latter part of the last century led to gradual governmental action on the local level. After Trudeau, with his pioneer work in the 1870's, proved the value of sanatorium treatment, tax-supported institutions developed so rapidly that today some 90% of beds for the treatment of this disease are under governmental auspices. Here was a disease so serious in its effects, yet so chronic, that its care was obviously beyond the means of the private individual to finance. This has, of course, become all the more true as the disease has gradually become more particularly an affliction of the low income groups.

So completely are these two groups of disease—the psychoses and tuberculosis—supported by government that they account for some 69% of all hospital beds in the country under government auspices. In addition, a growing number of general hospital beds are tax supported, either in institutions operated completely by municipal or county authorities or in voluntary hospitals in which a portion of the beds are supported by tax funds. The turnover, of course, for the predominantly chronic disease beds supported by government is naturally much less than for the predominantly acute illness beds supported by private funds or charity. It is significant, nevertheless, that the percentage of occupancy of privately supported beds tends to be considerably lower than that of governmentally supported beds—a reflection of the deterring influence of the cash barrier on the receipt of hospital care. The growth of group hospitalization insurance in recent years has been instrumental in raising the occupancy of general hospital beds.

Finally, of course, theories of contagion, taking their origin from Biblical notions about leprosy and applied to plague, smallpox, and cholera, gave rise to the " pest house "—the predecessor of the modern isolation hospital. In rural areas, isolation and quarantine of the sick individual in his home was considered adequate, but in the crowded cities special institutions had to be set aside. Temporary isolation hospitals or more accurately cabins were set up, therefore, in time of epidemics, as early as 1716 in Massachusetts. Thus began Bellevue Hospital, one of the earliest more or less permanent " pest houses " in the United States, in answer to an epidemic of plague in New York in 1794. There was little distinction between this type of institution and the poorhouse or mental hospital throughout the nineteenth century but, with the discovery of pathogenic micro-organisms, after 1870 most of the larger municipalities provided special isolation hospitals on the outskirts of the community. Today these institutions provide the bulk of hospital care for the acute communicable diseases of childhood, usually with municipal or county funds.

Public Health Services

The most commonly understood role of government in health services has probably been in the field of public health. The menace of pestilence has at all times demanded community efforts for control. Indeed, nearly all the early local boards of health in our country had their origins in popular reactions to a particular epidemic—yellow fever, cholera, small-pox, typhoid fever, or others. At the very birth of the new Republic local boards sprang up here and there in the towns, though they were often short-lived. After about 1830, however, permanent local boards were established increasingly, and by 1860 most of the larger cities were supplied with official boards of health.

With such beginnings the functions of boards of health became obviously the control of communicable disease and—insofar as disease was spread by certain of the utilities of community life—the control of environmental sanitation. It is highly significant that the medical care of the poor, from the beginning, was not in the hands of public health authorities but rather under poor relief administration—a separateness which largely prevails to this day.

The part played by official public health agencies, relative to all health and medical services, has on historic appraisal not actually been great until the recent period. Rugged individualism tolerated only a minimum of governmental services, for other than the indigent, and for almost all matters of personal or community health, the individual physician was looked to for nearly exclusive guidance. The great conquests of plague, cholera, typhoid fever and other enteric diseases, tuberculosis, or malaria, have probably not been chiefly referable to the work of individual physicians but neither can they be credited mainly to the operations of health departments as such. General improvements in housing, diet, living standards, and general civil engineering have probably played the chief role. In day to day affairs, health departments generally were called on for little, except in the event of epidemics, and the usual pattern was domination by narrow partisan interests with little special education or training in the incumbents. There were virtually no full-time salaried medical officers of health until a decade after the Civil War.

Epochs such as were marked by Shattuck's Sanitary Survey of Massachusetts were decidedly exceptional and, as we know, it was twenty years before this survey was acted upon with the establishment of the first permanent State Board of Health in Massachusetts in 1869. At about the same period as Shattuck's Survey, the federal government had unsuccessfully attempted to survey the health conditions of the nation in the manner of the then recent humanitarian surveys of the large European cities. The American Medical Association, a rebellious young organization of medical leaders, mostly from academic circles, did the job of revealing squalid conditions in a dozen larger cities, but nothing further came of it.

Federal Public Health Services

Because of the special structure of our constitutional government, maintaining the state as sovereign and granting only specified powers to the federal government, the role of federal authorities in health services was quite different from that of the states or local communities. The origin of our present United States Public Health Service was in a function that provided not public health or preventive services but rather hospital care for merchant seamen. In fact, since this service was supported by compulsory monthly contributions by the seamen themselves, by Act of Congress in 1798, it represented actually a form of compulsory health insurance, for a special group. A later Act of Congress changed the support for the service entirely to tax funds so that compulsory health insurance was, in effect, modified into complete " state medicine."

Except for quarantine functions to keep communicable diseases from crossing our borders, the health functions of the federal government were confined to the medical care of certain legal beneficiaries and to some small amount of research in infectious diseases until the present century. An attempt was made to organize a true national department of health in 1879, to cope with communicable diseases within our borders, like the yellow fever then common in the South, but Congress discontinued it after four years. The federal government had no specific health prerogatives granted by the Constitution, and it was a long time before the " common welfare " clause was interpreted to mean the promulgation of measures for the health of the population.

Development of Public Health Functions

The era of bacteriology is often regarded as marking the real beginnings of the public health movement throughout the world. This is true only in the sense that the discovery of pathogenic micro-organisms provided a scientific basis for sanitary measures, the importance of which had previously begun to be recognized on purely empirical grounds, and in providing measures for developing immunity in the individual without complete elimination of the external offenders. It is true that, with a more firm scientific basis for sanitation and communicable disease control, health departments grew rapidly. Yet before the bacteriological era, it must be recalled that considerable progress had been made in the control of smallpox and typhus fever, malaria and yellow fever, on an empirical basis. And what is less commonly recognized has been the deterring influence of the laboratory sciences, by which preoccupation with vaccines and serums came to substitute for a wholesome regard for the social and economic aspects of community welfare.

The expanding functions of official public health agencies since the turn of the century have been assumed mainly as a result of pressure from voluntary groups. The very origin of the public health nurse, the member of the modern health department giving most direct community service, has been in the visiting nurses' association supported typically by private philanthropy. From the days of Sir William Rathbone on, the " visiting nurse " has given nursing care to the poor in their homes although many new functions have been assumed by the nurse in the official agency. The entire movement for tuberculosis control was started by voluntary agencies at the end of the last century (now organized into the National Tuberculosis Association) and the American Social Hygiene Association was exerting its pressures long before venereal disease control became a key part of our public health efforts. Maternal and child health protection efforts long antedated the extensive program of the Children's Bureau, and it is significant that the first assumption of responsibilities for these functions in the federal government was by the Department of Labor rather than the established health agency. The mental hygiene movement, of course, arose from the indignation of private individuals and groups over the treatment of the inmates of " insane asylums," beginning with the pioneer efforts of Clifford Beers. Industrial hygiene had its beginning in private industry and in state and national departments of labor, only lately coming into the bailiwick of conventional public health work.

The usual course of events has been for needs to be demonstrated through the efforts of voluntary groups, with gradual assumption of responsibility for the new functions by government agencies. Not always have voluntary agencies promptly given up the responsibilities they have initially assumed, however, and entrenched interests have sometimes become developed. With increasing governmental responsibility for health matters, nevertheless, the relative importance of voluntary agencies in community health and welfare has gradually waned.

The entire role of public health in the national picture of medical service remains, on the whole, still pitifully small. Of the $30 per capita estimated expenditure on all medical services in prosperous 1929, only $1 was spent for public health services, including the aggregate of all federal, state, and local expenditures. This was far below the outlay, for example, for unprescribed patent medicines and below the outlay for the services of chiropractors and other cultist practitioners. The greatly expanded federal subsidy for state and local public health activities that came with the New Deal and the social security program after 1935 has altered the picture a great deal. Hundreds of new full-time county health departments have been set up under the stimulus of grants-in-aid provided by the U. S. Public Health Service and the Children's Bureau. The relative allowance for preventive public health services, however, is still only a small fraction of the vast sums spent on therapeutic medical services.

Medical Research

The role of American government in medical research has been even more limited than its role in the applications of science. The first hygienic laboratory to investigate the diseases of man and animals was established by the federal government in 1902, although its chief work was the standardization of biological products made by private manufacturers. The National Institute of Health, as the hygienic laboratory later was called, saw very little expansion until the 1930's when its appropriation was greatly increased and the research in certain communicable and industrial diseases was expanded. Intensive research in cancer was begun in 1937 with the founding of the National Cancer Institute. The federal health service produced the epochal work of Goldberger on pellagra and the discoveries of McCoy and Francis on tularemia and of Spencer and Parker on Rocky Mountain spotted fever, but relative to the whole of American medical research its scope has been somewhat limited.

On the state level, exclusive of the state universities, governmentally sponsored research has been even more limited. In the very recent period, the conception has developed that a good state or large municipal health department must keep itself alert with field research proceeding at all times, and state health departments, like those of New York or Massachusetts, have contributed some significant work in epidemiology. The vast bulk of medical research, however, has—under the American pattern—come from private universities and commercial interests. With the present war, great strides have been made in the coordination and organization of research—carried on in non-official centers throughout the nation—through the federal Office of Scientific Research and Development and the National Research Council.

Laws Governing Medical Practice

Government has had its influence on medical services, of course, not only through direct performance of health functions but also through laws governing the practice of private medicine. The day to day relations between physician and patient are theoretically governed by certain contractual understandings, in which the physician is under obligation to render service to his patient in good faith and without negligence or malicious intent and the patient, of course, is obliged to pay for the services rendered according to agreement or understanding. The confidential nature of the physician's findings is strictly protected by law, and divulgence of these findings before a public court cannot be compelled except when the public welfare is endangered. These physician-patient relationships are governed by state laws entirely.

Most important, by far, of the laws affecting private medical practice are those governing the licensure of various practitioners to follow their art. The history of licensure laws in the United States is a complex story of its own, reflecting particularly the flourishing growth of numerous marginal medical sects. America, with its deep-rooted freedom from governmental restraints and its wide area for pioneering of every sort, provided the ideal soil for such cults.

As early as 1760, irregular practices of various sorts became recognized as a problem and in that year New York passed the first law requiring the examination and licensure of all who would practice medicine. A few other states followed suit, but the laws were difficult to enforce and with the Revolution they became dead letters. After the Revolution, following the European custom, the medical schools were empowered to grant licenses to practise to the successful graduates. With the expansion of the new country, especially through the opening of the west, medical schools sprang up everywhere like the proverbial mushroom. The issuance of medical diplomas was a good business. Obviously, large numbers of quite inferiorly trained physicians were foisted on the public. After 1835, the states began to set up examining boards with representatives of each of the local sects on them. These soon became impotent and were dissolved. In the seventies, with the coming of age of more scientific medicine, state boards of medical examiners were again established, functioning at the present time.

The policy in establishing these boards, however, was deeply influenced by the fact that several different schools or systems of medicine existed side by side, and the state, in a spirit of liberalism, took the position that it coulo not discriminate against one or another art of healing but must license them all. As a result, chiropractors were licensed to practise chiropractic just as physicians were licensed to practise medicine. The Committee on the Costs of Medical Care estimated in 1930 that Americans spent about $125,000,000 annually on the various cultist services—or about $1 per capita. In recent years a handful of states have specifically withheld licenses from the several cultists (except Christian Science, which is protected under the cloak of freedom of religion), but the majority of states still grant cultist licenses.

Medical Education

The quality of the medical schools has been so greatly elevated in the present century that the basis for licensure by the state—to protect the public from the graduates of inferior schools—has largely ceased to exist. For this reason it has been advocated in recent years that licensure privileges be returned to the schools and that the level of the schools be upheld by government regulation. More direct control of the medical schools by government, furthermore, might serve the public welfare by providing for the training of adequate numbers of physicians, rather than tolerating any limitations on admissions in the interests of minimizing competition in the private profession. With the war emergency, we have seen the great expansion possible in our medical school enrollments, with little increase of facilities.

In medical education as such, government has played an indirect role, of course, through its licensure laws. More important, however, an increasing share of the total costs of medical education has been assumed by government bodies. This has been mostly on a state level through the operation of medical colleges in numerous state universities. In 1940 about 20% of the annual $21,000,000 bill for medical education was contributed by government sources. During the war period, of course, practically all our medical schools have been direct outposts of the federal government, with 80% of the students being enlisted in the armed services. The great majority of nurses being trained today, moreover, are subsidized by the federal government through the Cadet Nurse Corps.

Food and Drug Control

The history of governmental controls over food and drugs in the interests of the public health is another story of its own. The passage of the first national Pure Food and Drug Law in 1906 was the victory in a long struggle over private commercial interests claiming the " freedom " to sell anything that they desired. With the development of mass-scale advertising, the limitations of the 1906 law, restricted to proper labeling requirements as it was, soon became apparent. It was not till 1938, however, that the law was amended to include regulation of advertising and to bring cosmetics within its scope. It took the tragedy of " elixir sulfanilamide " with its toll of deaths to bring Congress to legislate that *any* new drug before being launched in interstate commerce had to receive the stamp of safety of the federal government. The current law retains many loopholes and weak points, but what is far more important, the greatest abuses of America's drug consumption are due to factors that cannot be legislated away. They depend rather on an inadequate provision of medical care that forces people to resort to the corner drug store as a cheap substitute for medical attention.

Medical Care for the Indigent

With respect to future trends, the most significant developments in governmental concern for health in the United States, have probably not been in public health programs, nor in specific legal controls, but rather in the field of medical care of the sick individual. For, despite the basic importance of preventive measures, the province of greatest need into which government may be expected to expand is that of medical care for the general public. In fact, one of the most important problems in the administration of government health services today springs from the artificial separation between preventive services rendered by departments of public health and therapeutic medical services—albeit to the indigent only—traditionally rendered by departments of public welfare.

We have noted how the care of the tuberculous and the insane fell relatively early to local government units in the counties and the states. We have noted also the development of the institution of the " town doctor " for the poor, a practice which still survives in many sections, though often the service is perfunctory and seldom used. While the role of government in medical care has been confined particularly to low-income or other specially dependent groups and to the care of certain high-cost illnesses, there can be no doubt that this role is continually broadening. As the cost of adequate medical services has risen, with advances in medical science, complete medical care has become financially inaccessible to a larger proportion of the population. The notion of "medical indigency" has developed, under which varying proportions of the population—well above the level of general indigency—require governmental assistance if needed services are to be received.

The more modern substitute for the "town physician" system of medical care to the indigent is the public clinic. Since the first out-patient clinic in the Pennsylvania Hospital in 1786, dispensaries have become a customary adjunct of most voluntary, non-profit hospitals. While these institutions do not, of course, represent government facilities, the share of their service that includes out-patient care to the indigent is often partly supported by tax funds and, in the larger cities, many entire general hospitals and clinics are operated exclusively by local government agencies. The rural areas are not nearly so well served but in metropolitan areas clinic service of this type has, for the lowest income groups, largely supplanted the services of the erstwhile private "family doctor." Numerous clinics are, of course, conducted by departments of public health for the management of venereal diseases, tuberculosis, maternal and infant hygiene, or other special problems. As medicine has become more complex, it has become increasingly more difficult for the private physician to render the needed services to all persons in his private office. Public clinics represent an efficient and economical method of rendering services to a large number of people, and it is natural that their number should increase by hundreds each year.

Governmental medical care of the indigent patient *at home*, however, has undergone little improvement through the years. With the Great Depression of 1929 and the occurrence of unprecedented mass unemployment, the relation between sickness and unemployment became better recognized. The treatment of the unemployed individual who was sick was appreciated as a measure necessary to put him in shape again to work. Moreover, medical care was coming to be recognized as a fundamental human right, no less than food, clothing or shelter.

While larger sums, both absolute and relative to total national income, were probably spent for government medical care in the home during this period than ever before in our history, the system of organization was far from economical. Faced with a new task, the federal government developed a program of home medical care for "relief clients" in 1933, which in effect carried over nearly all the patterns of private practice. Under the Federal Emergency Relief Administration program, the federal government allotted funds to local communities, through the states, to pay physicians on a private fee-for-service basis for care rendered to relief clients. Fee schedules were established by local medical societies in connection with relief authorities, and local physicians were appointed to advisory committees to prevent abuses. Rendered on such an individual basis, high costs relative to services rendered were inevitable. Services were more or less restricted, furthermore, to acute illnesses, and limitations were placed on drug coverage or other features of service. Despite the inadequacies, this was the first time that the federal government had directly financed medical care for the indigent. There can be no doubt that a greater volume of services were thus rendered than could have been on a local basis.

With the passage of the Social Security Act in 1935, this program came to an end and direct responsibilities for relief medical services were returned to the states and local communities. To avoid " pauperizing " the individual, federal funds granted to the special categories of public assistance cases (aged persons, dependent children, and blind) must be given in cash and not in kind. Cash allotments may be made to cover medical services, privately purchased, but all direct medical services must be financed out of state or local governmental resources. The administration of welfare medical services is unfortunately characterized by a polyglot of separate agencies and separate responsibilities in local government which reflects the faltering, piece-meal development of this segment of governmental health services. Because of this, total expenditures for public assistance medical services in the nation are almost impossible to estimate, but in many communities they undoubtedly exceed the budget for all organized preventive services.

Care for Special Dependent Groups

Quite apart from public welfare medicine, government—on federal, state, and local levels—has long felt responsible for the medical care of certain public wards such as orphans or prisoners. The medical care provided in the average county jail is on a pitifully low level, though here and there, as in the Essex County Jail in New Jersey, a model program for the promotion of both physical and mental health is conducted. In most of the state prisons, however, except in the less prosperous southern states, the medical care provided is on a level considerably higher than that enjoyed by the convicts before their incarceration, and in federal penitentiaries a well-rounded medical care program is generally conducted, under the supervision of the U. S. Public Health Service. The management of venereal disease therapy, for example, in Sing Sing Prison, New York, has established a level of performance that might well be emulated in any private institution. Where governmental units operate homes for the feeble-minded, the blind, the deaf and dumb or other such dependents, general medical services are, of course, provided.

Medical care for the Indians has been a responsibility assumed by the federal government through the Indian Service since about 1900, though an over-all organized health program was not set up until 1924. About $3,000,000 a year has been spent for the care of the 220,000 Indians living on government reservations in recent years. The medical care provided for merchant seamen has been indicated under the duties of the United States Public Health Service. The student health programs in state universities, such as the University of Michigan which initiated this service in 1913, or the University of Wisconsin, are essentially governmental medical functions. Employees of special federal governmental projects, such as the Panama Canal or the Tennessee Valley Authority, have received governmental medical services since the inception of these engineering programs. The TVA health program has developed special patterns of organized health services for whole communities springing up in isolated areas at the sites of the dams on the Tennessee River. A special program of direct tax-supported medical services for migratory farm workers has been sponsored by the Department of Agriculture since 1937. Clinics attended by public health nurses and local physicians have been maintained at points of seasonal labor concentration around the nation, providing care to the wandering Joads, whose lack of state residency makes them ineligible for local medical relief.

Perhaps the largest established programs of medical care to a specially dependent group have been the medical services to members of the armed forces. From the organization of the Army Medical Corps under men like Morgan, Rush, and Shippen in the army of the rebellion, military medical organization has had a somewhat fitful history, in line with the history of the nation's wars. Our ambulance system in civilian life owes its origin to the pattern for carrying wounded to hospitals in the rear developed during the Civil War. The growth of group practice clinics after the first World War was undoubtedly related to the military experience of the returning medical veterans. Always in time of war, the pressure of circumstances induces increased efficiency in the organization of medical services for fighting men.

Finally, an extensive program of medical services for United States veterans has been sponsored by the federal government since the end of the first World War. The Veterans Administration operates a chain of governmental hospitals, containing in 1942 about 90,000 beds, which provide bed care and ambulatory care for service-connected disabilities in any veteran and bed care for a non-service connected disability in a veteran unable to obtain this care privately. The great majority of admissions have, in fact, been of the latter type and over half the beds are for mental disorders. With some 13,000,000 veterans expected to be eligible for service after the present war, this governmental medical program is rapidly expanding and will undoubtedly take on tremendous importance, although much controversy surrounds its expansion. The advisability of physical facilities for so large a segment of the population, separate and apart from facilities for their families or the rest of the nation, is open to serious question, although everyone agrees that the *financial* burden of medical care for veterans should be borne by the government.

Medical Care Through Social Insurance

Despite all the medical services for the indigent or for special population groups or for high-cost illnesses, for which the government has taken responsibility for one reason or another, the rank and file of the population have depended for their health care primarily on the private medical practitioner. The great bulk of the $4,500,000,000 Americans were estimated to spend on medical care in 1940 comes from private pockets in payment to private physicians and dentists, voluntary hospitals, or private drug manufacturers. The principle of governmentally planned budgeting for medical costs on an insurance basis, which marked European medicine from the 1880's on, has gone little beyond the stage of controversy and debate in the United States.

We have noted the compulsory health insurance system for merchant seamen set up in 1798, but on the whole, with per capita income relatively high in a confident expanding economy, it is natural that social insurance should not have entered the public scene here until recent times. Under the influence of German social democracy, however, a class-conscious labor movement began to take root in the United States toward the end of the last century. The most obvious type of disablement against which protection should be afforded by society was injury on the job. For years cases had been wrangled in the courts between worker and employer, each in essence charging negligence on the part of the other, with the worker usually coming out as loser. In 1908 a federal law was passed granting compensation to certain federal employees injured while at work, and the first state workmen's compensation laws were passed in 1911 by New York and Wisconsin.

A large part of the compensation insurance funds, maintained usually in commercial companies, go for the payment of medical services incident to compensable injuries—some $80,000,000 annually in the 1930's. Today every state but Mississippi is covered by an act. Most state laws, however, remain restricted in their conception of "accidents," with only about 25 granting compensation for occupational diseases and most of these limited to a few specified conditions (lead poisoning, silicosis, etc.).

In the same period, about 1912, attempts were made in numerous state legislatures—largely through the efforts of the American Association for Labor Legislation—to enact state health insurance laws for wage earners in the lower income groups. The combined opposition of employers, workers, and the medical profession spelled failure for these attempts. The opposition of employers and the profession was on the same grounds as are familiar today—fear of higher taxes by the former and fear of regimentation by the latter. The position of organized labor, however, has changed from opposition in this early period based on fears of paternalism, led by the Samuel Gompers conception of independent unionism, to a current support of all types of social welfare legislation including health insurance.

Voluntary Health Insurance

The movement for health insurance after this period—as it was initially in most of the European nations in which compulsory legislation was subsequently enacted—was predominantly on a voluntary level. Industrial groups, particularly in isolated mining and lumbering sections, were the first to organize significant periodic prepayment plans, financed usually out of wages. In certain firms, of which the Endicott-Johnson Company is the classic example, the management paternalistically supplied rather complete medical services to employees, but the commonest pattern has been financial support by both workers and employer. Fraternal orders developed plans for cash indemnity during sickness and for certain limited types of medical service. Commercial insurance companies began to sell insurance to industrial groups, providing cash benefits during illness, and "mutual benefit associations" were organized in hundreds of plants to promote this type of policy.

More recently trade unions have become involved in health insurance plans for certain categories of ambulatory service for their workers.

Special medical groups have launched plans in the larger cities providing complete service on a prepayment basis to certain occupational groups, typically illustrated by the Ross-Loos Clinic in Los Angeles. A few independent prepayment plans were developed in rural areas, the most successful being at Elk City, Oklahoma, as part of a farmers' cooperative. With the war, as a measure of manpower economy, some significant prepayment plans have been developed in war industries, as in the Kaiser ship yards on the West Coast. Increasingly in the last ten years, the medical profession, viewing the trend of the times, has organized its own prepayment plans for low and middle income families in about a dozen states. Most of these plans have limited their protection to surgical and obstetrical care.

Finally, the voluntary health insurance movement reached its height in America by way of voluntary group hospitalization insurance. From an inauspicious beginning in Dallas, Texas in 1929, Blue Cross plans have grown to cover nearly 17,000,000 persons in almost every section of the country. This voluntary health insurance program has flourished because it has met a need and because it has had the strong support of the nation's hospitals, which naturally stood to profit from the guaranteed payment of their bills. Its significance, however, will not be overemphasized if it is recognized that hospital expenses account for only about 15 percent of the medical bill and the total membership comes to less than 15 percent of the nation's population—the bulk of these concentrated in a few industrialized states.

The history of the changing attitudes of the medical profession towards the voluntary health plan movement has reflected changing public pressures. Conviction of the American Medical Association in 1941 for violation of the Sherman Anti-Trust Act, because of its opposition to certain voluntary group prepayment plans, heightened the issue to a matter of Supreme Court judgment. The significant point in relation to governmental medical services is that the growth and judicial sanction of voluntary plans has indicated broad public interest in health insurance and has provided a basis for legislative proposals.

Thus, the Wagner National Health Bill of 1938 would have provided federal grants to the states for the development of " medical care plans " which were generally understood to mean health insurance plans, although the term " health insurance " was not mentioned in the bill. With the war brewing in the late summer of 1939 the bill never reached the floor of Congress for debate and met the fate of other so-called " non-essential " welfare measures of the same period. The question had, in any event, become a political issue of national proportions.

Governmentally Sponsored Health Insurance

One federal program of health insurance was set under way in 1935 with the almost complete approval of the physicians involved in rendering the services. This was the subsidized program of voluntary health insurance of the Resettlement Administration, later the Farm Security Administration, under which low income farm families were granted loans with which to join county prepayment plans. Arrangements were made through local medical societies for physicians to accept for their services on a prorated basis as much money as was available in the fund, which on the average represented about 70 percent of their fees. Similar plans were worked out for dental service, for hospitalization, and for prescribed drugs.

This program grew rapidly until, wartime pressures, associated with shortages of practitioners and raised farm income, set in but at its height over 600,000 farm people in over 1100 counties were covered in these plans. Through this program, rural physicians, with none too substantial incomes, have been provided with a source of remuneration from many farm families who before were treated free, at greatly reduced fees, or who were not seen at all. It is no surprise that, despite the traditional conservatism of country doctors, the program should have received their support. The decline of these plans under wartime pressures, however, reflects many of the innate weaknesses of health insurance plans limited to low-income families, on a voluntary basis, at the county level.

State bills on compulsory health insurance were again introduced throughout the thirties, but none ever became a major public issue. In 1942 in his budget message to Congress, President Roosevelt requested the enactment of legislation to provide federal hospitalization insurance and wage benefit compensation during illness. To implement this, Representative Eliot of Massachusetts introduced a bill in Congress on hospitalization insurance, but it did not leave committee. In 1943, with the war having reached a stage at which statements of war aims and formulation of post-war plans were fitting, a new major bill was introduced into the federal legislature by Senators Wagner and Murray and by Representative Dingell. The Wagner-Murray-Dingell bill called for the extension of the social security program to include broader sections of the population, to expand public assistance benefits, to federalize unemployment compensation programs, to provide disability and maternity benefits, and to provide medical care and hospitalization to all insured persons. About 100,000,000 persons would be covered by a system of federal compulsory health insurance. A storm of debate followed the introduction of the bill, promulgated chiefly by its opponents in the organized medical profession—but the chief reason the bill did not pass at the Congressional session in which it was raised was preoccupation with the task of winning the war. Similar broad proposals had been introduced before the parliaments in Great Britain (the Beveridge Plan) and in Canada at about the same time.

On the question of wage benefits during illness, one state actually broke the ice. This was Rhode Island which in 1942 passed legislation providing cash benefits when a Rhode Island worker, covered by the State Unemployment Compensation Act, is away from work due to sickness of more than seven days' duration. The contributions forthcoming under the Unemployment Compensation Act were considered adequate to sustain these additional benefits, since under favorable wartime economic conditions huge reserves had been built up. Severe drains on these reserves, however, may reasonably be expected in the post-war period so that one must probably anticipate the need for supplemental taxing legislation in Rhode Island or any other state that establishes a wage-benefit-during-sickness program. Sickness benefits, of course, are only half the story—an essential half though it is; if the worker is to be returned to his job in the shortest possible time, with minimum drain on the insurance funds, medical service benefits are necessary. In 1944 California—repeating with modifications a proposal of ten years earlier—considered in its state legislature several bills calling for statewide compulsory health insurance. Although all these bills failed, the issue is still under active debate in California and is winning the attention of the nation.

Whether or not future developments in health insurance will be predominantly on a state or a federal level is, of course, one of the critical questions of the day. The trend of social welfare legislation in all other categories has certainly been toward increased federalization. The nation's highest court has more and more arrived at a broadened interpretation of the Constitution's guarantee of state sovereignty, granting increasing prerogatives to the federal government in its authority to " provide for the general welfare." The current temper of our Congress seems to be somewhat in the opposite direction, but the long-time trend will probably not be reversed. As noted at the outset, Jeffersonian democracy, translated into modern conditions, calls for increased resort to federal administration and guidance. It would be foolish to expect a nation of the expanse and diversity of the United States to be developed to the same social, economic, and cultural level in all parts. If we are to grow as a free nation, the wealthier sections must help the less prosperous and the benefits of advanced medical and engineering science must be enjoyed by all sections. It is coming to be recognized that this can be best accomplished through national leadership, with proper decentralization of actual administration and constant democratic regard for the freedom of all individuals.

Health Departments and Medical Care

Historically, it has been observed that official public health agencies were confined to matters of environmental sanitation and the control of acute communicable and epidemic diseases. General day-to-day medical care, on the other hand, has been predominantly the province of welfare and relief agencies for the indigent sections of the population, except for special wards of the Government. Medical service was essentially given incidental to poor relief. As a result of this background, interest in the promotion of the health insurance movement in the United States has come primarily from social welfare rather than public health circles. Public health agencies, in fact, have customarily maintained a strictly "hands off" policy and in some instances have aggressively opposed health insurance plans even on a voluntary basis. Admittedly, this attitude has been dictated by the desire of public health personnel to maintain amicable relations with the private medical profession.

When the Wagner National Health Bill of 1938 was first drafted, it is reported that the administrative agency for the "state health plans" initially indicated was the state health department. Before reaching Congress, however, this significantly was changed to put the medical plan administration under an independent agency. In the last few years, however, on the federal level and in a few states, the situation has begun to change and public health agencies are starting to show an active interest in the general problems of medical care. An important reflection of the change is seen in the provision of the Wagner-Murray-Dingell bill of 1943, calling for the United States Public Health Service to act as administrative agency. To what extent the administration of widespread health insurance programs, under either state or federal auspices, will lie with health departments, however, to what extent with welfare or labor agencies, and to what extent with private medical societies, will depend to some degree on the interest and leadership forthcoming from each of these groups.

Some public health leaders have called attention to the pattern of affairs in other nations in which strong health insurance programs have been in effect: a pattern in which the public health department is reduced to a somewhat secondary role. It is clear that the more the individual's needs are provided for by health insurance, the fewer are left for the public health agency, as we now know it, to encompass. With an extensive health insurance program, covering dependent mothers and children, as well as wage earners, public health functions might be largely reduced to the earlier level of environmental sanitation and certain (not all) aspects of communicable disease control. If public health agencies are to maintain a significant role in the coming period, therefore, they would seem compelled to develop interest and devote attention to the general social security movement of which health insurance is one phase.

The resolution on medical care of the 1944 convention of the American Public Health Association, though long overdue, would seem to be a first important step in this direction. It remains for public health leaders in the states, counties, and municipalities to act upon this statesman-like declaration of principles. Otherwise major responsibilities for over-all medical care administration might fall, by default, to public agencies less skilled in the sciences of health or to private groups less vested with the public interest.

Continued Expansion of Government's Role

The general trend of government medical services in the United State, on both the local and the federal level, has been clear. Increasingly, government has widened its sphere of responsibility for both the prevention and the care of illness. So far as public health services alone are concerned, the line of division between therapeutic medicine under private auspices and preventive medicine under public auspices is rapidly being obliterated. The *treatment* of gonorrhea in a public health clinic helps to prevent the occurrence of new cases, just as the *prevention* of intestinal obstruction is accomplished when a surgeon performs a hernial repair.

The day when the private family doctor was the sum and substance of all medical service has passed as certainly as the horse and buggy that carried him. The relative contraction of private medicine, moreover, comes from deeper causes than the extension of governmental medical services as such. The broader conflict lies actually between private medical services and *socially organized services*, whether organized by government or by industry or voluntary lay groups or professional bodies. In fact, in a sociological sense, government represents merely the most highly organized expression of group action. Before the present war, the number of physicians working on full-time salary in the United States exceeded 15 percent of the total number; the percentage had been gradually increasing since 1900. The number on some form of part-time salary was even greater. The war, even exclusive of the medical personnel in the armed services, has probably accentuated the trend.

The influence of the current war, finally, on the role of American government in medical services is a story familiar to everyone. All wars, of course, have had their profound influence on medicine although least important have probably been the specific technical or administrative innovations of military mobilization and most important have probably been the long run effects on medicine of the political and economic outcome of the war.

The immediate effects of the war are apparent on every side with a severe depletion of civilian professional personnel, coupled with an increased effective demand by people for medical services, due to the economic prosperity of the wartime boom. In numerous areas of concentrated war production or military mobilization the strain on local health personnel and facilities has been tremendous, and the failure of death rates or disease rates to rise significantly throughout the nation can only be attributed to the beneficial effect of full employment and elevated incomes on general levels of living.

Under the pressure of the war, of course, new health responsibilities have been assumed by government. Recognizing local health problems generated by war production or military activities as national in origin, the federal government has provided federal public health personnel for local communities, through the United States Public Health Service. To recruit medical and dental personnel for the armed forces and to attempt to maintain an equitable civilian distribution of such personnel, the Procurement and Assignment Service was set up in the War Manpower Commission. While this program suffered from the inadequacies of any administrative function based on purely voluntary action, the principle of governmental concern for the distribution of professional personnel throughout the nation was at least established. To train professional personnel for the armed forces, the specialized training programs of the Army and Navy were set up, financing the education of thousands of young physicians and dentists, and the Cadet Nurse Corps was established under the U. S. Public Health Service to increase the supply of nurses. Maternity and infant care was provided out of government funds to the wives and infants of servicemen in the lower pay grades, through the Emergency Maternity and Infant Care program under the Children's Bureau. Scientific research, as observed above, has enjoyed a new level of governmental coordination to serve wartime needs.

It is evident that the war has accelerated the trend of governmental assumption of responsibilities for health services. But, as observed above, the influence of the war will probably be far greater through its ultimate social and political consequences. The probable outcome of the war has been predicted by many, from those who envisage the arrival of the " American Century " to those who look forward to the " Century of the Common Man." Whatever may happen in the United States, no one expects to see a return to the *laissez-faire* economic and social policies that led to worldwide depression and finally to the present world conflict. The Four Freedoms can hardly be assured by such a course. In the field of health, it is more than likely that we will see a wider extension of preventive and therapeutic services under governmental auspices than we have ever seen in the past.

Federal Public Health:

A Reflection of a Changing Constitution

MORRIS KAGAN[*][1]

I⊤ has long been accepted that protection and promotion of the public health are duties and privileges of any responsible government. Yet, our federal constitution does not provide a single reference to health. This does not mean that the founding fathers were not concerned with the public health, but it does indicate that they did not consider it a responsibility of the national government. They drew a distinction between "nation-wide" problems and "national" problems. For more than three quarters of a century following the founding of this nation, the federal government refrained insofar as possible from assuming responsibilities for the public health. The reasons were deeply rooted in a philosophy of government contained in Article X which reserved for the states those powers which had not been delegated to the federal government. In short, the major police powers were retained by the several states.[2] The powers of police permit the exercise of those actions necessary for the preservation of the government, maintenance of order, and the health and welfare of the inhabitants. The major responsibility for insuring the public health would then be within the province of state government, except as it might be delegated by the state to lesser units of government. The federal government would retain police powers directly pertinent to public health in areas where it exercised exclusive jurisdiction such as federal properties and territories. The main entry, therefore, of the federal government into the field of public

* Austin, Texas.
1 The writer was supported by a traineeship from the Public Health Service (No. 58-432) during a portion of the period spent in the preparation of this paper.
2 An antithetical view is supported by evidence that states per se did not delegate power to the federal government. Quite the contrary, the Union is older than the states which were, in fact, formed from royal colonies by a national Declaration of Independence. It should be noted that the delegates to the Constitutional Convention met under the Articles of Confederation "for the sole purpose of revising the Articles." The delegates dismissed such purposes and without authority and in defiance of the Articles proposed a new Constitution of national government. Further, the Constitution would become operative when approved by Conventions elected for that purpose in nine states. It by-passed assent of the Congress of the Confederation and the legislatures of the several states under whose authority the meeting was convened and went directly to the one-seventh of the adult male populace having the property qualifications for the franchise. See John R. Rood, *The history of building the Constitution of the United States,* Detroit, Michigan, Detroit Law Book Co., 1948, pp. 23 ff.

health was contained in its enumerated powers. These powers were expanded subsequently by interpretations which recognized the existence of certain powers implied from the original delegation of authority. Thus, the majority of federal enactments concerning public health would be indirect and incidental to the exercise of federal responsibility in more clearly defined areas.

The field of public health, as many other areas of government, has reflected directly the changing concepts of federal-state-local government authority. Its main significance for public health has been the synonymity of centralization of authority at higher units of government with the improvements in character and scope of public health programs. Concurrently, it emphasizes and perhaps exaggerates fear that loss of local and state autonomy coincident with expansion of centralized authority will result in arbitrary rule and loss of our liberties. However, the principle of democracy demands merely that government be constituted in accord with the will of the majority. Minorities, as individuals, remain protected by virtue of legislative limitations contained in the Constitution which guarantee basic liberties. The fact that authority may be placed in the federal government whereas it had previously resided in state government does not remove the basic repository of power from the people. The test of democracy relates to the extent to which the least assertive, the most underprivileged, the weakest member of society can participate in and receive the protection and benefits of the land. It is obvious that Rousseau's concept of individual liberty, practised in 1961, would result in anarchy and tyranny. As humanity becomes condensed in populous communities, restrictions on individual liberties become necessary in order to maintain the protection of the group. It is thus somewhat paradoxical that, through restraint, liberties are protected for group members as a whole. It has been observed that in an increasingly complex society of growing population, state governments are often unable to provide their citizens with adequate protection and the responsibility is assumed on a governmental level commensurate with the problem.

Social and Economic Factors of Change

The current role of the federal government is vastly different from the role it exercised in the initial stages of our national existence. Legally, this change has occurred as an integral part of constitutional development through the process of amendment, the enactment of legislation applying in detail the general principles of the Constitution, judicial review interpreting the principle of implied powers, and custom or usage. Since the Constitution is regarded as an organic document determining permissable behavior in 1961 although composed in 1787, it is apparent that great changes have occurred because external facts to which the document is applied are different.[3] The provision for federal public health services, then, is one of many derivatives of these changing facts.

Rosen points out that the history of public health deals with two components: (i) the development of medical science and technology, and (ii) the application of such knowledge which is dependent upon economic and social factors.[4] This writer would prefer to view the development of medical science and technology as a part of general scientific and technical developments which affect society and are affected by it. This is likely incidental, for Rosen clearly illustrates an interrelationship between technology and society, and between socio-economic factors and provisions for the public health.

At the time of the Revolution two and one-half to three million colonists occupied thirteen Atlantic seaboard beachheads facing a border of one-thousand miles of Appalachian wilderness. A number of communities occupying sparsely populated sections, connected by questionable roads and suitable waterways, were sustained largely by agricultural pursuits. The social and economic conditions of these communities were as diversified as their geographical isolation. Unity was more nominal than practical. Consequently, the maintenance of local independence or state sovereignty became a necessary part of the national Constitution. Yet the states did possess a common concern about foreign intervention, protection of commerce, exploitation of the frontier and other natural resources, and promotion of the general welfare. Their inhabitants typically were small farmers, although a small wage-earning class of citizens and unskilled labor existed in the towns. The leaders, an aristocracy of wealth and breeding, were the land proprietors, plantation owners, and seaboard merchants.

Regardless of the individual reasons for their presence on this seaboard, English mercantilism dictated their general arrival. The

3 See Arthur W. Machen, Jr., "The elasticity of the Constitution," *Harvard Law Rev.,* 1900, *14,* Nos. 3 and 4.
4 George Rosen, "Economic and social policy in the development of public health," *J. Hist. Med.* 1953, *8,* 406-430.

conflict of mercantile interests with the mother country was a precipitant of the Revolution, and mercantilism served as a basis for a dominating concern of the ruling class for a strong central government. Thus, a second part of the Constitution sought to establish an increase in national sovereignty. The compromise between states' rights and national sovereignty was a federal instrument in which no party was fully content.

The increase in the power of all government, and in the power of the federal government in relation to the states, was inevitable. The movement of our population to the frontier, which began with our first settlers and continues to the current concept of the New Frontier, produced a fluid, dynamic society whose problems could be met and resolved only through federal intervention. The westward expansion demanded improved means of communication and transportation, and these were provided by an industrial revolution which began prior to the Civil War. This revolution produced rapid and profound changes in manufactures and agriculture during the latter portion of the 19th century. These have continued at an accelerating rate and have resulted in a new society with new facts, problems, solutions, and *Zeitgeist*.

In contrast to our national beginnings, our population has increased sixty-fold; thirteen poor and isolated colonies have grown to fifty wealthy states connected by slivers of concrete and high grade steel, airways, and instant communications; gross national production has jumped several hundred-fold; towns and wilderness sites have become metropolises with populations greater than the entire United States of 1787 (the migration to the West has been succeeded by a migration to the city); agriculture has extended and become mechanized, but the agricultural character of the population has been submerged by greater urban industrial development; sectional social and economic interests and differences have been softened, fused, and tempered into a national mold. These are merely suggestive, rather than exhaustive, of the changes which separate today and yesterday.

In relation to the public health, it is apparent that the "same process that created the market economy, the factory and the modern urban environment also brought into being the health problems which made necessary *and possible* new means of health protection and disease prevention."[5] Many of the new means of

5 *Ibid.*, p. 422 (Italics added).

health protection and disease prevention could be exercised only by the national government.

The assumption of such responsibilities by the federal government has been challenged primarily on the bases of trespass of states' rights and trespass of individual rights. The principles for interpretation of state and national relationships reached a state of maturation before the War of Secession which was fought to preserve rather than change these relationships. This War proved conclusive on the question of constitutional law. The doctrines so important in controlling the relationship of private and corporate persons and the government were largely developed antecedent to the growth of big business and monopoly capitalism. This had been the period of *laissez-faire,* propounding a distorted version of natural law, extolling individualism, and reducing government to the role of handmaiden and facilitator of individual fortunes at public expense. Corwin writes:

> The *laissez-faire* theory . . . was not the gift solely of the Manchester School of Political Economy—it also owed much to the biological doctrine of Evolution. Adam Smith's great work, *The Wealth of Nations,* appeared the same year as the Declaration of Independence—Mill's Political Economy was published in 1857, to be followed two years later by Darwin's world shattering *Origin of Species.* As elaborated particularly by Herbert Spencer and his American disciple John Fiske, the evolutionary conception reinforced the notion of governmental passivity immensely. It was certainly reassuring to know that competition in the economic world was matched by "the struggle for existence" in the biological world, and that those who survived the latter struggle were invariably "the fittest," since that showed that those who were most successful in economic competition were likewise "the fittest."[6]

According to the proponents of *laissez-faire,* government regulation of public health intervened in the process of natural selection. The opponents of Social Darwinism could point out that *laissez-faire* substituted a private collectivism for individualism which was "characterized by monopolistic control very similar to that from which the theory of *laissez-faire* was originally devised to rescue freedom."[7]

An approximate conformity to the theory of *laissez-faire* was sustained in the face of rising industrialism by the reconstruction administrations. The 20th century introduced an era of social welfare and public health legislation which was opposed in part by

6 Edward S. Corwin, *Constitutional revolution, Ltd.*, Claremont, California, Claremont Colleges, 1941, pp. 82-83.
7 Benjamin R. Twiss, *Lawyers and the constitution: How laissez faire came to the Supreme Court,* Princeton, New Jersey, Princeton University Press, 1942, p. 258.

conservative administrations of the post-World-War-I years and by the Supreme Court of the Franklin D. Roosevelt administration in a last ditch defense of *laissez-faire*. Currently, it is generally accepted that the federal government has the responsibility for ensuring national health and social welfare.

JUDICIAL REVIEW

The continuing change in the role of the national government has been mechanically possible as a result of the generality of the powers given to the federal government by the Constitution. Their general nature requires continuous interpretation by the courts. The result is that many provisions of the Constitution can be known only by examining the list of decisions, i.e., Constitutional law. The process of judicial review is unique to this nation in that it permits the judiciary to declare acts of Congress unconstitutional. In actuality, the only original jurisdiction guaranteed to the Supreme Court pertains to cases affecting ambassadors, public ministers, consuls, and those to which a state is a party. Its appellate jurisdiction is subject to such exceptions and exercised under such regulations as Congress shall make.

The first claim to the right of judicial review was apologetically presented in 1792 when judges of several federal circuit courts indicated to George Washington that in their opinion an Act recently passed by Congress was not legal.[8] Two years later the Supreme Court declared an Act of Congress unconstitutional but supported their right to make this decision with no formal argument.[9] In 1803, John Marshall declared a Congressional Act invalid and laid down the principles which established the right of the Supreme Court to nullify Acts of Congress which it considered to be a violation of the Constitution.[10] "In this case in which a Congressional statute was held to violate the Constitution, the statute was written by men who helped to write the Constitution while the decision was that of a man who had not taken part in that historic process."[11] It could only be interpreted as a judicial version of the meaning of the Constitution and not a protection of original meaning or intent. It was bitterly resented by Jefferson,

8 *Heyburn's Case*, 2 Dall. 409.

9 *United States v. Yale Todd*, note to *United States v. Ferreira*, 13 How. 52.

10 *Marbury v. Madison*, 1 Cranch 137, 2 L. Ed. 60.

11 Benjamin F. Wright, *The growth of American constitutional law*, Boston, Houghton Mifflin Co., 1942, p. 37.

but the Court remained, with a few subsequent exceptions.[12] the final determiner of the law.

The lesson to be derived from a brief glance at judicial review is that the political philosophy of the Supreme Court does not always reflect the political temper of the times. A static, mechanistic, philosophical interpretation of the Constitution had been a deterrent to implementing broad social health legislation required by a dynamic society. Fortunately, the public of a dynamic and democratic society can reach into the legislative halls and judicial chambers and be heard. When the political climate demands changes, meanings of the Constitution also change. As Dunne's Mr. Dooley so aptly said: "Th' Supreme Coort follows th' illiction returns."[13] True, changes in accordance with the will of the electorate were often delayed but ultimately they did occur.

THE CONSTITUTIONAL DOCUMENT AND FEDERAL PUBLIC HEALTH

It is suggested that our attention be focused on specific clauses of the Constitution upon which federal health powers are based and note some of the changes which have occurred. Since the document contains no reference to health, each of these powers is viewed by inference. The Articles which have been of primary significance to federal public health are those which assign the national government power to: (i) regulate foreign and interstate commerce, (ii) establish a postal system, (iii) exercise exclusive jurisdiction concerning federal territories and properties, (iv) contract treaties with foreign nations, (v) provide for the nation's defense, and (vi) levy taxes and provide for the general welfare. It is also presumed that significant public health powers would be available to the national government through exercise of the census clause and full faith and credit clause of the Constitution, although no meaningful attempt to assert such power has been made.

12 In 1832 when the Supreme Court ruled that the State of Georgia had no jurisdiction over the Cherokee Nation within its borders, the State of Georgia refused to appear before the Court or obey its mandate. *Worcester v. Georgia*, 6 Wheaton 264. Jackson reputedly remarked, "John Marshall has made his decision, now let him enforce it." Marshall never did.

During the Reconstruction, Congress set up a military government in the South in violation of a Supreme Court decision. When the validity of the legislation was challenged, Congress deprived the Court of jurisdiction of the case. The Supreme Court held that this action was within the powers of Congress and refrained from judging the constitutionality of military reconstrutcion acts. *Mississippi v. Johnson*, 4 Wallace 475; *Georgia v. Stanton*, 6 Wallace 50; *Ex parte McCardle*, 7 Wallace 506.

In 1869 President Grant exercised his power to change the membership of the Supreme Court so that an Act of Congress declared unconstitutional was reversed. *Hepburn v. Griswold*, 8 Wallace 603, reversed by *Legal Tender Cases*, 12 Wallace 457.

13 Finley P. Dunne, *Mr. Dooley's opinions*, New York, Harper & Bros., 1906, p. 26.

ARTICLE I. SECT. 2, PAR. 3. The census clause stipulates that *enumeration shall be made . . . within every . . . term of ten years in such manner as [Congress] shall by law direct . . . .* Accordingly, the Bureau of Census has collected data relative to various health problems such as blindness, deafness, and mental disease. It would appear that if the nation has the power to collect such data, it must have the power to do so completely, i.e., the national government would have the right to collect information concerning the health circumstance of births and deaths, accident and morbidity statistics. Such vital statistics required for the book-keeping of public health are not collected now nationally; rather, some of this information is forwarded to the federal government upon the option of the states. This has resulted in a lack of uniformity and completeness in our national vital statistics. In short, it appears that although the federal government possesses Constitutional authority to exercise this function, it has not done so.

ARTICLE IV, SECT. 1. *Full faith and credit shall be given in each State to the public acts, records, and judicial proceedings of every other state. And the Congress may by general laws prescribe the manner in which such acts, records and proceedings shall be proved, and the effect thereof.* This means that an activity detrimental to the public health and illegal, for example, in Ohio, could not be practised in Pennsylvania specifically in order to evade Ohio laws. As an illustration, uniform marriage laws requiring premarital blood tests for syphilis might be made universal under this clause if this were considered desirable from a public health point of view. However, the federal government has not attempted to assert such authority. In practice, this means that interstate attempts to enforce uniform public health statutes would require interstate compacts. Such uniformity as now exists is traceable to federal control authorized by other Articles and influence exercised on the states by the nation through the grants-in-aid program.

ARTICLE I, SECT. 8, PAR. 3. The commerce clause empowers Congress *to regulate commerce with foreign nations, and among the several states and with the Indian tribes.* This power delegated to the U. S. represents one of the major purposes of the founding fathers—to establish a central government with adequate positive authority over the commercial life of the nation.[14] But governed

14 David Fellman, *Readings in American national government,* New York, Rinehart and Co., 1947, p. 214.

by the idea of states' rights which was then justified by existing economic conditions, Congress and the Supreme Court viewed national powers narrowly.[15] By 1820 it was necessary for the national government to make provision for communication between eastern and inland or Mississippi Valley states. Congress built roads and permitted them to be administered by the states. By 1824, in the first important case involving federal interstate powers, the Court held that the commerce power included authority to regulate navigation.[16] In later cases, the Court took the view that the power of Congress was not restricted to those instruments of commerce which were in use when the Constitution was framed, rather that it was an expanding power designed to "serve the needs of an ever changing society."[17] The definition of the terms "commerce" and "regulate" has been expanded accordingly. Commerce now includes physical instrumentalities by which it is carried on, transactions on which trade relations are based, and manufacturing where it is necessary to regulate effectively transactions or physical instrumentalities. This regulating power includes construction of routes, the right to make contracts, charter companies, issue licenses, prohibit commerce in certain articles and prohibit certain methods of commerce. These powers have diminished the distinction of commerce among states and within states so that the authority of the national government in the field of commerce is almost complete. It permits not only the promotion of commerce but its limitation as well for purposes of public health.[18] Inspection, embargo, and quarantine prohibit passage of persons and articles dangerous to public safety.

The change from the initial timid assertions of federal powers under the commerce clause to the present extensive assertions of federal powers can be seen by comparing the nature of the earliest public health legislation with current public health activities as carried on by law. Quarantine procedures serve as an apt illustration. The earliest public health legislation reflected the Congressional position that health control essentially resided in the states, except where the national government held exclusive powers regulating foreign commerce and powers within its territories. The first public health legislation in 1790 was not too important. It merely provided that each vessel of more than 150 tons

15 Frank Goodnow, "Constitutional foundations of federal public health functions," *Amer. J. Pub. Health,* 1919, 9, 562.
16 *Gibbons v. Ogden,* 9 Wheaton 1.
17 Fellman, *loc. cit.*
18 Goodnow, *op. cit.,* p. 563.

in voyage outside the limits of the United States would carry a medicine chest (1 Stat. L. 131). The second public health law enacted four years later authorized Congress to convene at a place other than the Capital in times of epidemic (1 Stat. L. 353). This was quite understandable since, at the time, Philadelphia was subject to a series of yellow fever epidemics. The important factor in this was that although Congress provided to remove itself from the scene, it proposed to do nothing about the epidemic. It would be a mistake, however, to infer that Congress was unconcerned about the situation; rather, it regarded the problem as one to be met by state action. In 1796, the first Quarantine Act was passed. It provided for federal cooperation with the states and localities in enforcing their quarantine measures in regard to shipping (1 Stat. L. 474). The original bill provided for federal authority in quarantine procedures on the basis that importing epidemic disease affected the entire nation, affecting not only the populace of cities but obstructing the commerce of several communities and injuring the revenues of the United States. The original bill had been defeated, 46-23, on the basis that each independent state had the right to formulate its own legislation.[19]

Epidemics were regular occurrences in the early days of the Republic. John Adams began his second annual message to Congress in 1798 by referring to the pestilence of yellow fever and urged federal laws to aid the health of the people within the states. It was nearly a hundred years before another President made such a direct recommendation. Despite the direct plea of the President, Congress merely enacted legislation in 1799 supplanting the Act of 1796 which did little more than recognize state rights over quarantine and again authorize cooperation (1 Stat. L. 619). Jefferson seems to have dodged the issue. In a message to Congress he mentioned epidemics in two cities but stated only that "although the health laws of the states should be found to need no present revisal by Congress, yet commerce claims that their attention be ever awake to them."[20] Monroe in 1825 related to Congress: "this being the seat of government, its protection against disease must form one of its principal objects."[21] Reminiscent of Philadelphia days, Congress took no action regarding quarantine. Van Buren,

[19] Harry S. Mustard, *Government in public health*, New York, The Commonwealth Fund, 1945, pp. 49-57.

[20] Thomas Jefferson, *Fifth annual message to Congress*, 3 Dec. 1805, in *Annals of the Congress of the United States, Ninth Congress*, Washington, Gales and Seaton, 1852, p. 11.

[21] James Monroe, *Message to Congress*, 17 Feb. 1825, in *Register of debates in Congress, 18th Congress, 2nd Session*, Washington, Gales and Seaton, 1825, Vol. 1, p. 623.

Tyler, Pierce, Johnson, and Grant sent messages to Congress concerning public health, but these were minor matters and not forcefully presented.

Congress passed an Act in 1832 which allowed the Secretary of the Treasury to aid the states in the enforcement of quarantine laws (4 Stat. L. 577). In 1866, an appropriation from the national treasury was authorized for the purpose of aiding the states in the enforcement of their quarantine regulations (14 Stat. L. 357). Neither Act provided for federal quarantine procedures. Thus, during the first three-quarters of the 19th century, public health quarantine procedure consisted merely of federal-state cooperation as provided by the Acts of 1796 and 1799.

In 1878, Congress permitted quarantine rules and regulations to be prescribed by the Surgeon General but within the same Act made this provision inoperative by stating that the rules and regulations "shall not conflict or impair any sanitary or quarantine laws or regulations of any state or municipal authorities now existing or which may hereafter be enacted." (20 Stat. L. 37). The national government carefully continued to avoid conflict with state authority but at great cost to the public health. President Hayes, spurred by the great yellow fever epidemic of 1878—the nation's worst recorded epidemic—finally recommended federal quarantine. Congress responded to Hayes's message by creating the National Board of Health in 1879 with power to enforce interstate quarantine measures in respect to cholera, yellow fever, smallpox, and plague (20 Stat. L. 484; 21 Stat. L. 5). National Board powers lapsed four years later, but the Board continued a rather jobless existence until 1893 when it was dissolved.[22] Public opinion continued to press for national quarantine control. In a court case during 1886 involving the right of a state to charge fees for quarantine services, the Supreme Court took the unusual step of criticizing Congress for not assuming federal responsibility in quarantine. The Court said:

> For the period of nearly a century since the government was organized, Congress has passed no quarantine law, nor any other law to protect the inhabitants of the United States against the invasion of contagious and infectious disease from abroad; and yet during the early part of the present century, for many years the cities of the Atlantic Coast, from Boston and New York to Charleston, were devastated by yellow fever. In later times the cholera has made similar invasions; and the yellow fever has been unchecked in its fearful course in the Southern cities. . . . During all this time

22 James W. Garner, "Federal activity in the interest of public health," *Yale Rev.* 1905, *14*, 195.

the Congress never attempted to exercise this or any other powers to protect the people from the ravages of these dreadful diseases. No doubt they believe that the power to do this belonged to the states. . . .

But it may be conceded that whenever Congress shall undertake to provide for the commercial cities of the United States a general system of quarantine . . . all State laws on the subject will be abrogated, at least so far as the two are inconsistent. But, until this is done, the laws of the State on the subject are valid.[23]

Congress belatedly accepted the suggestion after seven years in its enactment of the Quarantine Act of 1893 (27 Stat. L. 449). Although recognizing regulation of state and municipal authorities, it frankly stated for the first time that such regulation must conform with national law. It permitted national quarantine control to supersede control by the respective states although this power has been rarely exercised.[24] The Act also provided for the purchase of municipal and state quarantine stations if necessary to the nation. In 1920, the Port of New York became the last station absorbed (41 Stat. L. 875). Thus, our current quarantine program was established with the states administering interstate quarantine subject to national law and foreign quarantine being conducted by the national government.

The reluctance of the federal government to assume the quarantine function until the final quarter of the 19th century was merely a part of its general reluctance to assume interstate commercial regulatory responsibilities. However, when the Supreme Court in an 1886 decision[25] invalidated state regulation of interstate commerce as an infringement of the national government, legislative action became imperative. Congress responded by passing an Interstate Commerce Act in 1887 (24 Stat. L. 379), resulting in the first modern administrative board of the American government, the Interstate Commerce Commission. Administrative regulations were still alien to the American concept of government, and the federal courts insisted on the right to review orders of the Commission. By successive decisions of the Court, Interstate Commerce Commission powers were removed until the Commission became an ineffectual body.[26] Abandoned by Congress and ignored by three successive Presidents,[27] the Interstate Commerce Act of 1887

23 *Morgan's Louisiana and Texas R. R. and Steamship Co. v. Louisiana State Board of Health*, 118 U.S. 455, 6 S. Ct. 1114, 30 L. Ed. 237.
24 Plague in San Francisco during early years of the 20th century and in 1916 poliomyelitis epidemic in New York.
25 *Wabash, St. Louis and Pacific R.R. Co v. Illinois*, 118 U.S. 557.
26 Samuel E. Morison and Henry S. Commager, *The growth of the American Republic*, New York, Oxford University Press, 1942, Vol. II, p. 119.
27 Harrison, Cleveland, McKinley.

T. Roosevelt

ICC

was disinterred by Theodore Roosevelt. The Hepburn Act of 1906 authorized the national Executive branch to determine and prescribe interstate freight rates. There followed the introduction of other regulatory agencies of government so important to public health. Beginning with meat inspection and pure food and drug control in 1906, there were added, among others, agencies concerned with stream pollution, water rights, nuisance control, milk and food supervision, industrial conditions affecting health, animal diseases, narcotics, white slaves, false labeling, and misleading advertising.[28] The list is conglomerate and fragmentary, but it illustrates a few of the federal public health functions exercised under interstate commerce authority as permitted by a broadened interpretation of federal powers.

The public health purpose made no significant advance in the important area of child labor legislation. When the Supreme Court held in 1895 that the Sherman Anti-Trust Act could not apply to the manufacturing process, the pattern of constitutional interpretation of the commerce clause for the next four decades was established.[29] It meant the Court had drawn a fine line between commerce and manufacturing. In 1918 the Court invalidated a federal child labor law on the theory that it was actually a regulation of conditions of production.[30] A later attempt at enacting child labor legislation under taxation powers was also invalidated,[31] and constitutional amendment efforts came to naught. The National Industrial Recovery Act and the Guffy Coal Act were invalidated in 1935 and 1936, respectively,[32] on the same basis as the 1918 decision. In 1937 the Court reversed its previous position by its decision in the famous *National Labor Relations Board v. Jones and Laughlin Steel Corporation* case (301 U.S. 1), stating that the regulation of labor relations at the plant was within the scope of the commerce clause. This decision removes any constitutional hinderance to child labor legislation, but it is no longer a major public health issue. The importance of the decision is that it represents a victory for the modern dynamic interpretation of the Constitution and represents a turning point in the

28 "If administrative agencies did not exist in the federal government, Congress would be limited to a technique of legislation primarily designed to correct evils after they have arisen rather than to prevent them from arising." *Administrative Procedure in Government Agencies*, Senate Document No. 8, 77th Congress, 1st Session, 1941, pp. 11-18.

29 *U.S. v. E. C. Knight*, 156 U.S. 1.

30 *Hammer v. Dagenhart*, 247 U.S. 251, 38 S.Ct. 529, 62 L.Ed. 1001.

31 *Bailey v. Drexel Furniture Company*, 259 U.S. 20, 42 S.Ct. 449, 66 L.Ed. 817.

32 *Schechter Poultry Corporation v. U.S.*, 295 U.S. 495; *Carter v. Carter Coal Company*, 298 U.S. 238.

evolution of basic constitutional doctrine.[33] The notion of government as a necessary evil could be supplanted by an appreciation of government as a servant of the people and the instrument of national health and welfare.[34]

ARTICLE I, SECT. 8, PAR. 7: Congress shall have power *to establish Post Offices and Post Roads.* Federal postal authority has been a monopoly since its inception. It has operated as a monopoly, formulating such regulations as deemed necessary to providing mail services to the public on a beneficial basis. Thus, it has excluded from the mails such things as injurious foods, medicines, illegal drugs, misleading advertising, and other injurious substances and tracts. Court decisions have substantially reaffirmed postal authority in this area.

ARTICLE I, SECT. 9: *To exercise exclusive legislation in all cases whatsoever, over such District . . . as may . . . become the seat of government of the United States, and to exercise like authority over all places purchased by the consent of the legislature of the state in which the same shall be, for the erection of forts, magazines, arsenals, dock yards, and other needful buildings.*

ARTICLE IV, SECT. 2, PAR. 4: *The Congress shall have power to dispose of and make all needful rules and regulations respecting the Territory or other property belonging to the United States.* Federal power of exclusive jurisdiction is essentially concomitant with the power of police. It should be recalled that police powers were possessed by the separate states prior to the adoption of the Constitution and were not relinquished by them. Amendment X reserved police powers for the state subject to Constitutional limitations. However, since self-preservation is regarded as the first law of nature and *salus populi suprema lex est* are dicta recognized by common law, police power assumes precedence over the Constitution when necessary for the health and welfare of the people. Articles I and IV did not confer police power upon the national government for it is, in actuality, an inherent function of government necessary to its survival.[35] Rather, it mapped out an area in which federal police powers might be exercised. The awesome bounds of police power whose limits perhaps cannot be prescribed are attested to by the fact that state police has been deter-

[33] Fellman, *op. cit.*, p. 215.
[34] Henry S. Commager, *The American mind*, New Haven, Conn., Yale University Press, 1950, p. 641.
[35] Henry B. Hemenway, *Legal principles of public health administration*, Chicago, T. H. Flood and Co., 1914, p. 88.

mined as superior to the regulation of commerce.[36] It can be legally exercised even if it stops navigation[37] or interferes with a foreign treaty entered into by the United States.[38] The police power may override provisions of the Constitution which guard the sanctity of contracts,[39] freedom of person,[40] due process of law,[40] and property rights.[41] Ordinarily, private property may not be taken or destroyed without due compensation; or private individuals pressed into public service, especially without compensation. However, the Courts have upheld this action as proper when exercised for the protection of the community. This power cannot be exercised arbitrarily, all usual legal means being first exhausted or deemed inapplicable to the problem. In fact, whenever the health of the community is at stake, contrary rights of the individual are superseded. The only limits, if any truly exist, to such power are the necessity for reasonableness and validity in its exercise as a public health measure.

ARTICLE II, SECT. 2, PAR. 2: The President *shall have power, by and with the advice and consent of the Senate, to make treaties, providing two-thirds of the Senators concur . . . .*

ARTICLE VI, SECT. 2: *. . . and all treaties made, or which shall be made, under the authority of the United States, shall be the Supreme Law of the Land.* There have been two opposing views as to the extent and limits of treaty authority—one which asserts that arbitrary power exists; the other which limits the subjects of treaties to other delegated national powers. In practice there have been few instances in which federal-state conflict occurred or where due process of law has been questioned. When such conflicts have appeared, the Courts have found no limitations on the treaty power.[42] An early illustration of the use of the treaty power for purposes of public health is seen by the several treaties with Indian tribes committing the Federal government to provide certain health services to the Indians. The first such provision occurred in 1832 as a partial payment for Winnebago Indian property, and by

36 *Smith v. St. Louis and Southwestern Ry. Co.*, 181 U.S. 248.
37 *Leovy v. U.S.*, 177 U.S. 621; *Wilson v. Blackbird Creek Co.*, 2 Pet. 245; *Gilman v. Philadelphia*, 3 Wall. 713.
38 *Compagnie Francaise de Navigation a Vapeur v. Louisiana*, 186 U.S. 380.
39 *Boston Beer Co. v. Mass.*, 97 U.S. 25; *Stone v. Miss.*, 101 U.S. 814; *Boyd v. Ala.*, 94 U.S. 645; *Butcher's Union Slaughterhouse v. Crescent City Livestock Land Insurance Co.*, 111 U.S. 746; *Kreses v. Lyman*, 74 Fed. 765.
40 *Sears v. Gallatin County*, 20 Mont. 462.
41 *Bass v. State*, 34 La. Ann. 494; *Eldridge v. Trezevant*, 160 U.S.
42 See, for example, *Fairfax's Devise v. Hunter's Lessee*, 7 Cranch 603; *U.S. v. Curtis-Wright Export Corporation*, 299 U.S. 304; *Missouri v. Holland*, 252 U.S. 416; *Wilson v. Girard*, 254 U.S. 524.

1871 at least two dozen treaties provided for some kind of medical service to various tribes. Most of the Indian treaties limited medical services to five or ten years, but the government adopted the policy of continuing services.[43] The other major significant use of the treaty power in aid of public health was contained in a 1926 commercial treaty with Germany empowering the consuls of both nations to inspect all vessels at ports within their districts with a view to more effective enforcement of quarantine regulations (44-Part 3, Stat. L. 2155). However, if public health should become a matter of international regulation through conventions with foreign nations, the treaty power may become a very important basis for public health activity on a national level.[44]

ARTICLE I. SECT. 8, PARS. 11-14,16: Congress shall have the power *to declare war . . . to raise and support Armies . . . to provide and maintain a navy. To make rules for the regulation of land and naval forces . . . to provide for organizing, arming, and disciplining the militia, and for governing such part of them as may be employed in the service of the United States.* In time of peace this power has generally been restricted to providing the armed forces with medical protection and care for its personnel. It had been used as the basis for beginning federal health services for Indians. This began about 1802 or 1803 when Army physicians took measures to curb smallpox and other contagious diseases among Indians in the vicinity of the military posts.[45] In times of military conflict, the war power legalizes all acts of federal government related to gaining military success. The generous interpretation by the courts of the health aspects of the war power was well illustrated in 1919 when the Supreme Court upheld an order of the Secretary of War forbidding houses of ill fame within five miles of a military establishment.[46] During World War II the war clause served as a basis for extending health and medical care services to certain defense employees and servicemen's dependents. Views on the constitutional implications of this clause have remained rather constant, their application depending upon the exigencies of the military situation rather than changing political thought.

[43] U.S. Dept. of Health, Education, and Welfare, *Health services for American Indians* Public Health Service Publication No. 531, USGPO, 1957, p. 86.

[44] Robert D. Leigh, *Federal health administration in the United States*, New York, Harper and Bros., 1927, p. 73.

[45] U.S. Dept. of Health, Education, and Welfare, *loc. cit.;* and George S. J. Perrot and Margaret D. West, "Health services for American Indians," *Pub. Hlth Repts.*, 1957, 72, 565.

[46] *McKinley v. U.S.*, 249 U.S. 397.

ARTICLE I, SECT. 8, PAR. 1: *The Congress shall have power to lay and collect taxes, duties, imposts and excises, to pay the debts and provide for the common defense and general welfare of the United States.* This clause has been variously referred to as the taxation clause, welfare clause, and the appropriations clause. If we view the public health powers which this clause places in the federal government, it should be considered in terms of the taxation and appropriations aspects related to general welfare.

The delegation to Congress of taxing authority ranks with commercial regulation as one of the main objects of the framers of the Constitution. A major importance for public health resides in the levying of excise taxes. It is by way of excise taxation that the national government has authority to regulate goods and persons while it raises revenue. In this respect national authority is not limited to interstate jurisdiction. "If a commodity can be taxed at all by federal authority it may be reached anywhere."[47] However, limitations on federal taxing authority do exist. Although statutes may be regulatory or prohibitory, they must show "on their face" a revenue purpose. In 1886 Congress levied a tax on oleomargarine clearly attempting to discourage, if not to prohibit, its manufacture (24 Stat. L. 209). In 1904 the Supreme Court upheld the statute with the comment that it could not take judicial cognizance of the alleged Congressional intent.[48] It was thus regarded as a revenue measure "on its face." In 1912 a heavy tax was placed on poisonous white phosphorus matches and, although uncontested, this tax is legally analogous to the oleomargarine tax (37 Stat. L. 81). With the Narcotic Drug Act of 1914 (38 Stat. L. 785), the taxation clause was used with a control purpose similar to that in the oleomargarine and match taxes but with a distinctly different revenue aspect. It merely required a nominal tax of one dollar for registration of dispensers of narcotic drugs, but the Court, in *U.S. v. Doremus*, 49 U.S. 86, 94 (1919), was willing to read in the Act a revenue purpose. This meant that by means of nominal license taxes the public health agencies might extend their control to businesses injurious to health where possession of names and records provides a basis for effective legislation. By a curious quirk in logic, a regulatory tax on child labor employers enacted in 1919 (40 Stat. L. 1138) was declared invalid because it was not a bona fide tax,[49] i.e., an act for raising revenue. The

47 Leigh, *op. cit.*, p. 51.
48 *McCray v. U.S.*, 195 U.S. 27.
49 *Bailey v. Drexel Furniture Co.*, 259 U.S. 20, 42 S. Ct. 449, 66 L. Ed. 817.

exact point at which a federal tax law is a tax "on its face" and therefore bona fide has not been clearly defined. The change in political philosophy since the 1922 child labor law decision indicates that public health measures are not significantly limited by the concept of a bona fide tax. Currently, if they serve a public health purpose, they are likely to be regarded as a revenue measure "on their face."

The second aspect of this Article and Section of the Constitution pertains to appropriations. It has been assumed that if the nation possessed means to raise money, it could also expend money for stated purposes, i.e., the common defense and the general welfare. In the field of public health this has served as the basis of providing grants-in-aid to the states and direct health services for promotion of the general welfare. However, the boundaries of the term "general welfare" had not always permitted expenditures for the wide variety of services now current. The term "general welfare" does not define the purpose of the expenditure with reasonable clarity. Its current definition, thus, has evolved with the development of constitutional law.

Divergent views concerning the welfare clause existed in the very antecedents of the Constitution. Hamilton assumed the broad view that it was left to the Legislature to determine "objects which concern the general welfare." His views are clearly presented in *The Federalist* (Nos. 30 and 34) and his *Report on Manufacture,* 1791. Madison argues in *The Federalist* (No. 41) that the general welfare clause restricted objects of spending to the other expressly delegated powers contained in the Constitution. This latter view, or more properly a modification of it, appeared repeatedly to contest outlays for internal improvements up to the time of the War of Secession. Presidents Monroe and Buchanan, holding a modified view, accepted Hamilton's position that objects of expenditure under this clause were not confined to enumerated powers but concluded that they were limited by the Tenth Amendment. The modified view then denies the right of national spending to transgress the field of state sovereignty. Despite Presidential pronouncements of limited spending powers, there occurred a gradual expansion of national appropriations in areas not enumerated by the Constitution. Federal grants for roads, canals, and education were made prior to the Civil War, but the development of federal aid to public health was not an accepted principle.

Federal cooperation in quarantine procedure,[50] federal assistance to education having a public health by-product,[51] and direct federal aid to seamen,[52] general citizens,[53] and Indians[54] were individual events which aggrandized the national concept of the welfare clause but did not serve as an accepted precedent for federal expenditures for the internal improvement of public health. When, in 1854, Congress passed a bill providing land grants to the states for the purpose of providing hospitals and services for the care of the mentally ill, it was vetoed by President Pierce. Pierce's veto message repeated the modified view of the welfare clause stating that the government could not become thus involved in any cause, no matter how humanitarian, when it would usurp the powers of the individual states.[55]

In 1879, the first clearly intended grant-in-aid to state programs for the purpose of promoting public health came to an untimely conclusion. In the Bill creating the National Board of Health which had been passed by the House of Representatives there was contained a provision to extend $500,000 financial aid to the states. The clerk transcribing the Bill for Senate action failed to include this provision.[56] It was thus not until 1916 that public health grants-in-aid on a matching basis occurred. It was specifically designated for demonstration projects in rural sanitation, and the total amount for the program was a modest $25,000 (39 Stat. L. 21). The passage of the Sixteenth Amendment in 1913 established the federal income tax and opened the way for a tremendous expansion of national expenditures and grants. With the passage of the Venereal Disease Act of 1918 there seemed to be an acceptance of federal grants to states as a principle in public health (40 Stat. L. 886).

The gradual expansion of national appropriations in areas not enumerated by the Constitution occurred without being ques-

50 Quarantine Acts of 1796, 1799 and 1832.

51 Land grants for the establishment of the Connecticut Asylum for the Deaf and Dumb (1819) and for a similar institution in Kentucky (1826).

52 Act of 1798 establishing a Marine Hospital Service for the relief of sick and disabled seamen.

53 Act of 1813 which stated that vaccine was to be provided to all citizens at no cost upon receipt of their applications (2 Stat. L. 806). This was repealed nine years later (3 Stat. L. 677).

54 Act of 1832 which authorized vaccination for the Indian tribes (4 Stat. L. 514).

55 Roy F. Nichols, *Franklin Pierce*, Philadelphia, University of Pennsylvania Press 1931, pp. 348-349.
See also Albert Deutsch, *The mentally ill in America*, New York, Columbia University Press, 1952. Deutsch gives a graphic portrayal of the efforts of Dorothea Dix to secure passage of this legislation on behalf of the mentally ill.

56 J. L. Cabell, "Presidential address," *Amer. Publ. Hlth Aso. Papers & Rpts.*, 1880, 5, 1-23.

tioned in the Courts for more than a century and a quarter. This is understandable when one considers that it involved no direct interference with state activities; rather, it doled out benefits to the states and the individuals therein. But in 1923 the Commonwealth of Massachusetts challenged the legality of the Sheppard-Towner Act (42 Stat. L. 135).[57] A suit was also entered by a Massachusetts citizen against the United States for taking property by taxation without due process for the purpose of financing this Act.[58] The State claimed that rights guaranteed to them by the Tenth Amendment were usurped. The Supreme Court disposed of both cases without ruling on the legality involved. The Court merely stated that the Commonwealth of Massachusetts and the taxpayer were "without status in the premise" (having no basis for suit). The decision in the case of the Commonwealth hinted at the constitutionality involved. It held that the Commonwealth could not be a party to a suit unless its rights had been transgressed. The grant of funds did not take anything away from the state since the state was free to reject the funds. The obvious corollary that granting monies "with strings attached" exercised a power over the recipient was not deemed to be a case in issue. The method of federal grants then appears to be limited only by determination of public purpose and sanction by public opinion.

In the 1920's national grants to the states were slightly more than $100 million and confined to a few functions. About 75 per cent of the total grants were disbursed for highways.[59] Federal aid for state public health which had lapsed in 1929 was renewed in 1935 under Titles V and VI of the Social Security Act (49 Stat. L. 620). Successive Congresses have curtailed or eliminated certain funds and increased others, but federal financial aid to state public health no longer appears to be on a temporary basis. The present picture is radically different in size, scope, and activity than during the 1920's. The Department of Health, Education, and Welfare portion of grants to the states during fiscal 1960 was more than $2,730,000,000. Public health has shared in this expansion, receiving more than $200,000,000, which has resulted in vast changes in services.[60] It has been the basis of expanded and newly developed programs such as demonstration projects, clinic services for

57 *Frotheringham v. Mellon*, 262 U.S. 447.

58 *Massachusetts et. al. v. Mellon*, 262 U.S. 447.

59 W. Glen Campbell, "Decentralizing big government," *Amer. econ. Sec.*, 1953, *10*, 23-24.

60 U.S. Department of Health, Education, and Welfare, *Annual report, 1960*, Washington, D.C., USGPO, p. 9.

diagnosis and treatment, construction of hospitals and facilities, research, health education and training, and consultation.

Since the authority for providing direct health service to individuals is contained in the same Article permitting grants-in-aid, the development of direct health service has been, from a constitutional point of view, similar to the development of grants-in-aid. The same arguments for and against federal appropriations occurred. The familiar proponent of strong central government based on a broad interpretive view of the Constitution, Mr. Hamilton, in a 1792 report to Congress, suggested establishing hospitals for the care of seamen in the interests of navigation and trade. It was the first step in the creation of the U. S. Public Health Service. In 1798 a bill was introduced to establish federal Marine Hospitals for seamen.[61] The matter was referred to the Committee on Commerce and Manufacture as a problem concerning commerce, with health being considered solely as an aspect of the commercial problem. (This was the precedent for a pattern of federal handling of health and medical matters secondly and indirectly until recent years. This pattern has resulted in the wide scattering of health activities among various governmental units of administration.) The passage of the Federal Marine Hospital Act in 1789 (1 Stat. L. 605) has been used as proof that the principle was accepted that the Federal government should provide medical services and hospitalization for certain classes of independent, non-relief persons. It was among the first systems of compulsory insurance against sickness in the world. Yet it would be an error to attribute to the Fifth Congress any intent to institute any far-reaching medical insurance scheme. It was intended to remove from seamen a handicap by which they were unable to receive medical services even commensurate to the degree of care obtained by paupers in their home community. This lack of medical care for seamen posed a serious threat to the nation's commerce. Opposition to the hospital plan was primarily based on the philosophy that the problem was a state responsibility. But it was also clear to the thirteen seaboard states that it would be more practical to have a central plan for support of the endeavor. Practical considerations and exigencies of

61 This was the American counterpart of the earlier action of the British government in their establishment of the Royal Hospital for Seamen at Greenwich, England, for the purpose of providing care for sick and disabled seamen. Both governments, consistent with prevailing mercantilist values, were motivated toward the provision for such services in the interest of maintaining the economic strength of the nation. The view of British hospital services for seamen as a pattern for adoption by the United States is reflected in the Congressional discussion of the issue. See the remarks of Mr. Parker (H. of R.) , 10 April 1798 in *Annals of the Congress of the United States, Fifth Congress*, Washington, Gales and Seaton, 1851, p. 1391.

the situation did, as on subsequent occasions, exert sufficient pressure to modify meanings derived from the Constitution. Political thought still maintained the supremacy of state sovereignty, and the Act accordingly provided for medical and hospital service to be rendered through utilization of local facilities. The records between 1798 and 1870 are fragmentary and incomplete, but it is clear that the venture fared poorly.[62] Leigh states:

> During its first seventy years of activity, the Service had acquired practically all the administrative disabilities associated with Jeffersonian and Jacksonian democracy; its personnel was the subject of party spoils; its purchases of supplies was an adjunct to party machinery; its decentralization and lack of supervision were almost complete; its hospitals were a part of the annual distribution from the Congressional pork-barrel; as a mean of governmentally supervised sickness insurance it was a fiscal failure requiring annual doles from Congress to keep it functioning; on account of enforced parsimony it was also very far from offering any guaranty of medical aid to the sailors even at the principal sea ports.[63]

It was evident that unless far-reaching authority was assumed by the national government, the program would collapse completely. The 1870 revision reviewed the old discussion as to why the government should be uniquely concerned with seamen. In addition to the response concerning their importance to commerce, there had now been added a description of seamen as being the most improvident class of men on earth, a classification which had consequently always been treated somewhat as wards of the government. This argument heralded the application of a concept in federal government responsibility which previously had been exercised only in regard to the Indian population. (Assumption of wardship responsibility has been a matter of necessity or expediency rather than interpretation of the Constitution which is silent on this issue.) Before the end of the century the concept of national responsibility for health services was extended to lepers and immigrants.

As a result of the 1870 revision the new public health corps and its procedures were organized along military lines. The beginning knowledge of bacteriology resulted in a public health focus on research and on preventive medicine. Medical services became centralized in state programs. A program of federal-state co-operation on an organized, systematic basis was instituted. The ground work for the present program of public health medical care service was laid. It required only an extension of the principle of federal

62 Mustard, *op. cit.*, pp. 32-39.
63 Leigh, *op. cit.*, p. 92.

responsibility to other categories of individuals to "fill out" the 1870 framework.

In 1918 medical care services were broadly extended to veterans; in 1922 mothers and infants became recipients; in 1935 the dependent blind, dependent aged, and dependent children became eligible for some medical care; in 1950 the permanently and totally disabled were added. Concurrent with this development, outpatient diagnostic and treatment services became available for individuals with communicable diseases such as tuberculosis and venereal disease. In more recent years this has been extended to include various chronic diseases. With the advent of the New Deal there occurred also a federal acceptance of the reciprocal relationship between poverty and ill health. Consequently, the development of national participation in providing public assistance to needful categories of citizens and conducting other income maintenance programs paralleled the broadened extension of direct medical care services. This development was a recognition of the superiority of preventive to palliative measures, and restorative to custodial efforts, as common bases for complementary public relief and public health activities.

The fragmentary inclusion of certain categories of citizens and categories of diseases for certain public health benefits has been a less desirable mode of development than a unified, comprehensive program for the entire citizenry. But it is a natural outgrowth of democratic, constitutional government which brings the central government into the business of public health only at such times and in such particular instances as lesser units of government are unable to perform the general health and welfare duties of government. The increasing role of government, particularly national government, in providing social control for health and other purposes has presented the dilemma of reconciling individual liberty with the changing concept of government. For example, men have many rights, but among them is not included the right to ill health and the transmission of ill health to their neighbors. Katherine Lenroot, in her presidential address to the national social work body in 1935, remarked that "government may prove to be the only (agent) having range and power necessary for dealing with the most complicated and difficult situations." She considered a basic problem of the 20th century to be one of making government "an effective agency of social control."[64] If the state is

64 As quoted in Frank J. Bruno, *Trends in social work, 1874-1946*, New York, Columbia University Press, 1948, p. 347.

to be "an elected body whose duty was to impose the minimum restrictions and safeguard the maximum liberties of the people," as according to Kant, there would be placed on the state no other obligation than to protect men and police their liberties.[65] Although this is one of the primary attributes, the state must also be positive. The state should be a well-spring for the creative impulses in which all men can share. In public health, the Constitution has been the framework within which such impulses have been directed to effecting an increase in human well-being and dignity.

[65] As quoted in Robert Payne, *Zero*, London, Allan Wingate Publishers, Ltd., 1951, p. 253.

The Sarah Stout Murder Case:
An Early Example of the Doctor as an Expert Witness

ALBERT ROSENBERG*

"**H**ER face and her neck to her shoulders appeared black and so much corrupted that we were unwilling to proceed any further; but her mother would have it done, and so we did open her up."[1] The jury listened attentively to Dr. Coatsworth's testimony concerning the autopsy performed on the corpse of Sarah Stout six weeks after its burial. The Hertford Assizes were in session; it was 18 July 1699; Spencer Cowper and three alleged accomplices, John Mason, Ellis Stevens, and William Rogers, were on trial for the murder of Sarah Stout.

Spencer Cowper, the main defendant, was a young, successful lawyer, whose father and older brother were prominent Whig politicians. All four defendants were members of the legal profession traveling with the home circuit of the Assizes, which had arrived in Hertford that year on Monday, 13 March.

In Hertford Sarah Stout and her mother were living in very comfortable circumstances because of the industry and thrift of the late Mr. Stout, a maltster. Indeed Sarah, attired in a close white cape and poke bonnet, received considerable attention as the local heiress. Since the Stouts had supported the Cowpers in local elections and were good friends of the family, it was natural that Spencer should call there when he arrived in Hertford. It was also generally known that he had invested some money in mortgages for Sarah, and he declared that he called that evening to deliver to her a payment of interest on her money.

As is usual in trials of murder, the accounts of what happened varied. The main outlines of the case, however, were clear. At about eleven o'clock in the evening Cowper and Sarah Stout were alone together in the sitting room of her house. The maid had gone up to warm his bed, understanding that he was to spend the night there. The sound of a door closing was heard; and when the

* University of California, Davis, California.
1 *The trial of Spencer Cowper, Esq; John Marson, Ellis Stevens, and William Rogers, Gent. for the murder of Mrs. Sarah Stout, a Quaker. Before Mr. Baron Hatsell, at Hertford Assizes, July 18, 1699.* London, 1741, p. 48.

maid and Sarah's mother, anxious because no further sounds of activity were heard, came into the sitting room, no one was there. They waited up all night; their vigil was in vain. Early in the morning a neighbor brought the sad news. Sarah Stout had been found drowned in the pond by the mill dam.

The coroner's inquest was routine. In absence of any evidence of foul play and of any motive, the decision was that she took her life while *non compos mentis*.

Six weeks later Dr. Coatsworth, a surgeon, was summoned by Dr. Phillips to be present at the opening of the body of Sarah Stout. He was told that there was suspicion of murder. While in Hertford he lodged with the mother of the dead girl, who told him she would not rest until she knew whether her daughter had been with child or not. As he declared in court, he informed her that "we should find the parts contained in the abdomen so rotten, that it would be impossible to discover the uterus from the other parts."[2] Dr. Coatsworth then explained patiently that it would only be possible to tell if the embryo had already become bony. Still the dead girl's mother insisted on the autopsy.

The Stouts were Quakers, and the Quakers were the target of seemingly endless scurrilous abuse. Grub Street writers like Tom Brown and Ned Ward used the name Quaker as a synonym for hypocrite. And now rumors were circulating that Sarah Stout had not been as good as she might have been and that she took her life to avoid the shame of being pregnant and unwed. The entire Quaker community demanded that action should be taken to clear the name of Sarah Stout.

Dr. Coatsworth continued his testimony:

And as soon as she was opened, we perceived the stomach and guts were full of wind, as if they had been blown with a pair of bellows; we put her guts aside, and came to the uterus, and Dr. Phillips shewed it us in his hand, and afterwards cut it out, and laid it on the table, and opened it, and we saw into the cavity of it, and if there had been anything there as minute as a hair, we might have seen it, but it was perfectly free and empty.[3]

Satisfied that the Quaker girl had not been pregnant at the time of her death, the doctors and surgeons continued examining the body. They found that the stomach, lungs, and diaphragm were sunk flat and contained no water; and they were not putrefied. The surgeons and doctors present, with the exception of Mr.

[2] *Ibid.*
[3] *Ibid.*

Camlin, Spencer Cowper's surgeon, concluded and signed an affidavit to the effect that Sarah Stout could not have been drowned, since if she had taken in water, the water must have "rotted all the guts."[4]

Armed with this affidavit, they were able to bring a charge of murder against Spencer Cowper and his three colleagues. Mr. Jones prosecuted the case as Counsel for the King, while Cowper conducted his own defence. It was, as the King's Counsel stressed, really two trials: to clear Sarah Stout's name from the obloquy of suicide and to punish her murderers.

The prosecution's star witness was Sarah Walker, the Stouts' maid. She insisted that Spencer Cowper intended to spend the night at the Stouts' home, that she warmed his bed for him, and that she heard a door slam shut about eleven o'clock at night. This evidence placed Cowper in a very awkward situation; he was shown to be acting in a very suspicious manner and to have been the last person known to have been with Sarah Stout while she was still alive.

Next the prosecution called a series of witnesses, the people who removed her body from the pond, to establish that she was floating very near the top of the water. She was, according to their testimony, on her right side, with her right arm driven between two stakes (used to keep weeds from drifting into the mill) just below the surface of the water, which was about six feet deep. This testimony was intended to establish the fact that she was floating in the water and that nothing hindered her from sinking.

Mr. Jones then called to the stand the women who stripped the body of Sarah Stout. Elizabeth Hustler, Sarah Kimpson, and Anne Pilkington, who removed her stays and prepared her body for burial, agreed that the nude body revealed no swelling. They also declared that there were some bruises on the body, but no mark around her neck. This testimony was corroborated by John Dimsdale Jr., a surgeon, who was the first expert to examine her.

When Sarah Peppercorn, the next witness, appeared a wave of laughter spread through the court. Sarah was the local midwife; she had obviously been called to testify because of the malicious

---

4 *Ibid.*, p. 49. The affidavit read: "We, whose Names are here under-written, having examined the Body of Mrs. *Sarah Stout* deceased, do find the Uterus perfectly free and empty, and of the natural Figure and Magnitude as usually in Virgins; we found no Water in the Stomach, Intestines, Abdomen, Lungs or Cavity of the Thorax." A true copy of the affidavit was published in *Some observations on the tryal of Spencer Cowper, J. Marson, E. Stevens, W. Rogers, that were tried at Hereford, about the murder of Sarah Stout, together with other things relating hereunto.* London, 1701, p. 13.

rumors of Sarah Stout's pregnancy. She declared she found no evidence of pregnancy and no swelling of the body.

The prosecution then presented the evidence of the group of surgeons who had examined the body of Sarah Stout at the autopsy. They agreed with Dr. Coatsworth's contention that the absence of any quantity of water in the internal organs indicated that Sarah Stout had not been drowned, but had been dead before her body entered the water. They also agreed with Dr. Coatsworth that a body is drowned when it is suffocated by water passing down the windpipe into the lungs upon inspiration; and at the same time, the water pressing down upon the gullet, a great part of it is swallowed into the stomach.

The next witness, Edward Clement, a sailor, related some of his experiences at sea during bloody battles; he had seen many drownings and dozens of dead bodies flung into the sea. When he began narrating some difficult-to-believe tales of sea life, Mr. Jones interrupted him: "Then you take it for a certain rule, that those that are drowned sink, but those that are thrown overboard do not." The loquacious sailor gave what he considered both a witty and authoritative reply: "Yes, otherwise why should the government be at the vast charge to allow threescore or fourscore weight of iron to sink every man, but only that their swimming about should not be a discouragement to others."[5]

The evidence linking and implicating John Marson, Ellis Stevens, and William Rogers with Spencer Cowper rounded out the prosecution's case. The three lawyers had come to Hertford together and lodged together at the house of the Gurrey family. They were reported to have come in at eleven o'clock at night and to have engaged in some very suspicious conversation. One said to Marson: "She was an old sweet-heart of yours." "Ay," says he, "But she cast me off, but I reckon by this time a friend of mine has done her business." Another bit of discourse overheard was: "I believe a friend of mine is even with her at this time." Still more damaging was the remark attributed to one of the group: "Sarah Stout's courting days are over." Furthermore, there was some talk about money which seemed incriminating. "What money have you spent today," said one man. "Thou has had forty or fifty pounds for thy share." The reply was: "I will spend all the money I have for joy the business is done."[6] These three men were linked with Cowper,

5 *The trial of Spencer Cowper*, p. 69.
6 *Ibid.*, pp. 82-6.

for they all admitted that they met the next day, held several conferences, and left town together. The prosecution closed its case by presenting evidence that Cowper left Hertford early on the morning that the body of Sarah Stout was found. Furthermore, he left without calling to express his sympathy, despite the fact that he was a close friend of the family.

The evidence against Cowper and his fellow defendants was all circumstantial, but it was strong. As a lawyer he knew that many men, guilty or innocent, had gone to the gallows on circumstantial evidence. Cowper had to break down the case against him; to fail meant death.

In his opening speech Cowper complained that two factions sought to prosecute the case: the Quakers, especially their eminent Mr. Mead who thought the reputation of the sect was on trial, and the Tory opponents of the Whig Cowpers, who hoped to break the political stronghold the family had in Herefordshire. He was transported by his deep feelings on the subject and the Judge was forced to interrupt his flowery rhetoric, warning him: "Do not flourish too much, Mr. Cowper."[7]

Cowper's first objective was to establish that Sarah Stout's body was mostly under water when it was found, but he only succeeded in weakening slightly the evidence presented by the prosecution on this vital point. At this point the gallows were still a very disconcerting probability.

Then Cowper called to give testimony some of the most eminent physicians in England, who had come down from London especially for this case. The prosecution's medical witnesses were virtually unknown outside their home counties, but Cowper's physicians and surgeons were men famous throughout the kingdom. Dr. Hans Sloane, the first to testify, was noted both as a brilliant physician and a great collector of curiosities of natural history. As physician to Christ's Hospital and Secretary of the Royal Society, he was able to command respect as an expert witness in medical matters. He declared in an authoritative tone that the quantity of liquid taken in was of little importance in cases of drowning. It is the fact that some enters the windpipe that causes death in drowning cases, Sloane maintained. As proof of this statement, he told of people suffocating on a few spoons of medicine when they were too weak and were forced to take the medicine. In concluding his testimony Sloane struck another blow at the prose-

7 *Ibid.*, p. 108.

cution's case by asserting that water in the stomach would not cause putrefaction.

Samuel Garth, noted as a poet and wit as well as a physician, was now called upon to give evidence. Asked for his opinion of the testimony presented by the surgeons who were witnesses for the King, he answered in a methodical manner:

I observed in this Trial the first Gentleman called for the King, that spoke to this Matter, was Mr. *Coatworth;* he saith, he was sent for to open her, upon an Aspersion of her being said to be with Child. I agree with him in what he speaks as to that Point, but must differ with him where he infers she was murdered, because he found no great Quantity of Water in her, as also her Head extremely mortified, but not her Lungs.[8]

Garth then presented his reasons, based on his experience as a physician, for differing with the surgeon Coatsworth:

Now, my Lord, as to the Matter of Putrifaction, I think 'tis not much material whether there be any Water or no in the Cavities of the Body; if Water would hasten Putrifaction, it would do it as well in the Lungs as otherwise; there is always some Water in the *Lymphaducts* there, the breaking of which may be one Occasion of Catarrhs. As to what relates to the Putrifaction of the Head, it may happen from a Stoppage of the refluent Blood, which is staid there in a great Quantity, thro' the Suffocation of the Water, or from the Neatness of the Brain, which is observed often to mortify first.[9]

Next Garth considered the evidence concerning Sarah Stout's body being found floating in the water. He contended that it was impossible that the body should have floated, except if it were entangled among the stakes. All dead bodies not containing some extraordinary tumor, he believed, would sink in water. He reasoned:

The Witnesses all agree she was found upon her Side, which, to suppose her to float in this Posture, is as hard to be conceived, as to imagine a Shilling should fall down and rest upon its Edge, rather than it Broad Side; or that a Deal Board should rather float Edge ways than otherwise; therefore 'tis plain she was entangled, or else the Posture had been otherwise.[10]

Garth continued, this time considering the evidence that very little water was found in Sarah Stout's internal organs:

As to the Quantity of Water, I do not think it necessary it should be very great. I must own the Water will force itself into all Cavities where there is no Resistance. I believe, when she threw her self in, she might not struggle to save herself, and by Consequence not sup up much Water. Now there is not direct Passage into the Stomach but by the Gullet, which is

8 *Ibid.*, p. 124.
9 *Ibid.*, p. 125.
10 *Ibid.*

contracted, or pursed up by a Muscle in Nature of a *Sphincter;* for if this Passage were always open, like that of the Wind Pipe, the Weight of the Air would force itself into the Stomach, and we should be sensible of the greatest Inconveniences. I doubt not, but that some Water fell into her Lungs, because the Weight of it would force itself down, but if we consider the Wind Pipe with its Ramification, as one Cylinder, the Calculation of its Contents will not amount to above 23 or 24 solid Inches of Water, which is not a Pint, and which might imperceptibly work or fall out.[11]

There was a burst of laughter at Garth's mentioning a wager made at Garaway's coffee house on the liquid capacity of the windpipe. Then the Judge, Baron Hatsell, questioned Garth concerning the sailor's testimony and also Dr. Sloane's statement that water would not putrefy a body. First Garth declared he believed as his eminent colleague did, noting that in some places meat was preserved from corrupting by keeping it in water. Then he took exception to the sailor's testimony, asserting with disdain,

The Seamen are a superstitious People, they fancy that a whistling at Sea will occasion a Tempest; I must confess, I never saw any Body thrown overboard, but I have tried some Experiments on other dead Animals, and they will certainly sink; . . .[12]

Garth now referred to the experiments he and his colleagues had just completed which convinced them that dead bodies will sink in water. He then gave another reason for suspecting the sailor's evidence:

. . . he saith, that threescore Pounds of Iron is allowed to sink the dead Bodies, whereas six or seven Pounds will do as well. I cannot think the Commissioners of the Navy guilty of so ill Husbandry, but the Design of tying Weights to their dead Bodies, is to prevent their floating at all, which otherwise would happen in some few Days; . . .[13]

At this point Garth indicated that he thought the case against the defendants was very weak because no evidence had been presented that Sarah Stout had been strangled or had received a mortal wound. He ended his testimony by answering the question whether any quantity of water can enter into the cavity of the thorax:

'Tis impossible there should, till the Lungs be quite rotten, there is no Way but by the Lungs, which are invested with so strong a Membrane, that we cannot force Breath with out Blow Pipes through it, and there's a great Providence in such a Texture, for if there were any large Pores in this Membrane, the Air would pass through it into the Cavity of the Thorax, and prevent the Dilation of the Lungs, and by Consequence there would be an End of breathing.[14]

11 *Ibid.,* p. 126.
12 *Ibid.,* pp. 127-8.
13 *Ibid.,* p. 128.
14 *Ibid.,* pp. 128-9.

The testimony of Garth and Sloane was backed up by the evidence given by their eminent colleagues, including the pedantic Dr. Crell, who would not heed the Judge's objections and insisted on presenting the opinions of several ancient authorities on the subject of drowning.

Then the eminent surgeon, William Cowper, considered by many the outstanding anatomist of his age, was called to give evidence.[15] Cowper related experiments he had performed to determine whether a dead body would float in the water. First a spaniel with an abundance of long hair was used, but his hair prevented his sinking. Then a dog with short hair was employed, and the body sank immediately. Cowper then conducted an experiment to establish what quantity of water entering the body is required to cause suffocation. Three live dogs were plunged under water. Less than three ounces of water was found in their lungs and one in their stomach.

From his experiments, Cowper concluded that "Dead Bodies necessarily sink in water, if no Distention of their Parts buoy them up; . . ."[16] He also concluded that the "Contents of a dead body are discharged by the Mouth and Nostrils, so soon as it begins to ferment."[17] Therefore, little fluid would remain in a body after six weeks in a grave. Cowper ended his testimony by expressing his opinion that it was utterly ridiculous to expect water in the cavity of the thorax, unless some damage had been done to the lungs to permit passage of water into the thorax.

The prosecution's case was significantly weakened by the expert medical testimony marshalled by Spencer Cowper. However, it still remained for Cowper to show that some motive for the suicide of Sarah Stout existed. Even if the circumstantial evidence in the case was not strong enough to result in a conviction, it might be damaging enough to ruin his career. He had to prove that Sarah Stout's death was suicide and not murder.

When the medical aspects of the case were ended, several confidantes of the Quaker miss testified that she was often melancholy and that the cause of her disorder was unrequited love. One wit-

15 William Cowper (1666-1709) was not related to the defendant. At the time of the trial, although only 33 years old, he was a Fellow of the Royal Society and the author of two important anatomical works: *Myotomia reformata; or, a new administration of the muscles of the humane bodies,* . . . (London, 1694), and *The anatomy of the humane bodies, with figures drawn after life by some of the best masters in Europe,* . . . (Oxford, 1698).

16 *The trial of Spencer Cowper,* p. 137.

17 *Ibid.,* p. 138.

238

ness declared that Sarah Stout admitted being in love, but sadly insisted she would not change her religion for a husband. Another witness had extracted from her the admission that she was in love with a person she could not marry.

Now came the sensation of the defence's case. Two letters purported to be from Sarah Stout to Cowper were introduced as evidence. In presenting these letters, Cowper declared that it was done only to save the three men accused with him; if he alone were on trial, he would not introduce evidence which would show the weakness of a gentlewoman. These letters were sent to false names, but it was clearly established by comparison with known letters of Sarah Stout's that they were written by her. The first ended with a lover's plea:

When you come to H———D pray let your steed guide you, and don't do as you did the last time; and be sure order your Affairs to be here as soon as you can, which cannot be sooner than you will heartily welcome to——— your very sincere friend.[18]

The second letter was considerably more damaging to the reputation of the Quaker miss; for it indicated that she sought to live with him as a wife, though he was legally married to another woman:

I writ you by Sunday's Post, which I hope you have receiv'd; however, as a Confirmation, I will assure you I know of no inconveniency that can attend your cohabiting with me, unless the Grand Jury should thereupon find a Bill against us, but I won't fly for't, for come life, come death, I am resolv'd never to desert you. . . .[19]

Members of Sarah Stout's family denied vehemently that she had written these letters. Her brother, when questioned if he believed the letters to be in her handwritings, declared, "I don't believe it, because it don't suit her character."[20] But the jury and many of the spectators at the trial had formed a new concept of the character of the dead girl.

Cowper then skillfully examined Mr. Barefoot, who took in lodgers, to establish that he had arranged to spend the night at his house and that he did definitely spend the night there. Following this, Cowper explained away the damaging testimony given by Sarah Walker by insisting that he allowed her to believe he was going to spend the night at the Stouts' home, so that he could

18 *Ibid.*, p. 165.
19 *Ibid.*, p. 166.
20 *Ibid.*, p. 171.

talk privately with Sarah and tell her that he could not "cohabit" with her.

The testimony of the three alleged accomplices was now taken. Their conversations on the night of the murder were so vague and circumstantial that they had little influence on the outcome of the case. Then, as the trial was ending, Sarah Stout's brother desired to call witnesses to attest to his sister's spotless reputation; but the Judge, wearied by the excessively long testimony, prevented this by asserting: "I believe no body disputest that she might be a virtuous woman, and her brains might be turn'd by her passion, or some distemper."[21]

The Jury was out for half an hour; few people were surprised at the verdict—not guilty.

---

21 *Ibid.*, p. 202. Spencer Cowper's career was not impaired by the trial. Cowper served a number of terms in Parliament and held some important offices. At the time of his death he was Judge of the Common Pleas. The strange death of Sarah Stout was never forgotten. Shortly after Cowper's death, in 1728, a poem appeared entitled: *Sarah, the Quaker, to Lothario, lately deceased, on meeting him in the shades.* This poem champions Sarah in such poignant lines (p. 5):

> In vain his Guilt attempts to shun my Eye;
> From my Reproach he cannot, shall not fly;
> On earth, his Crimes his Eloquence might clear;
> I'll be Accuser, Judge and Jury, Here.

AN HISTORICAL VIEW OF THE M'NAGHTEN TRIAL *

JACQUES M. QUEN **

It was 3:45, Friday afternoon, January 20th 1843. Edward Drummond, private secretary to Prime Minister Sir Robert Peel, had just left his brother's bank at Charing Cross, when a young man, somewhat above medium height, thin, respectably dressed, walked up behind him, placed a pistol against Mr. Drummond's back, and fatally shot him. Except for a short struggle to fire a second shot, no resistance to arrest was offered.[1]

When arraigned the following day, the prisoner said, " The Tories in my native city have compelled me to do this; they follow and persecute me wherever I go, and have entirely destroyed my peace of mind. . . . I can get no rest from them night or day. . . . They have accused me of crimes of which I am not guilty; and they have [done] everything in their power to harass and persecute me, in fact they wish to murder me. It can be proved by evidence." [2]

That prisoner's name is one of the most famous in the history of Anglo-American jurisprudence of insanity: Daniel M'Naghten, The M'Naghten trial, The M'Naghten Rules. They are but the middle of a story that began centuries ago and which continues to stumble along its way today. How to determine the criminal responsibility of the mentally ill remains a difficult, complex, and vexing problem. One of the earliest recorded evidences of society's recognition of it is attributed to the *Babylonian Talmud,* where it is written, " A deaf-mute, an Idiot, and a minor are awkward to deal with, as he who injures them is liable, whereas, if they injure others they are exempt." [3]

Our present laws regarding the insane are derived from the Judaeo-Christian heritage, as well as Roman law and the moral philosophies of Plato and Aristotle.[4] English common law [5] is an amalgam of pre-Nor-

---

* Read at the fortieth annual meeting of the American Association for the History of Medicine, New Haven, Connecticut, April 28, 1967.

** From the Department of Psychiatry of the New York Hospital (Payne Whitney Clinic)—Cornell Medical Center, New York, N. Y. 10021.

[1] *The Times* (London), 21 January 1843, p. 5.

[2] *Ibid.,* 23 January 1843, p. 5.

[3] Cited in A. Platt and B. L. Diamond, " The origins of the ' right and wrong ' test of criminal responsibility and its subsequent development in the United States: an historical survey," *California Law Rev.,* 1966, *54*: 1227-1260.

[4] This presentation of the development of English common law through 1724 is based on the work of Platt and Diamond cited above (n. 3); A. Platt and B. L. Diamond,

man conquest sectional laws and Canon law. It was Canon law which insisted upon moral guilt, or guilty intent, as a necessary component of crime. Common law crimes have two essential elements, the act and the intent. Fundamental to any definition of intent is the assumption of free will and freedom of choice.

In the thirteenth century, Bracton, the ecclesiastic and common law judge, wrote of children and the insane, " They lack sense, reason and no more do wrong than a brute animal." [6] Three centuries later, Lambard, the Elizabethan jurist, wrote, " If a mad man or a naturalle foole . . . or a childe y apparently hath no knowledge of good or evil, do kil a ma [sic], this is no felonious acte nor anything forfeited by it . . . for they cannot be said to have any understanding wil [sic]." [7] The necessity to have knowledge of good or evil, to be able to differentiate between right and wrong, now becomes explicit. Without the intent, or will, to do wrong or evil, there is no crime in the common law.

In the seventeenth century, Sir Matthew Hale, in his *History of the Pleas of the Crown,* observes that " most persons that are felons . . . are under a degree of partial insanity. . . . It is very difficult to define the invisible line that divides perfect and partial insanity; but it must rest upon circumstances duly to be weighed and considered by both judge and jury." [8] One can distinguish, without question, the difference between night and day, but who can say where dusk begins and dusk ends? Hale chose to solve this dilemma by removing it from consideration; only *total* night, or the *total* absence of the light of reason would be a bar to punishment.

In 1724, Edward Arnold, while delusional, shot and wounded Lord

"The origins and development of the 'wild beast' concept of mental illness and its relation to the theories of criminal responsibility," *J. Hist. Behav. Sc.,* 1965, *1*: 355-367; R. H. Dreher, "Origin, development and present status of insanity as a defense to criminal responsibility in the common law," *J. Hist. Behav. Sc.,* 1967, *2*: 47-57; and J. Biggs, Jr., *The Guilty Mind,* New York: Harcourt, Brace, 1955.

[5] By common law, I mean the body of traditional law, that is non-legislated, which arose and continues to develop and evolve from the accumulation of judicial decisions and precedents. ("The unwritten law of England, administered by the King's courts, based on ancient and universal usage, and embodied in commentaries and court cases," *The Shorter Oxford English Dictionary,* London: Oxford Univ. Press, 1964.) For another definition, see Dreher, *op. cit.*

[6] Quoted in Platt and Diamond, ". . . 'wild beast' concept . . .," *op. cit.,* n. 4 above, p. 357.

[7] Biggs, *op. cit.,* p. 84.

[8] Quoted in Isaac Ray, *A Treatise on the Medical Jurisprudence of Insanity,* Boston: Little and Brown, 1838, p. 13. Reprint edited by Winfred Overholser, Cambridge, Mass.: Belknap Press of Harvard Univ. Press, 1962.

Onslow. In this first of the commonly referred to "insanity trials," Justice Tracey told the jury that "A man must be totally deprived of his understanding and memory, so as not to know what he is doing, no more than an infant, a brute, or a wild beast." [9] Arnold could read, write, make purchases, and obtain employment. He had functioned in the community without being incarcerated, without a guardian, and without the care of a physician. He could not, therefore, be included in the legally non-responsible group of the "perfectly insane." He was found guilty and sentenced to be executed, but his victim interceded for him and his sentence was changed to life imprisonment. This trial established the "total insanity" or "wild beast" standard in English criminal law for more than seventy-five years. [10]

The first time that this precedent was successfully challenged in a criminal trial of major importance was in 1800. James Hadfield, discharged from the Army for insanity, entertained the delusion that mankind was about to be destroyed but could be saved by the sacrifice of his own life. He could not bring himself to commit the moral crime of suicide. His death had to be brought about by others. He decided that attempting to murder King George III would result in his own execution and, thus, the salvation of mankind. At his trial he was defended by Lord Erskine.

Of perfect insanity, Lord Erskine said, ". . . no such madness ever existed in the world. It is idiocy alone which places a man in this helpless condition. . . . In other cases, Reason is not driven from her seat, but distraction sits down upon it along with her. . . . Delusion, therefore, where there is no frenzy or raving madness, is the true character of insanity. . . . I must convince you, not only that the unhappy prisoner was a lunatic, but that the act in question was the immediate unqualified offspring of this disease." [11] Charging the jury at this trial, Lord Chief Justice Kenyon said, "If a man is in a deranged state of mind at the time, he is not criminally responsible for his act." [12] Hadfield was acquitted.

This trial overrode the authority of the Arnold trial of 1724 and marked a radical change in the attitude of the court. Heretofore, the state had to show only one shred of reason in the defendant to establish his legal

[9] Quoted in Biggs, *op. cit.*, p. 88.

[10] See n. 4 above.

[11] Quoted in R. Hunter and I. MacAlpine, *Three Hundred Years of Psychiatry, 1535-1860*, London: Oxford Univ. Press, 1963. See also George Dale Collinson, *A Treatise on the Law Concerning Idiots, Lunatics, etc.*, London: Reed, 1812, vol. 1, pp. 469-510; p. 480.

[12] Quoted in Biggs, *op. cit.*, p. 89.

responsibility. In Hadfield's case, the jury could decide whether the defendant was exculpably insane, not by one standard alone, but by several. It was no longer *only* the presence or absence of reason, but the presence of delusion or of a deranged state of mind, which the jury was to take into account.

Twelve years later, John Bellingham shot and killed Spencer Percevale, First Lord of the Treasury and Chancellor of the Exchequer. A request for a delay in the trial to allow witnesses time to come and testify to Bellingham's mental state was denied. He shot Percevale on May 11th and was executed on May 18th, exactly one week later.[13] The refusal to allow time for the arrival of witnesses, the prejudicial and emotionally inflammatory opening of the judge's charge to the jury, and the complete exclusion of any reference to the precedents set in the trial of Hadfield were flagrant abuses of judicial function and prerogative. The jury was told that the *only* question to be decided was whether, at the time he committed the act, Bellingham was capable of distinguishing between right and wrong, good and evil, and whether he knew murder was a crime against the laws of God and man.[14]

In 1840, Edward Oxford attempted to assassinate Queen Victoria. At his trial, Lord Chief Justice Denman charged the jury, " If some controlling disease was in truth the acting power within [the defendant], which he could not resist, then he will not be responsible. . . . The question is, whether the prisoner was . . . under the influence of a diseased mind, and was really unconscious at the time he was committing the act, that it was a crime." [15] Oxford was acquitted. This was another attempt to divest the law of its constricting dependency upon the right-and-wrong test. In fact, the trial of Bellingham was now explicitly disclaimed as legal authority because of the questionable propriety of its conduct. Lord Chief Justice Denman reaffirmed the primacy of the question of the determining or responsible factor for the act: the disease or the individual?

Three years later, the twenty-seven year old wood-turner, Daniel M'Naghten, fatally shot Edward Drummond. The symptoms described at the trial indicate he was suffering from paranoid schizophrenia. Unlike

[13] *The Times* (London), 14 March 1843, p. 3, quoting Lord Brougham in a debate in the House of Lords.
[14] Quoted from *The Times* (London), 28 January 1843, p. 5. A report of the trial can be found in Collinson, *op. cit.*, n. 11 above, vol. I, pp. 636-674.
[15] Quoted from Biggs, *op. cit.*, pp. 94-95. A report of the trial can be found in *English Reports*, Edinburgh: Green, 1928, vol. 173, pp. 941-952.

Bellingham, M'Naghten was given adequate time to prepare his defence and arrange for witnesses.[16]

M'Naghten's sanity was the crucial question. The Solicitor-General, Sir William Follett, tried to prove that M'Naghten had intended his bullet for Prime Minister Peel. This would provide the missing element of *reason* for the crime. Follett could offer only the unsupported testimony of a police inspector that M'Naghten had told him that he thought he had shot Sir Robert Peel. The Glasgow *Chronicle* reported that M'Naghten's acquaintances (apparently he had no close friends) were quite certain that he had seen and heard Sir Robert Peel in the House of Commons too often to make such a mistake.[17] Dr. E. T. Monro, testifying for the defense, reported M'Naghten as saying to the medical examiners, that " the person at whom he fired gave him as he passed a scowling look. At that moment all the excitings of months and years rushed into his mind, and he thought that he could only obtain peace by shooting him." [18] This type of thinking is common in paranoid schizophrenia.

Alexander Cockburn, counsel for the defence, followed the lead of Lord Erskine and attempted to establish a more flexible test of exculpable insanity. He made extensive and almost exclusive reference to the work of the American physician, Isaac Ray, in his attempt to demonstrate that legally exculpable insanity should include more than disease of the intellect. " What," he asked the jury, " was the result of the investigations of modern science? . . . It was this—that [the mind of a person who] was sane upon many points might be under the influence of morbid passion, . . . which made him the creature and the victim of . . . ungovernable impulse." [19] Cockburn's task was made the more difficult because M'Naghten had been successful in business, had a reputation for being intelligent, and had carried out the assassination without appearing to be a raving or frenzied maniac. Eight physicians testified that there was

[16] The discussion of the M'Naghten trial is based on: 1) *The Times* (London), 4 and 6 March 1843; 2) J. E. P. Wallis (ed.), *Reports of State Trials, New Series,* London: Eyre and Spottiswoode, 1892, vol. 4, cols. 847-926; 3) R. M. Bousefield and R. Merrett, *Report of the Trial of Daniel M'Naughton, at the Central Criminal Court, Old Bailey, (on Friday, the 3rd, and Saturday, the 4th of March, 1843) for the Wilful Murder of Edward Drummond, Esq.,* London: Renshaw, 1843.

[17] *The Chronicle* (Glasgow), quoted from *The Times* (London), 28 January 1843, p. 3. See also trial testimony of William Gilchrist.

[18] Quoted from the report of the Trial in *The Times* (London), 6 March 1843. The wording differs slightly from that reported in *State Trials* but the substance is essentially the same.

[19] Quoted from *The Times* (London), 6 March 1843.

no doubt that M'Naghten was insane. Four testified, specifically, that M'Naghten's disease deprived him of control over his actions.

The trial was interrupted by Lord Chief Justice Tindal after the testimony of the eighth physician. When the Solicitor-General admitted that he had no witnesses or evidence to refute the medical testimony offered by the defence, the Lord Chief Justice said, " We feel the evidence, especially that of the last two medical gentlemen . . . who are strangers to both sides and only observers of the case, to be very strong, and sufficient to induce my learned brother [sic] and myself to stop the case."

In charging the jury, he said, " If he was not sensible at the time that he committed the act that it was a violation of the law of God or man, undoubtedly he was not responsible . . . or liable to any punishment flowing from that act." [20] No reference was made to delusion, mono-mania, moral insanity, or loss of control over one's actions because of a diseased will or mind. In short, none of the points argued by Cockburn from Isaac Ray's *Treatise,* nor those in the medical testimony, were in any way acknowledged by the judge.

Following M'Naghten's acquittal, the Chancellor of the House of Lords addressed the House on the law of England regarding the responsibility of the insane. He reviewed the legal precedents and previous trials to show that the law had been properly executed in the case of M'Naghten. The mood of the House was such that he offered, gratuitously, to convene the judges of the land, so that the House, if it desired, could " hear their opinion on it . . . to operate in all time, for the guidance of the courts of justice, and to direct, with more force than is attained by the influence of a single judge, the verdicts of justice.[21]

Three months later, fifteen judges of the Queen's Bench assembled to define the law. This they did with one dissenting voice. Of the M'Naghten Rules, as the judges' answers, unfortunately, are called, the major one states that " to establish a defence on the ground of insanity, it must be clearly proved, that, at the time of the committing of the act, the party accused was labouring under such a defect of reason, from disease of the mind, as not to know the nature and quality of the act he was doing, or, if he did know it, that he did not know he was doing what was wrong." [22] Applying this to the case of Hadfield makes the inadequacy of the rule obvious. Hadfield knew the nature and quality of his act, knew it was wrong, that it was attempted regicide and against

[20] *Ibid.*
[21] *Ibid.*
[22] See *State Trials, op. cit.,* n. 16 above, cols. 847-848; 926-934.

the law of his land; in fact, it was *precisely* because he knew all this that he made the attempt! Yet there is little doubt that Hadfield should not have been held responsible.

Few criminal trials have been referred to as often as that of M'Naghten or have generated as much emotional heat, distortion of fact, or confusion. Symbolic of this, perhaps, is the observation by Hunter and MacAlpine that M'Naghten's name is found " misspelt in sixteen variants." [23] The intended victim of the assassination is almost always identified as Sir Robert Peel.[24] This speculation was never proved. Coupled with the testimony of Dr. Monro, M'Naghten's symptoms make it far more likely that he *knew,* intuitively, that if he shot the person who gave him that look, it would stop the persecution. Another common and persistent distortion is that the verdict for acquittal was a directed one. The judge's charge included ". . . but if on balancing the evidence in your minds, you think the prisoner capable of distinguishing between right and wrong, then he was a responsible agent and liable to all the penalties the law imposes." [25] This was not a charge for a directed verdict.

I believe these errors persist because the trial had such little intrinsic importance that its proceedings have not received careful attention. Certainly, it had far less legal import, as a trial, than had those of Hadfield and Oxford, or even that of Bellingham. What is it then that would lead a modern student of medico-legal history to call it " the most important sanity trial of all time? " [26] Like the famous shot fired at Concord, it was important because of what it symbolized in its setting, and because of the end and the beginning that it marked.

M'Naghten's act took place against a backdrop of violence and profound national unrest. England was in a state of social, political, and economic ferment. There were the Chartists and the Anti-Corn Law

[23] *Op. cit.,* n. 11 above, p. 919. I misspell it differently from the way they misspell it (i. e. McNaughton). See also B. L. Diamond, " Correspondence," *Am. J. Psychiat.,* 1954, *110*: 705.

[24] See Biggs, *op. cit.,* n. 4 above, pp. 97-100; Hunter and MacAlpine, *op. cit.,* n. 11 above, p. 919; and F. C. Redlich and D. X. Freedman, *The Theory and Practice of Psychiatry,* New York: Basic Books, 1966, p. 785.

[25] The origin for this error may well lie in the report in *State Trials, op. cit.,* n. 16 above, where the headnote (pp. 847-848) says, ". . . Tindal, C. J., finding that the Crown was not prepared with medical evidence to contradict them [i. e. defence testimony], stopped the case, and the jury, *under his direction,* found the prisoner Not guilty on the ground of insanity." (Italics added.) Reading his charge makes it quite clear that it was not a directed verdict. See also Biggs, *op. cit.,* n. 4 above, pp. 101-102.

[26] B. L. Diamond, " Isaac Ray and the trial of Daniel M'Naghten," *Am. J. Psychiat.,* 1956, *112*: 651-656.

League, agitation for extending suffrage, radical demands for reform of child labor practices, and various schemes for experimentation in providing welfare relief. Radicals were rife and appeared to be threatening the structure of England. The temper of the time appeared to require the reassurance of definite and explicit rules. It was a time of violent ideas, violent feelings, and violent acts. Three years earlier, Oxford had attempted to assassinate the Queen and had been acquitted. M'Naghten had killed someone close to the Prime Minister and had been acquitted. The anxiety about lawless violence found a target in the M'Naghten verdict. Like a lens, it focused attention on the violent and the criminally insane, and on what protection the law offered society. That protection was seen as directly proportional to the stringency of the law.

This then is the importance of the trial of Daniel M'Naghten. It inspired the House of Lords to convene the judges to define the legal responsibility of the criminally insane " for all time." Under the national stress of the time, the British judiciary redefined the common law of insanity so as to constrict it and to deny to it the flexibility necessary for its adequate functioning. They appear to have begun with the law as it was, and to have pared it down to its leanest possible form consistent with the expressed philosophy of Sir Matthew Hale and with the least concession to the decisions of the Hadfield and Oxford trials.

The English common law, by its precedents, had allowed flexibility for individual cases. An understanding will, delusion in the presence of reason, mind or will overwhelmed by disease, ungovernable delusions, irresistible impulse—all these had been present in the law before the judges' answers. With their answers, all had been stripped away but " knowledge of the nature and quality " of the act and " knowledge of right and wrong." Then, as now, there was heated controversy as to the meanings of these phrases.[27] Partial insanity was a valid plea, but only if the defendant, accepting the details of the delusion as fact, behaved as a thoroughly reasonable man would in those same circumstances.[28]

The M'Naghten trial served another purpose. Earlier, there was only a desultory interest in the medical jurisprudence of insanity among

[27] See, for example, Lord Brougham's comments in debate in the House of Lords, *The Times* (London), 14 March 1843, p. 3, and editorial " On MacNaughten's trial, and the plea of insanity in criminal cases," *Legal Observer*, 1843, *26*: 81-89. For a twentieth-century discussion of the meanings of these phrases, see M. S. Guttmacher and H. Weihofen, *Psychiatry and the Law*, New York: Norton, 1952, pp. 403 ff.

[28] Isaac Ray is at his peppery Yankee best in his discussion of the judges' answers. His treatment of this last point is particularly incisive. *A Treatise on the Medical Jurisprudence of Insanity*, 3rd ed., Boston: Little, Brown, 1853, pp. 43-51.

248

British physicians. The legal and Parliamentary reaction to the trial focused their attention and concern on this subject. Just before the M'Naghten trial, Forbes Winslow published *The Plea of Insanity in Criminal Cases*,[29] in which we find him restrained, even equivocal, in his criticism of the right-and-wrong test. Eleven years later, he dismisses the test as " worthless and practically inapplicable." [30]

In America, the M'Naghten Rules are still being debated.[31] These debates have emphasized the dissatisfaction with present practices and laws in the complex problems posed by the criminally insane. One result of the increased attention to the neuropsychiatric aspects of criminality has been the finding of significantly high incidences of psychiatric and electroencephalographic abnormalities among " responsible " criminals. It would appear that, as Lord Hale said 300 years ago, " most persons that are felons . . . are under a degree of partial insanity."

Bernard Diamond suggests that we deal with the problem of determining criminal responsibility by abolishing the need for the determination. This need could be abolished, he says, be revising our penal philosophy and system so that all violators of the law, insane or otherwise, would have their sentences determined by rehabilitative planning, rather than a primary concern for punitive measures.[32] This interesting and controversial approach, offered by a psychiatrist who is also a professor of law, gives one the feeling that we have come full circle back to Lord Hale. Let us hope that we shall proceed, this time, on a more constructive and satisfactory course.

[29] F. Winslow, *The Plea of Insanity in Criminal Cases,* Philadelphia: Littell, 1843.

[30] F. Winslow, *Lettsomian Lectures on Insanity,* London: Churchill, 1854, p. 107.

[31] See Guttmacher and Weihofen, *op. cit.,* n. 27 above, p. 406, n. 4, for a list of references. See also J. Hall, " Psychiatry and criminal responsibility," *Yale Law J.,* 1956, *65*: 761-785; and " Mental disease and criminal responsibility—a symposium: Part I," *Catholic Lawyer,* 1958, *4*: 294-332, 368.

[32] B. L. Diamond, " From M'Naghten to Currens and beyond," *California Law Rev.,* 1962, *50*: 189-205.

EARLY HISTORY OF LEGAL MEDICINE

ERWIN H. ACKERKNECHT

"There is a kind of medical knowledge which is not so much concerned in the cure of disease as in the detection of error and the conviction of guilt." Thus is legal medicine defined in the opening words of one of the first treatises on the subject in English (Farr, 1788). Representative of more modern, formal and scientific definitions is that of J.J. Reese: "Medical jurisprudence, or Legal, or Forensic Medicine, as it is sometimes called may be defined to be the science which applies the knowledge of medicine to the requirements of Law."

Whether judge and court avail themselves of medical expert testimony depends essentially on two sets of factors: on a sufficiently high development of the law, and on a sufficiently high development of medicine. A study of the history of legal medicine must therefore follow both trends: the attitude of courts and the technological perfection of medicolegal methods. Our historical survey will show that under certain circumstances even a highly developed medicine is not used by the courts, while in another setting a rather inadequate medicine might be employed.

Obviously the existence of legal medicine is an indication of an advanced stage of civilization. In exposing the true malefactor, and at the same time absolving the innocent and the mentally deranged, it protects society and the individual, and provides a more equitable, more effective and more humane jurisdiction. It is therefore not surprising that legal medicine is a very late product of civilization. In the search for criminals, primitives, especially in Africa and Asia, will, like our barbarian forefathers, much rather rely on information from supernatural agencies obtained through divination and so-called "ordeals" than on naturalistic examination by medical practitioners. Ordeals consist in fire walking, casting into water, poison tests, confrontation with the corpse and similar practices. The absence of legal medicine in our sense of the word and the use of ordeals in primitive societies is easily explained through their general supernatural orientation and the absence of a developed medical art, of formulated laws and an organized state. A great many actions, prosecuted today, are not recognized as crimes at all, or are left to private settlement by the families involved.

In none of the materials concerning early high civilizations, such as those of Egypt or Babylonia, is there any evidence that judges consulted medical persons in assessing crime, while for the ancient Jews such consultations are reported from the Hellenistic period (1st-3rd centuries A.D.).

No document exists that provides evidence for the use of medical experts in ancient Greece, despite high development of a rational medical art. Many factors may have contributed to such an attitude, such as the low social status of the medical profession, or the predominantly private character of the prosecution of crime. Acts like abortion and infanticide which later played a great role in legal medicine were not regarded as criminal among the ancient Greeks.

An equal lack of documentation exists for the Roman period. It is true that the inexhaustible Galen (131-201 A.D.) also wrote a treatise on simulation and malingering. But nothing shows that such knowledge was applied by doctors in court. Only the late law collections (codices) of the Roman Empire, especially those that bear the name of the emperors Theodosius (438) and Justinian (533), contain considerable medical information on different forms of insanity, impotence, premature births, and so forth, suggesting that medical experts, at least midwives, were used in court.

Paradoxically enough, the first clear evidence of the use of medical experts is found in the law books of the Germanic barbarians who overran the Roman Empire. It would be out of place to romanticize the judicial practices of these invaders. Some of their supernaturalistic "tests," akin to the methods of the Australian aborigines, such as the ordeals by fire and water, the judiciary duel (opposed eventually by St. Louis, King of France, in the 13th century), "cruentation" (a confrontation based on the belief that the corpse of the victim would start bleeding again at the approach of the murderer—practised far into the 17th century!) were certainly no welcome contributions to Western culture. But their rulers, in a laudatory attempt to abolish the disruptive custom of blood revenge, instituted increased intervention of the State and the principle of monetary compensation (Wehrgeld) for wounds, determined in court. Courts thus became dependent on medical experts for an assessment of wounds that were classified and described in painstaking details in some of these laws. Whether in this respect these laws reflect old customs of the barbarians, or on the contrary represent new inventions to deal with law situations and the influences of Byzantine law, cannot be stated with certainty. In view of the fact that these laws were mostly written down by clerics, unfriendly toward pagan traditions, and that professional medical men of a rational complexion were far more familiar to the Greco-Romans than to the barbarians, I am inclined toward the latter hypothesis. These laws were composed and were valid between the 6th and 10th centuries. Laws like those of the Alemanni, Longobards and Salian Franks contain clear reference to medical expertise in the case of wounds. How limited in scope this medicolegal effort was, is, on the other hand, obvious from the merciless attitude of these laws toward the mentally ill.

We hear about the use of surgeons as experts in Godefrey of Bouillon's Kingdom of Jerusalem in 1073 and 1250. Such evidence is also reasonably frequent in the French homeland after the 12th century. It is contained, for example, in Norman laws of 1207, decrees of St. Louis (1220), and Philip the Bold (1278). Philip the Handsome speaks, in 1311, of his "well beloved surgeons, sworn experts in his court of Paris." Original reports of surgeon experts are extant for the same period, one by Master Henri Tristan of 1332, another by Master Jehan Le Conte of 1390. While the French increasingly were using surgeons as experts since the beginning of the second millennium of our era, English law made provision for the lay coroner, an institution, which, whatever its merits, has been to a large extent responsible for the inferiority of Anglo-Saxon countries in legal medicine up to very recent times.

Legal medicine is also indebted in its growth to legislation of the Popes in

Italy as reflected in the Canon Law. An edict of Pope Innocent III of 1209 stated that the character of the wounds (the occasion was the case of a thief slain with a spade) must be determined by medical experts. Gregory IX called for medical experts, especially in the case of torture in 1234. The medicolegal expert thus acquired a most unpleasant function which for many centuries constituted one of his main tasks. The establishment of the Inquisition in this period involved ecclesiastic institutions in the practice of judicial torture, which to the detriment of justice, lasted in secular courts well into the 18th century, and has a tendency to recur wherever the standards of civilization are lowered. Canon law also called for medical experts in cases of impotence and leprosy. The diagnosis of leprosy was of the greatest juridical importance as the leper was therewith banned from society. Numerous medicolegal documents concerned with leprosy (*Lepraschaubriefe*, mostly around 1400) have survived.

In 1249 the great Italian surgeon, Hugh of Lucca, famous for his anticipation of the antiseptic treatment of wounds, took an oath as medicolegal expert of the city of Bologna. Numerous declarations of Bolognese medical men, dealing with the inspection of deathly wounds, exist from the end of the 13th century. In 1302 Bartolomea da Varignana of Bologna performed a medicolegal autopsy in a case of suspected poisoning of a nobleman called Azzolino. A medicolegal postmortem is also credited to William of Saliceto (about 1201-1280), another famous Bolognese surgeon. It will be realized that these dissections are among the earliest recorded in modern history, that they took place in Bologna, which was outstanding because of its law school and which with Mondino de Lucci (*c.* 1270-1320) became an early center of the anatomical revival on which all modern medicine is based. Charles Singer has made a good case for the theory that the modern study of anatomy grew out of the first medicolegal dissections.

Bologna is by no means the only one of the medieval Italian cities that incorporated into their laws detailed rules for medical experts. Such rules are also found, *e.g.*, in the city statutes of Padua (1316), Genoa (14th century), Mirandola (1386), Bassano (1389), Florence (1415), Verona (1450), Brescia (1470), Milan (1480), Ferrara (1506), Genoa and Urbino (1556). These cities that played such a tremendous role in the genesis of modern economics, political thought and art, must therefore also be regarded as among the most influential factors in the establishment of legal medicine.

Increasing use of medicolegal experts in the late Middle Ages may be attributed partly to the greater specialization and secularization of learning. The judge was no longer an omniscient cleric whose general education also included a smattering of medicine. The university-trained doctor on the other hand enjoyed a higher social standing (though no greater abilities) than his tradesman-predecessor in Antiquity.

In Germany, forensic medicine received its first strong legal foundation in the so-called *Bambergische Halsgerichtsordnung* of J. von Schwarzenberg (1507), and in the *peynliche Gerichsordnung* of the German emperor, Charles V, also called the Carolina (1533) which are likewise milestones in the development of law in general. Both laws asked for "serious examination and, if necessary, opening of the body" in the case of violent death. They prescribed the use of medical experts in case of infanticide, abortion, or medical malpractice. They increased the medicolegal importance of suicide by making it a crime (which it has remained in some countries up to this day). The Carolina, imitated, though not equaled, in other countries like France, created the legal foundation for the development of forensic medicine as a special discipline and a science in the late 16th and early 17th centuries.

China had long preceded and excelled the West in this way. An official text for coroners called *Hsi Yüan Lu* (Collected Excerpts Concerning Injustice Eliminated), written by Wang in Hoai in the middle of the 13th century, but obviously based on earlier sources, has been transmitted to us. In a first book it deals with wounds, tabulating the location of mortal and non-fatal wounds, the signs of death (putrefaction and rigor mortis), the age of infants found dead (also tabulated), and identification. The second book deals with violent death, whether wounds were inflicted before or after death; strangling, suicide, drowning and burning, true and simulated. The third book deals with doubtful cases, especially poisoning. The fourth book describes first aid in accidents and poisoning, and gives a form for writing medicolegal reports. Like all books on legal medicine the *Hsi Yüan Lu* provides a great many insights into the morals and customs of the society from which it emanated.

Western reviewers of the work have usually insisted on the many absurd notions and practices it contains (such as ascertaining relationship through the union of blood drops in water, or through being absorbed by the bone of a dead parent; a blow upon the cord by which a man is hanging indicates by the manner of its vibration either suicide or murder, and so forth). In view of what European writers produced along these lines up to the 19th century, some greater tolerance might be advisable.

LEGAL MEDICINE IN TRANSITION
(16th-18th CENTURIES)

The Italian city laws, the Carolina of 1533 and its imitations, which made medical expertise a large scale routine procedure, called for a science of legal medicine. The tremendous progress of medical science in the 16th century, the medical renaissance symbolized in the names of Vesalius, Fernel, Fracastorius, Paracelsus and Paré, made the birth of such a science possible.

A number of monographs produced during the 16th century threw new light on important problems that faced the medical expert continually. We mention only the treatise of J.B. Sylvaticus of 1595 on simulation; of Pineus (1550-1619) on virginity and pregnancy, 1598 (Pineus knew about the possibility of cohabitation with an intact hymen); of H. Augenius (1527-1603) on the duration of pregnancy, 1595) Augenius fought the Hippocratic superstition that eight-month babies are less viable than seven-month); the treatises on poisons and poisoning by Cardanus (1563), Stuebing (1561) and Mercurialis (1584).

The greatest single accomplishment of medical men in the field of legal medicine in this period was their fight against the superstitious belief in witchcraft and sorcery which annually sent thousands of mentally ill persons to the stake. The greatest of these fearless fighters for humanity, and protagonists of modern psychiatry, legal and general, was undoubtedly the Dutchman Jan Weyer (1515-1588), a pupil of Cornelius Agrippa (1486-1535). Despite the flood of abuse and menace that were Weyer's compensation for his great book, *De praestigiis daemonum* (1563) and the fact that witch hunting was practiced in some parts well into the 18th century, it left a deep impression on many judges and medical men. It is typical that Paré's pupil, P. Pigray (1532-1613), was able in 1595 to save fourteen sorcerers from execution, although his master still believed in sorcery.

The first more systematic treatise on legal medicine seems to be the little book on "Reports in Court" by the great French renovator of surgery, Ambroise Paré (1517-1590). Published in 1575, it is written as deftly, honestly and intelligently as the other works of this most remarkable character. As a surgeon Paré, of course, paid the greatest attention to wounds, their size, their prognosis, the signs of skull fracture, the lesions of the esophagus, trachea, the lungs and other internal organs. Paré insisted on the moral qualities of the medicolegal expert, and into his book inserted model reports for the young surgeon. He discussed abortion and infanticide; the signs of death by lightning; how to differentiate between wounds, hanging or submersion inflicted before and after death. His chapter on poisoning was superior to the views of most of his contemporaries. Particularly interesting is his discussion of accidental death by "coal-gas" (CO), and on intestinal changes caused by corrosive poisons. Paré was extremely sceptical whether virginity or its absence could be actually proven. Among the tests of sexual impotence, he vigorously rejected the validity of so-called "congress," that is, the obligation for the couple to cohabit in the presence of judges and experts when one partner, accusing the other of impotence, had asked for annulment of marriage. Paré's treatise, short as it is, deals extensively with two essential problems of legal medicine: violent death and disputed sexual relations.

Another short early treatise on legal medicine was the *Methodus testificandi* (Method of testifying), of G.B. Condronchi of Imola, Italy, published in 1597. Condronchi dealt briefly with the phenomena most often giving occasion for medical expert opinion, such as wounds, poisoning, simulation, impotence, virginity, pregnancy and abortion. He also gave models for expert reports. He was superior to his countrymen, Zacchias and Fidelis, who otherwise overshadow him, in denying the possibility of bastards (monsters) issuing from the intercourse between witches and the devil.

In the *De relationibus medicorum* (On the relations of doctors, 1598) of Fortunatus Fidelis of Palermo (1551-1630), we encounter the first full-fledged treatise of legal medicine. We omit here discussion of those parts of Fidelis' work that deal with what is now called public health, and which was often contained in works on legal medicine up to the end of the 18th century. "Legal Medicine" was then understood in a wider sense: not only as that part of medicine which helps in the application of laws, but also that which helps in the formulation of certain (sanitary) laws. The tremendous development of public health in the 18th century brought about the development of this field as an independent discipline separate from legal medicine proper.

Fidelis' discussion of sexual data pertaining to legal problems was realistic, except that he admitted duration of pregnancy up to 23 months. He showed that bleeding after cohabitation is not necessarily an index of virginity. In his excellent discussion of wounds, Fidelis made a plea for complete autopsies in legal cases, which found general acceptance only in the 18th century. Till that date, inspection or local dissection still prevailed. Fidelis felt that stifling and strangling were popular methods of murder because these left few traces. He gave a number of signs on bodies killed by drowning or lightning. Most cases of sudden death he attributed to heart accidents, thus preceding Lancisi in this matter by one hundred years. He dealt with malpractice, and in consonance with the customs of his time with the medical aspects of torture, prison organization, and petitions of dismissal for medical reasons. Discussion of psychopathology is conspicuously absent from Fidelis' book.

In 1614 one of the many brilliant Jewish refugee doctors from Portugal who are so characteristic of the period, Rodrigo a Castro (1545-1627), who was the favored physician of kings, bishops and dukes, published in Hamburg a treatise called *Medicus politicus* (The political doctor). The book contains many chapters on legal medicine, covering wounds, the signs of poisoning, virginity, impotence, and so forth—and examination of slaves, a procedure which in its content has been compared to a modern life insurance examination.

Despite Fidelis, it is usually Paul Zacchias (1584-1659) of Rome who is crowned with the title of the "father of legal medicine." It is true that Zacchias' monumental *Questiones medico-legales* (Medico-legal problems, 1621) was far more extensive, comprehensive and incomparably more influential than the book of Fidelis, which almost had to be rediscovered in the 19th century. Zacchias, who was the body physician and medical confidant of Popes Innocent X and Alexander VII, based his book on decades of experience as an expert at the highest papal court of appeals, the Rota Romana. Zacchias was a most fascinating personality, equally learned in law and medicine, a gifted painter, musician and poet. He wrote a special treatise on mental diseases, and like other papal physicians (for instance G.M. Lancisi, 1654-1720) was an outstanding public health man.

In the relevant chapters of the first book of his treatise, Zacchias divided human life into seven ages, with different degrees of legal responsibility. He tried to determine the age of the fetus beyond the criteria established by the jurisconsults, but was hampered by the rudimentary embryological knowledge of his time (Fabricius, Arantius). He opposed the Hippocratic legend of the greater viability of the seven-month compared to the eight-month fetus. He still believed that monsters might be the result of intercourse between man and animal, though the usual cause of this phenomenon was, according to him, "corruption of the sperm." He was more critical than Fidelis concerning the signs of pregnancy, and felt that a reliable diagnosis is hardly possible before the fourth month. Even then differentiation from "moles" (ovarian cyst, fibroma) is difficult. Although the duration of pregnancy judged possible by Zacchias still exceeded our present-day opinions, his narrowing down of the maximum period represented considerable progress. He believed in the possibility of superfetation. In discussing abortion, fixation of the time when the embryo receives a soul was of great concern to him as punishment would change accordingly. In a chapter on physical similarity, besides paternity cases, Zacchias reported interesting cases of assumed identity, and of true identity not recognized after long absence.

Zacchias' second book starts with a discussion of mental disease, and similar states implying legal problems, such as inebriety, somnambulism and deafmutism. Zacchias is not too advanced in his psychiatric ideas and leans heavily on the confusions of older writers. Only "total" mental disease was recognized as absolving from responsibility. While Zacchias' analysis of love as a mental disease might be regarded by some as realistic, and his denial of the existence of the so-called devil's mark (insensible spot) in sorcerers and witches as progressive, the same cannot be said of his general belief in demons, the evil eye, possession, conjuration, and so on, though on the other hand it must be stated for the sake of justice that he shared these beliefs with the overwhelming majority of his educated contemporaries.

As the 17th century was one of the most poison-ridden in human history, as evidenced by the incredible de Brinvilliers and La Voisier scandals which involved the French court and Louis XIV's own mistress, Mme. de Montespan, it is but logical that Zacchias should have paid great attention to the problem. Unfortunately, the undeveloped state of chemistry reduced him to identification of poisons chiefly through smell, taste and feeding the suspected matter to animals. Zacchias, unlike Fidelis, believed in the legend of Pliny that poisoned bodies do not putrify. He knew about original methods of poisoning per vaginam or through clysters. Under the heading of miscellaneous malformations, eunuchs and particularly hermaphrodites were discussed at length, as both states implied serious legal limitations (impossibility to marry, fill public office, take holy orders). Hermaphrodites, also the subject of monographs such as that by Duval in 1612, were regarded as a "third sex" at the period. Zacchias denied the contemporary belief in the existence of individuals possessing simultaneously an equally developed male and female sex apparatus.

The third book of Zacchias starts with an extremely detailed account of impotence. The great importance of impotence as a medicolegal problem during this period must be understood from the fact that legal divorce was nonexistent, and the only way to dissolve an unbearable marriage was to have it annulled by the Church on some physical basis, the foremost of which was impotence of one partner. The medical expert had therefore to pronounce himself on innumerable accusations of impotence, usually proffered by wives against their husbands. We cannot follow Zacchias in his detailed discussions, which include the characterization of a marriage between two extremely obese partners which is dissolvable, while obesity of only one partner allows for other technical solutions consistent with the procreative goals of marriage.

Zacchias differentiated between natural and accidental impotence, the latter category including impotence caused by sorcery and spells. Against the authority of Aristotle, St. Thomas and Averroes, Zacchias defended the ability of frigid women to conceive. He also observed conception in non-menstruating women. In a chapter on simulation which, besides a long list of simulated diseases, includes discussion of the techniques of simulating virginity and simulation among slaves, our author states that the simulation most difficult to unmask is that of mental disease. In a chapter on contagion, the following chronic contagious diseases are admitted as reasons for the annulment of marriage: phthisis (pulmonary tuberculosis), alopecia; leprosy and syphilis.

The chapter on miracles in the fourth book was necessitated by the need of the Church for the aid of the medical expert in dealing with false miracles and those produced by sorcerers. Zacchias again appears as a great realist in his chapter on virginity. He was sceptical in regard to such strange tests as the "bee test" (bees don't sting virgins!) or certain fumigation tests. On the other hand, he defended the normal occurrence of the hymen, not yet recognized as a standard element of female anatomy by such authorities as Vesalius, Paré, Riolan and de Graff. He regarded rape as extremely difficult in the case of normal, adult women, while he knew of cases of rape in boys. Zacchias formulated the anatomical signs of "sodomy" (homosexual intercourse) that were held valid till exploded by Casper in 1852.

Zacchias' chapter on wounds in the fifth book shows him less experienced in this field than in others. This is not surprising in view of the nature of the court with which he was associated. Much of his material on premortal and postmortal wounds, drowning, hanging and other standard items is taken from Fidelis or Sebitz. It is obvious that he practised inspection rather than autopsy. His opposition to cruentation and the concept of critical days in wounds is noteworthy. Legal reasons (succession and so forth) obliged him to create complicated standards for the determination of the person to die first and to die last in a deadly accident involving several persons. For the same reasons he also created medical rules for the recognition of the first born in multiple births. A chapter on mutilations is again much concerned with the effect of mutilation on marital competence. In the field of torture Zacchias tried at least to protect the very young and the old and diseased. The last chapters of his book, with the classic Hippocratic title, *De aere, aquis et locis,* deal with problems of public hygiene. This very fragmentary survey of his work nevertheless shows the fundamental characteristics of the "Father of Legal Medicine," a man of an unusual breadth of knowledge and experience, and great dialectical ability, subject to many of the errors of his time, but not rarely ahead of his contemporaries through his realism and sincere human sympathies.

Nicolas de Blegny (1642-1722), a remarkable adventurer, founder of the first medical journal, court surgeon from 1678-1693, but dying in dire poverty after many years in prison, in 1683 produced a *Doctrine des rapports en chirurgie,* centered, of course, around the examination of wounds. Much inferior to Zacchias as a whole, many passages of his book are of considerable cultural interest, for instance, his rules for an expert:

I. You must resist the offers of seducers and the begging of your friends.
II. You must examine everything yourself, and not be influenced by your colleagues.
III. You must confirm nothing on the basis of subjective signs.
IV. You must beware of simulation (injected blood, painted contusions).
V. You must make your prognosis as uncertain as the events are doubtful.
VI. You must measure with the utmost precision length, breadth and depth of wounds.
VIII. You must see whether the wounds are the real cause of death.
IX. You must describe the functional capacity of the wounded in clear terms, without Arab, barbaric and scholastic terms.

The other French 17th century author in our field, Jean Devaux (1649-1729), in his *Art de faire des rapports en chirurgie*, also deals primarily with wounds, but offers interesting reports on syphilitic infection of babies by their nurse, and vice versa, on poisons, on rape (he regarded a narrow vagina as the most reliable sign of virginity). Like Paré and Blegny he is conspicuously silent on homosexuality, despite its prevalence in the French upper class of the time. Devaux produced a long catalogue of local causes of impotence in both sexes. He opposed the "congress," like Guy de Chauliac, Paré, Tagereau (1611), and Blegny before him, and called the replacement of ordeals by congress in the 16th century "the change from cruelty to infamy." Congress was officially abolished in France in 1677, after the scandal of the Count of Langey who, recognized impotent by this method in 1659 and divorced, produced no less than seven children in a second marriage.

The laws of Henri IV (1604) and Colbert (1670) strengthened considerably the legal foundations of forensic medicine in France. The great tradition of Weyer in defense of unfortunate psychotics, tortured and burned as witches, was continued by Yvelin in Louvier (1642), Grangeron and F. Bayle in Toulouse (1681) and De Rhodes in Lyon. Valuable monographs of the period are those by Benedetto Sinibald of Rome (1594-1658), and M. Sebitz (1578-1671) of Strasbourg on virginity (1642 and 1630). Sebitz also did valuable work on wounds (1638). The voices against torture became louder and louder (Spee 1631, Bekker 1694, Thomasius 1705), and the gradual abolition of the disgusting practice made a science of legal medicine all the more necessary. The 17th century provided one of the basic tests in legal medicine: the sinking of the lung of the deadborn child that had never breathed versus the floating of the lung of the newborn that had lived and was likely to have been a victim of infanticide (Docimasia). (So far, infanticide had been "proved" primarily through torture.) The phenomenon was first observed by the anatomists Bartholinus (1663) and Jan Swammerdam (1667), but first introduced into medicolegal practice in 1682 by J. Schreyer of Zeitz, who paid for his invention with a protracted law suit. The test has survived despite all criticism and limitations, while later lung tests like those of C.F. Daniel (1714-1771) and W.J. Ploucquet (1744-1814), or the bladder test of Arnisacus (1650) have not stood the test of time. Insight into infanticide also improved greatly through the demonstrations by the obstetricians H. van Deventer (1651-1724) and J.J.

Roederer (1726-1763) that skull fractures in the newborn are not absolute proof of violence, since they may occur spontaneously in cases of protracted and difficult labor.

The science of legal medicine had arisen—logically enough in view of the positive medieval traditions in both countries—in France and Italy, but as the 17th century progressed, became more and more a German monopoly which it remained up to the end of the 18th century. One of the earliest German treatises was Suevus' *De inspectione vulnerum lethalium* (1629). G. Welsch (1618-1690), of Leipzig, opened a long line of distinguished Leipzig medicolegal experts with his *Rationale vulnerum lethalium judicium* (Rational judgment of deadly wounds), in 1660. Welsch tried to establish some standards for legal autopsies. P. Amann (1634-1691), also of Leipzig, dealt mostly with the problems of sudden death and wounds in his *Praxis vulnerum lethalium* (1690). His *Medicina critica* (1670) is a witty satire on the many legends and errors surviving in legal medicine. Johannes Bohn (1640-1718) of Leipzig is probably the most outstanding of the earlier German authors; a keen observer, and a highly educated and widely traveled man, bringing to his impoverished and provincial country the new creed of Harveian experimental medicine. In the field of legal medicine he leaned heavily on Zacchias (for example, in his *Specimen medicinae forensis,* 1690, or his *Dissertatio de officio medici,* 1704). Still he was quite original in the field of wounds, cultivated with such zeal by all German authors, and rightly so, as up to the present this remains the most current problem in legal medicine (see Bohn's *De renunciatione vulnerum,* 1689). His division of wounds into those deadly by themselves, and such as are deadly only through accidental circumstances, has been followed widely. Bohn still saw in putrefaction the only certain sign of death. Like Haller and Morgagni, he was very critical in regard to *docimasia* (lung-test by floating). His fight for obligatory and complete autopsies vs. mere inspection—a wish which eventually became law in 1720—for medical control of prisons, and against the "expert" activities of ignorant midwives, was most progressive. With his disbelief in possession and magic he stayed far above his predecessors, his contemporaries and most of his successors.

After Bohn, there was in Germany during the 18th century an almost uninterrupted production of treatises on legal medicine. Of these only a few can be mentioned here. Unavoidably this routine production caused a lot of mutual copying and reproduction of errors. The customs of the country, the influence of the lawyers, and the spirit of the period—this is the classic epoch of medical "systems" from Linné to John Brown—make for a lot of empty dialectics and formalism. Backward opinions on general issues reflect the unhappy situation of a country, divided into hundreds of miniature despotisms, and still anemic from the Thirty Years' War. On the other hand, the industry of the authors and continuous cultivation of the field makes for exhaustive treatment and speedy assimilation of the progress in rapidly expanding related fields such as surgery, obstetrics, pathological anatomy and embryology. The adoption of many of these treatises by an otherwise more developed English and French medicine prove that they competently filled a widely felt need.

In 1706 J.F. Zittmann (1671-1758) published his *medicina forcensis*, based on a collection of expert opinions of the Leipzig Medical Faculty from 1650-1700. B. Valentini (1677-1729) of Giessen, who also introduced the use of quinine in Germany, authored a *Corpus juris medicolegalis* in 1722. In 1723 H.F. Teichmeyer (1685-1746) of Jena, father-in-law of the famous physiologist, Albrecht von Haller, published his *Institutiones medicolegales*, based on Bohn, the standard textbook for many years. In his own lectures on legal medicine (1782), Haller followed his father-in-law rather closely. By calling the Strasbourg obstetrician, J. Roederer (1726-1763), known for his work on spontaneous fetal skull fractures, to Goettingen, Haller created there a center of legal medicine, which was still active in the 19th century. Like his successor, F.B. Osiander (1759-1822), remembered for his work on virginity, Roederer typifies the great role which obstetricians played in 18th century legal medicine. None of these obstetricians limited himself to the medicolegal problems arising from his own specialty. Osiander worked much on suicide (1813), Roederer on drowning. Drowning was also experimentally explored by the pathological anatomist, G.B. Morgagni, who found water in the lung rather than, as traditionally assumed, in the stomach of the victims. Morgagni also made observations on strangulation and hanging, and illustrates the continuous deep influence of pathological anatomy on legal medicine.

Other German medicolegal treatises of the 18th century are those of A. Goelicke (1723), C. Eschenbach (1712-1788), of Rostock (1746), E.B.G. Hebenstreit (1753-1803), of Leipzig (1775, popular in France), and Plenk of Vienna (1781). In 1782 the first of the many medicolegal journals was published by Uden and Pyl in Berlin. The treatises of Roose (1800) and Autenrieth (1806) of Tubingen made a special attempt to refine and standardize medicolegal dissections.

The Systema jurisprudentiae (1736) of M. Alberti (1682-1757) of Halle is rather typical for the period in its queer mixture of backwardness and progress. Old Alberti was still in favor of torture, even cruentation, and like Zittmann, Teichmeyer, Haller or Eschenbach believed in demons and magic. On the other hand, he gave a competent discussion of wounds, showed that suggillations of the head are not reliable signs of infanticide, and even explained a case of attempted suicide and supposed sorcery as mental disease.

In 1731 German legal medicine had to weather a last desperate onslaught against autopsies by the leading German jurisconsult, Polycarp Leiser. The hangman was still used in some parts as "medical expert" during the 18th century.

Credit for the "discovery" of spontaneous combustion of chronic alcoholics, a scientific legend surviving into the second half of the 19th century, is usually given to Le Cat (1750) though it can be found already in René Moreau of Lyon in 1604 and in Bartholinus in 1663. At the end of the 18th century the Germans were still as fiercely discussing character and classification of lethal wounds as in its beginning; see for instance the discussions between W.J. Ploucquet of Tubingen (1744-1814) and J.D. Metzger (1739-1805), an Alsatian whom Frederick II brought to Königsberg. Metzger, also the author of a "system" (1793), opposed the belief in demons vigorously and successfully, and showed remarkable insight into the psychopathological character of simulated insanity.

The English contribution to legal medicine in the 18th century is practically nil. Samuel Farr's (1741-1795) treatise of 1788 was an abstract of the German Faselius (1767). Thomas Percival's *Medical Jurisprudence* is a misnomer, and was actually a first version of his famous *Medical Ethics*.

The only noteworthy works in 18th century France were several memoirs by the great surgeon, Antoine Louis (1723-1792), for example, on drowning (1748), rigor mortis (1752, thus established as another definite sign of death), and hanging (1763, differentiation of murder and suicide). Louis taught also legal medicine in the College of St. Còme, and played a most salutary role in the trials and rehabilitation of Baronnet, Calas, Chassagneux, Montbailly and Siren.

LEGAL MEDICINE BECOMES A MODERN SCIENCE
(19th Century)

Together with clinical medicine, legal medicine entered its decisive stage of development at the end of the 18th century. Its "appendix," public hygiene, consciously omitted for the first time in Eschenbach's treatise of 1746, had by that time established itself as a flourishing and independent discipline, especially through the work of Johann Peter Frank (1745-1821). In legal medicine, as in general medicine, the formalism of systems was more and more replaced by concentration on scientific and technological detail. As in general medicine, we encounter two subsequent stages of this development: first the prevailingly *observational* stage, then the *laboratory* or experimental stage. While in clinical medicine observation proceeded mostly in the wards of the great hospitals of Paris, Dublin, London, and Vienna, the role of the "hospital" in legal medicine was played by the morgue, as indicated by Alphonse Devergie, one of the protagonists of this development. As in general medicine the new trends appeared most strongly and prevailed first in the France of the Great Revolution where the gigantic and violent floods of the popular uprising had removed all medieval obstacles and released new energies.

The surgeon and obstetrician, François Chaussier (1746-1828) no longer aimed to establish any "system" of legal medicine. He concentrated on the different degrees of subcutaneous hemorrhages, and the establishment of a systematic autopsy technique. Like Orfila and Devergie, he did experimental work on postmortal wounds. His greatest accomplishment is perhaps the erection of chairs of legal medicine in Paris, Strasbourg, and Montpellier, when called in 1794 by Fourcroy to collaborate in the reorganization of medical studies.

Through his treatise, *Les lois éclairés par les sciences physiques ou Traité de médicine légale et d'hygiene publique*, 1797 (3 vol.; the 1813 ed. has 6 vol.), Francois Emmanuel Fodéré (1764-1835), a native of Savoy, professor of legal medicine in Strasbourg from 1814 to his death, became the leading figure in this medicolegal revival. The field covered in Fodéré's great work is about the same as in Zacchias, even the sequence of subjects is similar. But what a difference in approach and materials between the 17th century papal court physician, and the pupil of Antoine Louis, the child of the Enlightenment, the former surgeon of the revolutionary armies. Fodéré also contributed monographs to the medicolegal problems of insanity in 1817 and 1832. Fodéré's medical importance is not exhausted by his gigantic medicolegal work. It was preceded by outstanding studies on scurvy, goiter, medical statistics, and followed by others on epidemiology, public health and economics. As a character, Fodéré is one of the most attractive in medical history. Never taking advantage of his family relations with the dictator Napoleon I; always putting his work, built up in the turmoil of wars, above self-promotion; disregarding officialdom to the point of assisting the imprisoned Spanish royal family during the Franco-Spanish War, Fodéré appears as a character of truly classic greatness. That Fodéré was only a member of a movement, however, is shown by the fact that almost simultaneously with his treatise those of P.A.O. Mahon (1752-1801), and J.L. Belloc (1730-1807) also made their appearance (in 1802 and 1807 respectively).

The new scientific trend of exact measurement was introduced into legal medicine with the identification "tableaux" (tables of body proportions in different ages based on averages of large series) of Sue, Orfila, and later Quetelet. The new activities in pathological anatomy produced the discovery of the ossification center in the lower end of the femur in the thirty-fifth week by Bichat's pupil, P.A. Béclard (1785-1825) in 1819, a discovery which gave an inestimable criterion for determining fetal age. The new invention of auscultation, likewise acquired tremendous medicolegal importance through the discovery of fetal heartsounds by Kergaradec in 1821. That the new *Code Napoléon* provided a framework for medicolegal consultation, superior to all previously existing laws, was emphasized by C.C.H. Marc (1771-1841), the German-trained physician of Louis Philippe. Marc, author of a treatise on legal psychiatry in 1840, is of particular historical importance as the editor of the *Annales d'hygiène publique et de médecine légale*, founded in 1829 and soon the leading journal in the field. The names of its editorial board illustrate the quality of French legal medicine and public hygiene at the time. They were Adelon, Andral, Barruel, D'Arcet, Devergie, Esquirol, Kerandren, Leuret, Marc, Orfila, Parent-Duchatelet, and Villermé.

Probably the most influential man in this group as far as the development of scientific legal medicine is concerned, was the naturalized Spaniard, J.M.B. Orfila (1787-1853), physician of Louis XVIII, dean of the Paris faculty 1830-1848. His *Traité de Toxicologie* of 1813, introducing the new experimental methods and the new chemistry into one of the most important branches of legal medicine, opened a new era. His *Leçons de Médecine Légale* (1823) are demonstratively modern through omission of a historical introduction. They contain interesting experimental work on putrefaction and postmortal wounds.

Legal toxicology was, of course, no invention of Orfila. Fr. Hofmann, for instance, had been able, in 1716, to unmask a case of "sorcery" as CO poisoning. But one need only look at the poison "test" of the great Boerhaave (throw the suspected material on fire), or the unspecific pictures of poisoning of older authors in order to appreciate the change brought about by Orfila through application of quantitative chemical methods and the experimental approach of a Magendie. No less brilliant as a speaker than as a scientist, Orfila attained the fame or notoriety of a modern movie star through his appearance in the great poison murder trials of the period, especially in the Affaire Lafarge in 1840, when he had to fight the equally brilliant chemist and radical Raspail. By 1840 Orfila was able to use a test that has almost ruined a whole branch of crime: the arsenic test of J. Marsh (1795-1846) of 1836, based on Trommsdorf's test of 1803. The curve of Brouardel that was drawn without any intention to support our point, illustrates with its dramatic decline of poisoning trials in the 1830-1840 decade better than any words what the Marsh test did to the "gentle art of poisoning." Important landmarks in legal toxicology were the method of extracting alkaloids from the cadaver found by the Belgian, J. Stas (1813-1891), in 1851 in the "Affaire Bocarmé," and the discovery of ptomains, alkaloids produced in the body by putrefaction, by F. Selmi (1812-1881) of Bologna in 1872. Notable British contributions to legal toxicology were those of Sir Robert Christison (1797-1882), (poisoning with calabar beans, oxalic acid, etc.) and A.S. Taylor (1806-1880).

Another branch of legal medicine that owes its rise mainly to the French medical revolution is legal psychiatry. Again we enter no original field. Remember Weyer, Bohn, Metzger and Fodéré. E. Platner (1744-1818) of Leipzig had made vigorous attempts to obtain psychiatric consultation in the courts; Hopfengärtner (1792), Malfatti (1809), Henke, Osiander had fought against the legal responsibility of children. But eventually only a new psychiatric science, possible only after the total disappearance of the possession superstition, and a new legal attitude, in terms of which the problem of responsibility was no longer approached in an absolute either-or manner, but in a more relativistic way, could open the path for a more frequent and willing use of psychiatric insight by the courts. This new psychiatry is essentially the work of Pinel, Esquirol and their pupils in France, of men like Batties and Perfects in England, J.C. Reil in Germany, and Benjamin Rush in the United States. The main problem of the legal psychiatrist has always been to convince the court of the existence of mental disease in persons who are not deteriorated intellectually or who might reach the court in a stage of remission. (The classic raving madman or demented individual could always be identified without expert help.) Pinel tried to characterize such cases through the concept of "*folie raisonnée*"; Esquirol, Georget, Marc and Leuret by speaking of "*monomania,*" or "*manie sans délire,*" Trélat and Morel of "*manie avec conscience,*" Bernheim of "irresistible will," Pritchard of "moral insanity" and Tuke of "inhibitory insania." The vigorous and tenacious opposition of many men of the law to legal psychiatry found a very articulate expression in Elias Regnault's *Du dégré de competence des médecins dans les questions judiciaires rélatives aux aliénations mentales* (1828). In the field of mental disease doctors seemed no more competent to Regnault than judges or other laymen.

The English were dramatically faced with the problem of the insane criminal and his disposal by the attack of the schizophrenic Hadfield against

George III in 1800. From this period dates the foundation of criminal lunatic asylums. John Haslam (1764-1844) produced a fine early treatise on *Medical Jurisprudence as it relates to insanity* in 1817. For awhile Cesare Lombroso's pseudo-anthropological work on "criminal man" (1876) excited the public like, in later times, Spengler, Freud or Kinsey. The best known German forensic psychiatrist of the 19th century was probably Richard von Krafft-Ebbing (1840-1902), author of a treatise on the subject in 1875 and of the classic *Psychopathia sexualis* in 1886.

The mantle (although not the chair) of Orfila as the leader of French legal medicine fell to Alphonse Devergie (1798-1879), author of a monumental treatise in 1835, most assiduous collaborator of the *Annales* and discoverer of innumerable valuable details, founder of the medicolegal society in 1868, and above all, promoter of practical medicolegal instruction in the Morgue, where he was followed by P.C.H. Brouardel (1837-1902). Brouardel and Ambroise Auguste Tardieu (1818-1879), pupil of Orfila and like his master a courtroom "star" of many "causes célèbres," were essentially casuists. They no longer produced "treatises," but series of monographs on limited problems such as hanging, abortion, poisoning, wounds, and so forth. Tardieu also did outstanding work in the field of industrial hygiene.

Transition from the old to the new legal medicine was much slower in Germany than in France for obvious reasons. Their glorious traditions now became rather a liability for the Germans. The two most famous German medicolegal authors of their period, C.H.A. Henke (1775-1843) of Erlangen, and the obstetrician J.C. Mende (1779-1832) of Greifswald and Göttingen, belong rather to the 18th than to the 19th century. It is hard today to understand Henke's tremendous popularity, except through his extraordinary industry (publication of a textbook in 1812, collected essays in 1815, a journal in 1821). It is true that Henke tried hard to overcome the formalism of older authors, especially in the field of the classification of wounds. Objectively he became even more deeply involved in judicial formalism than many of his predecessors. Bookishness in the discipline probably reached its apogee with him. Casper tells about this most famous teacher of legal medicine of his age that "he had never performed one judicial dissection, never stepped across the threshold of any prison, never examined any woman said to have been deflowered, never investigated the doubtful mental condition of even one criminal or of a single case of malingering, or ever stood as an expert before any court."

With Johann Ludwig Casper (1796-1864) of Berlin, who started publishing the results of his practical observations in 1825, the new period of legal medicine actually started in Germany, and was represented by Casper with no less brilliance than by Orfila, or Tardieu in France. Casper was essentially a practical man and casuist, and rightly called his great textbook that began appearing in 1851, a *clinical treatise on forensic medicine*. Some quotations from the preface to the third edition of his textbook in 1860 will give some idea of his intellectual complexion:

"In this book as in all my lectures in the last thirty-six years I have striven especially against the prime failing of most authors on forensic medicine, viz., the separation of it from general medicine, and have endeavored to purify it from all irrelevant rubbish, which has been so copiously accumulated in it by tradition, want of experience in forensic matters, and therefore ignorance of the proper relation which the medical jurist bears to the judge, as well as mistaken ideas as to the practical object of the science. . . .

"The correct appreciation of a simple dogma, which is as unquestionably correct as it is to be unalterably maintained, leads of itself to the necessary reform in treating of juridical medicine. I mean the dogma that a medical jurist is—*a physician*—nothing more, nothing less, nothing else, and, as this simple dogma has been grossly misunderstood, to make it still more plain, I again repeat, he is a *physician*, and not a lawyer, etc. Just as a technologist, artist, or any other craftsman must hold his knowledge or experience in his art or trade at the service of justice in the interest of the common need, so must the physician, and nothing else is required of him. . . .

"This erroneous blending of medical and legal ideas and objects is also combined with another greater and more consequential error in the practice of forensic medicine. I mean the tendency to endeavour to obtain strict apodictical proof, such as was required by the practice of the older penal courts. . . . I demand in what other branch of general medical diagnosis, of which the forensic is but a part, is such indubitable certainty required, or where can it be attained?"

Casper was also the great promoter of the practical methods of instruction in legal medicine that had been fathered by Devergie in Paris, Tourdes in Strasbourg, and Joseph Bernt (1770-1842) in Vienna. Passing mention might be made here of the fact that Bernt's successor J. Kolletschka (1803-1847), through his tragic end from septicemia, involuntarily stimulated his friend Semmelweis' immortal discovery of asepsis in obstetrics.

The large scale application of the so-called basic sciences (physiology and biochemistry, histology especially applied to pathological anatomy and embryology, pharmacology, toxicology, bacteriology and serology) to medical problems brought about a new era in clinical medicine, the reign of the laboratory, specialization and unheard of progress. The application of the same disciplines to the problems of legal medicine led to the solution of not a few of its knottiest problems. These applications are on the other hand so numerous and detailed that in the limits of this survey they and their authors cannot be listed—a listing which like many modern discoveries would also involve numerous priority controversies—with the comprehensiveness that has been applied to the events of the past. Only a few examples will be given.

It is obvious what pathologico-anatomical histology was bound to accomplish in the specification of such processes as putrefaction, premortal and postmortal wounds, and so forth. It also helped greatly in the identification of doubtful tissues and spots (semen, blood). The latter problem was tackled microscopically by the master of modern pathological anatomy, Rudolf Virchow (1821-1902). Virchow also established the standard autopsy procedure. The progress of embryology through the application of microscopy allowed greater accuracy in the field of doubtful sexual relations.

What the advances in toxicology through the use of modern chemistry and experiment meant to the explanation of criminal poisoning has already been mentioned above. Chemistry also helped greatly in the identification of doubtful stains and spots as evidenced by an early treatise on the subject (1848) by

Carl Schmidt (1822-1899) of Dorpat, the famous biochemist and collaborator of Bidder. The discovery of haemine crystals, in 1853, by Ludwig Teichman Stawiarski (1823-1895) of Gottingen and Cracow, advanced the doubtful blood stain problem one further important step.

Its final solution in the Uhlenhuth-Bordet complement test of 1901 grew out of the adoption of bacteriology-serology by legal medicine. The application of bacteriology changed again the whole field of wound appreciation, putrefaction studies, and cleared up several toxicological riddles.

A great improvement in identification methods was the use of a combination of measurements worked out by Bertillon ("Bertillonage") in 1886. It was largely superseded after 1892 by *dactyloscopy*, a method based on the uniqueness of fingerprints. This method, known already to the ancient Chinese, was suggested by J.E. Purkinjě (1787-1869) and Francis Galton (1822-1911).

Legal medicine speedily and successfully applied every new major scientific discovery to its own special problems. We mention only spectroscopy, photography, the X-ray, and the discovery of blood groups by Landsteiner in 1901, the latter used now in paternity cases.

Legal medicine grew not only insofar as its own methods were concerned, new fields also opened through technical and social developments where the courts stood in need of expert help: the large scale use of insurance, private or state-sponsored, brought about numerous court actions of a new type.

During the last hundred years legal medicine has undoubtedly come closer to its goal of helping to reduce legal errors to a minimum than in any previous period of history.

TRANSLATIONS OF EARLY REPORTS
BY MEDICAL EXPERTS

THE THREE EARLIEST EXISTING MEDICOLEGAL REPORTS (from the Latin texts in G. Bohne: Die gerichtliche Medizin im italienischen Statutenrecht des 13-16. Jahrhunderts, Vierteljahresschrift f. ger. Med. 3 ser. 61: 79-81, 1921)

Bologna 1289

Master Albertus Malevoda and Master Amoretus, physicians, who, on the injunction of Albertus of Gandino, judge, have seen and examined Jacobus Rustighelli in the Church of St. Catherine of Saracocia, wounded and dead, state in concordance, after having seen and examined, to have found the following:

  in the thorax: seven deadly wounds
  in the neck: one deadly wound
  in the middle of the forehead: two deadly wounds
  in the occiput: one deadly wound
  in the upper jaw: one non-fatal wound

Sworn to be true on Saturday, February 12th.

Bologna 1289 (February 11th)

Master Bertolacius and Master Angellus, physicians, who, at the indication of the said judge, went to see Cambius Venturella of Castel del Vescovo, on the above-written day, have reported and sworn, to have seen and examined the said Cambius and found: that he has two wounds, one in the posterior part of the head and one above the hip, and have stated on the basis of the signs that they have seen, that he will entirely recover if nothing else intervenes.

Bologna 1289 (April 5th)

Master Angelus and Master Primiranus, charged by Albertus de Gandino, judge, have seen Simon, dead, and having fifteen wounds, nine of them deadly. They also have seen Hubertus, brother of the above mentioned Simon, having three non-fatal wounds, one in the arm, with a doubtful prognosis especially as to the future debility of the arm, and two in the right hip.

AMBROISE PARÉ (Oeuvres complètes, ed. by J.F. Malgaigne, Paris, 1841, vol. 3, pp. 651 ff., 666)

Deadly Wound

I, Ambroise Paré have gone today on the order of the court of parliament to the house of X, Rue St. Germain with the ensign of S, and have found him in his bed having a wound on the left part of his head over the temporal bone with fracture. Several parts of this bone have broken through the two membranes and entered the substance of the brain. Therefore the above-named had lost all consciousness with a convulsion, the pulse is very small, and the sweat cold. He neither drinks nor eats. I therefore certify that he will soon die. Testified by my seal, etc.

Invalidity Through Wound

I, Ambroise Paré, have gone on the order of the Attorney of the King to the house of Mr. X, which is situated on Rue St. Pierre aux Boeufs, on whom I have found a wound on the right ankle joint, great about four fingers, with incision of all cords or tendons that move the foot together with incision of the veins, arteries and nerves. Therefore, the above-named is in danger of death because of the accidents which often follow such wounds like extreme pain, fever, inflammation, apostema, convulsions, gangrene, and others. He therefore has to keep a good regimen and must be well and duly bandaged and drugged. And when he will escape death, he will nevertheless always remain crippled in the part. Certifying this to be true by putting my seal, etc.

Sudden Death from Wounds

We, the undersigned, certify that today in the presence of the Chief of Police and the Attorney of the King we have seen, and examined the cadaver of a nobleman on whom we have found a wound made with a sword near the left mammilla, large about two fingers, passing through the body from one side to the other, and passing through the heart. Furthermore one other great wound made with a sword about three fingers large and long on the left shoulder joint, penetrating into that joint with incisions of the nerves, ligaments, veins and arteries of the said region. Furthermore, one other great wound made also with the sword under the left axilla about four fingers long and large, penetrating into the axilla with incision of the veins, arteries and nerves. Furthermore, two other wounds also made with the sword, in the thorax, one somewhat lower than the left mammilla, long and large about one finger, and penetrating into the thoracic cavity. Another great wound made with the sword situated near the right mammilla, long and large about four to five fingers, penetrating only to the ribs. Another cutting wound on the right elbow, about three fingers great, and two large, cutting off the ligaments of the joints. Another wound also made with the sword on the right side, a thumb long and large about, and not very deep. Another wound also made with the sword on the right hand on the finger called medius, with total incision of the first joint and penetrating the metacarpals. In view of all these wounds we certify that sudden death had occurred.

Signed, Sunday, the 7th August, 1543.

Ambroise Paré, Jean Cointeret,
and Jean Charbonnel.

Abdominal Wound Resulting in Abortion

I, Ambroise Paré, have come on the order of the great Provost to the Rue St. Houbré, to the house of Mr. M., where I have found a lady called Margaret in bed with a high fever, convulsions, and hemorrhage from her natural parts, as consequence of a wound that she has received in the lower abdomen situated three fingers below the umbilicus, in the right part, which has penetrated into the cavity, wounded and penetrated the uterus. She has therefore delivered before term a male infant, dead, well formed in all its limbs, which infant has also received a wound in its head, penetrating into the substance of the brain. Therefore the above-mentioned lady will soon die. Certified this to be true in putting my signature, etc.

Report on a Confirmed Leper

We, sworn surgeons of Paris, have been nominated by order of the Attorney of the King on August 28, 1783, to make a report whether G.P. is a leper. We have examined him as follows. First we have found the color of his face reddish, bluish and livid and full of blue spots. We have torn his hair and his beard, and his brow and have seen that at the roots of the hair a little portion of flesh was attached. In the brow and behind his ears we have found small glandular tubercles. We have found the forehead full of wrinkles, his expression fixed and immobile, his eyes red, brilliant, the nostrils wide outside and narrow inside, almost stuffed with little crusty ulcers, the tongue swollen and black, and above and below we have found little grains as one sees them in measly pigs, the mouth corroded inside, and the teeth denuded and the breath quite stinking, the voice hoarse, speaking through the nose. Also we have seen him naked, and have found all his skin crisp and unequal like in a badly-plucked goose, and in certain regions several spots. Then we have penetrated rather deeply with a needle at the Achilles tendon; he has hardly felt it. On the basis of these signs, clear ones and equivocal ones, we say that G.P. is a confirmed leper. Therefore it would be good that he should be separated from the company of the healthy because this evil is contagious. We certify the truth of this in signing the 6th May, 1583, etc.

MIDWIVES

Pretended Loss of Virginity Through Rape

We, Jeanne de Mon and Jeanne Verguire and Beatrice Laurade, from the parish of Espoire in Béarn, matrons and midwives examined and approved, certify to whom it may concern that by order of the Judge of Espere, we, the undersigned matrons, have found, visited and seen, on May 15, 1545, Mariette de Garrigues, age 15, and the said Mariette said to have been raped and deflowered and devirginized. Therefore, we the undersigned midwives have examined and observed everything in the light of three candles, touched with our hands and examined with our eyes, and turned over with our fingers. And we found that neither was the vulva deformed nor the carunculae displaced, nor the labia minora distended, nor the perineum wrinkled, nor the internal orifice of the uterus opened, nor the cervix uteri split, nor the pubic hair bent, nor the hymen displaced, nor the breasts wilted, nor the margin of the great labia changed, nor the vagina enlarged, nor the membrane that connects the carunculae returned, nor the pubis broken, nor the clitoris in any way damaged. All this we, the above-mentioned midwives, state as our report and direct judgment.

Signs of Rape

We, Marion Teste, Jean de Maux, Jeanne de la Guigans, Madeline de la Lippue, matrons of the city of Paris, certify to whom it may concern that on the 14th of June, 1532, by order of the Police Chief of Paris or his Lieutenant in the said city, we have gone to the Rue de Frepaut, where hangs the ensign of the slipper, and we have seen and visited Henriette Peliciere, a young girl, age about 15, who has complained in court against Simon the Boaster, who, she says, has raped and deflowered her. We have all seen and examined with the finger and the eye and we have found that she has the pubis excoriated, the labia minora distended, the hymen retired, the vulva gaping, the breasts descended, the caruncles formed, the perineum wrinkled, the internal orifice of the uterus opened, the cervix split, the pubic hair bent, the clitoris sore, the labia majora pealed, the vagina enlarged, and the labia minora hanging. Having all seen and examined we have found that there were traces of visitation. And this we, the above-mentioned matrons certify to be true to you, Monsieur, Chief of the Police under the oath that we have sworn to the above-mentioned city.

DEVAUX

False Accusation of Malpractice in Bleeding

After haveing examined with much care the party pretending to be sick, we have found the wound well united without hardening, unusual pulsating inflammation or any other accident which could induce us to judge that the arteries and nerves, the tendons and membranes, or any other part which one has to avoid in bleeding should have received any detrimental damage. We have found that the woman makes with her supposedly wounded arm all the movements that one can ask of this organ unless the patient opposes a voluntary resistance to the action of the muscles that serve to move it. All things thus having returned to normal in the external disposition of the mentioned part, we conclude that there is a false pretension in the spirit of the Madeleine A, that there is no disorder in the part of which she complains and that certainly she has not received a wound in the last bleeding. We confirm this by our signature, etc. Paris, October 17th, 1691.

Insane Prisoner

Guillaume Bidart seems to us to have an atrabilious temperament. We judge from his short and restless sleep, from the disordered character of his look, from his sudden movements of joy and sadness, and from his attacks of fury and audacity that he is clearly suffering from a kind of delirium that is called mania, the cure of which is very difficult. Therefore we judge that he should be retained and observed closely in order to prevent annoying consequences of his fury which he could direct against himself or other persons (April 22, 1684).

Syphilis Given by Husband to Wife

We have seen and visited the said Catherine La Febvre who complained to us of several symptoms and venereal accidents contracted by the impure contact with her husband. And we have found in the said woman La Febvre a tumor in the right groin of the size of a pigeon's egg which can be regarded as a venereal bubo. Furthermore we have found the whole vulva inflamed, ulcerated and secreting a yellowish liquor which runs continually and stains her shirt with a yellowish matter. We have also observed on the head a little ulcerous and painful tubercle in the hair, and the whole throat seems to us inflamed and ulcerated especially on the right side. She furthermore complains of nocturnal pains and that she loses her hair. That she has had for six weeks an obstinate diarrhea which has made her lose much weight. We have found her pulse small and frequent.

We judge that all these accidents are venereal and contracted by impure and contagious contacts. Therefore the said Febvre must be treated promptly with specific remedies, otherwise her beginning syphilis will become more generalized and more difficult to cure because of the delicacy of her constitution and the violence of the remedies (September 16, 1666).

Infant and Second Nurse Infected by
Syphilitic Nurse

We have seen and visited Toussaint Jean, gardener at Surene, in whom we have found a venereal pustule in the middle part of his penis which seems to us old, dry and crusty. The said Toussaint Jean has told us that this pustule had been preceded by several similar pustules distributed all over the skin of his body to the hairy part of his head although we have seen none. He has told us that he has contracted the pustules from his wife who was covered with them all over.

Then we have seen and examined Margaret Poussin, wife of the mentioned Toussaint Jean, who has complained to us to suffer from syphilis. This seems true to us on account of lack of hair on different places of her head and on account of the brown venereal pustules which we have found around the labia of her vulva and all over her behind. They seem to us old, hard, and of a bad color. When we inspected her breasts we have found a red spot of the size of a silver dollar around her left mammella which she says itches much. The right mammella seems intact.

Thereupon we have gone to the Rue St. Honoré, opposite the Hotel de Vendome, to the apartment of Mr. Gestard, whom we have examined in all the parts of his body which we have found very healthy, especially his genital parts on which we have found no marks nor traces of any venereal symptoms. And the same holds good for Antoinette Madeline Colletet, his wife, whom we have seen and examined in all her parts and especially her genital parts where we have found no symptoms of venereal disease. The said Gestard and his wife appeared to us of very good disposition and of perfect health.

We then have gone to the apartment of Jacques Nauroy, opposite cloister of the Jacobins, in the same street, Rue St. Honoré, where, in the presence of the said Poussin, first wet nurse of the little daughter of the said Gestard, and in the presence of Mr. Lénon, her attorney, we have seen and visited a little girl aged from 9 to 10 months, in whom we have found the region of the behind filled with venereal pustules, red and inflamed. Then we have opened her mouth and we have found that the throat was inflamed and ulcerated, and considering her whole body, she seems to us well nourished and of a rather good disposition.

Thereupon we have seen and visited Jacqueline Saule, wife of the said Nauroy in whom we have found two or three venereal pustules around the left mammella which she told us to have contracted in nursing the daughter of the said Gestard of which she is presently the nurse. All her genital parts and others appeared to us healthy and without venereal disease. Therefore the said Saule, presently wet nurse of the daughter of the said Gestard, has received the venereal disease through the pustules which are on her mammella while she nursed the little Gestard. And the said little Gestard has contracted the venereal pustules and the ulcers in her throat from the impure and venereal milk of her first nurse Margaret Poussin whom we have found infected with an old syphilis, while one cannot suspect the little Gestard of bad congenital principles, being of good disposition and born of a very healthy father and mother. (Paris, August 13, 1663.)

Corpse Found Hanging

We have found the corpse of a woman, aged about 50 years, hanging from a rafter which we were told was the body of a certain Jeanne Souchet. As this corpse had the face in no way discolored, nor any foam at the mouth, no black tongue, no nostrils filled with mucous excrement nor even the slightest redness, wound or other change of color round the neck at the place where the cord by which it had been suspended had made its impression we have decided to make an exact examination of all the other parts of the corpse. Whereupon we have found a very small wound at the anterior right part of the thorax, hidden under the breast and where a small probe could hardly enter. Having dilated this opening we have found that it penetrated between the sixth and fifth rib. Whereupon we have opened the thorax in order to study the progress of the said wound. We have found that this little wound has been produced by a round, very narrow piercing instrument and traversing the heart from one side to the other had caused a great, very extensive hemorrhage into the thorax. In summarizing all these observations we conclude that the wound in the thorax has preceded the suspension of the corpse of the said Souchet woman and has been the only and true cause of her death. (February 23, 1663.)

Corpse Drowned After Poisoning

I have seen and examined the body of a man about thirty years old who had been removed from the water several hours before. I have found his face purple and swollen, the tongue black, swollen and hanging out of the mouth about two fingers, no swelling of the lower abdomen, and no scratches at the extremity of the fingers. Whereupon I have opened the lower abdomen where I have found the stomach showing a reddish-brown at the exterior and cauterized inside at the bottom on two places. Furthermore I have found a little black liquid in the lower abdominal cavity which had blackened the intestines on those places where it had touched them. All these signs are more than sufficient to judge that this man had been thrown into the water after his death. (June 29, 1685.)

CO Poisoning

I have found the named Olivier Graville and Jacques Usart motionless, the face of a leaden pallor, speechless, and cold all over, and as I have perceived that the gases of coal had brought them into this state on account of the bad odor with which this little room was still infected, I have made promptly bring one of them outside, that is the said Jacques Usart, who still showed some kind of life, that is a very feeble movement of the heart, while Olivier Graville was already dead beyond help. To help the said Usart who was still alive I have opened his mouth with an appropriate instrument, I have made him swallow a strong emetic, and I have blown into his nostrils the euphorbus powder in order to provoke sneezing. These remedies have worked, the said Usart has opened his eyes, recovered speech, and has complained of a great heaviness of the head, and of extreme tiredness and weakness. (Paris, January 16, 1681.)

BLEGNY

Child, Choked to Death

Being ordered to examine the cadaver of René Poron who had died the preceding night at the age of 10, I have found his face purple, mouth and nose covered with slime, and after opening the body we found the lungs full of spongy air. Therefore and on account of the good state of all the other parts of his body, external as well as internal ones, we have judged that he has been suffocated during the night by some sleeping person or in some other similar way which judgment has been confirmed through the fact that several persons present at this examination have declared that the child was still in excellent health on the preceding day.

CLAUDE DU PRADEL

Poisoning

After having found all the external parts of his body in their natural order we have then proceeded to opening the body, and beginning by the lower abdomen we have found it cauterized at the bottom which contains about an egg full of a black, sandy liquid, which produced, after having been put by us into a zinc vessel, the stains characteristic for acid and corrosive liquids, and which when given in a small quantity to a dog, had strong effects on the dog as we judge from his cries and barking. We therefore judge that the said Pernel has been poisoned with arsenic or sublimates or another such corrosive mineral poison. We have been confirmed in this through the good state of all the other internal parts of his abdomen as well as his thorax and head which we have opened and where we have found no cause of death. (Lyon, September 28, 1682.)

AUBERT

Dead Infant

Today, June 14, 1707, I the undersigned, Anthony Aubert, master surgeon of the suburb of Sissone, official expert, certify to whom it may concern that on the order of the State Attorney de la Sehie which has been delivered to me today by Jean Dovay, police sergeant, after having sworn before the police lieutenant I have proceeded to the examination of a little corpse at the house of Paul Charpentier, truck driver, where I have gone. Having seen and examined the cadaver of the newborn, delivered by Elizabeth Charpentier, daughter of the above-mentioned Ponce, I have found the head of the cadaver fractured and livid, which in my mind has occurred during delivery, be it that he was too long in the passages or that he was delivered too brutally as there was nobody knowing the operation. And I certify that the little infant is between seven and eight months according to its size. And having opened the thorax I have not found any blood there nor in the heart. I herewith certify that what I have said above is truly given this day and year.

Signed, Aubert, surgeon.

HENRI GUEYT

Epilepsy

I the undersigned, Henri Gueÿt, master surgeon, sworn royal expert to report in this city and its surroundings, certify that today the 17th November, 1713, I have seen and examined in a shop the said Anne Legahaignou, daughter of Anne Marec, born in the village of Kalloren, parish district of Plouzanec, suffering from epilepsy who has had an attack while in my room. During this attack which lasted about ten minutes, she has had convulsions. Ordinarily this kind of disease tends to increase. Her parents who were with her have told me that ordinarily she has five or six attacks per day, that in addition she is not in her senses and has no judgment and is almost completely invalid, unable to use her limbs and consequently unable to gain a livelihood. I certify this to be the truth. Brest on the day and year mentioned above. Gueyt. Received three pounds, four shillings.

THE FIELDING H. GARRISON LECTURE *

THE GROWTH OF MEDICINE AND THE LETTER OF THE LAW

BENJAMIN SPECTOR

I wish to express my deep appreciation for the honor of being chosen the Garrison Lecturer of the American Association of the History of Medicine for the year 1952. The influence of Garrison on American medicine is deep and unquestionably of timeless validity. Garrison's distinction does not consist alone in the proved worth of such a work as his *Introduction to the History of Medicine* (1st ed. 1913; 4th ed. 1929). His distinction consists also in revealing to the American medical profession and to the intelligent lay public a breadth of concept, a new method of approach, and a liberal-minded quality of thought. A re-reading of his writings clearly shows an amplitude of mind and a felicity of phrase which are both rare and precious. It is the special privilege and pleasure of a Garrison Lecturer to acknowledge with grateful thanks the great scholarship of the man for whom this Lectureship has been established.

For many years I have studied the growth of medicine in relation to

* Read at the twenty-fifth annual meeting of the American Association of the History of Medicine, Kansas City, Kansas, May 1, 1952.

the evolution of the law. It was with the assistance of Mrs. Spector (LL.B.; LL.M.), that I was able to survey certain areas of medical history in which the letter of the law fostered the growth of medicine.

The historian of medicine must turn his attention at times to the Hammurabi Code, to the common law, to the commentaries of Coke (1552-1634) and Blackstone (1723-80), (the great English jurists), to statute and positive law as well as to Imhotep, Hippocrates, Galen, Avicenna, da Vinci, Harvey, and Jenner if he is fully to understand the growth of medicine. For without law we should not have standards of medical practice; without law the health of communities would be at a low level; without law, instead of enjoying the advancement of medical progress, we should be uncivilized. In other words, any development in the history of medicine which affects the health of peoples must have its counterpart in law. When medicine was essentially an art with but a mere sprinkling of scientific fact the problem of defining it precisely was like Pilate's question, " What is truth? " Yet the question, " What is medicine " is not academic, and in the field of law, at least, it has become an important practical problem. As medicine advanced to the point where a cluster of closely allied sciences induced its growth and development, law became one of the important hinges upon which medicine had to turn to make effective newer discoveries for the general welfare of communities. Law indeed became a directive force in socio-medical problems. One comes to see that, historically considered, the medical and legal rules governing health and sickness are not of today, nor of yesterday, but are a part of a rich stream of inheritance which goes back through the centuries. The broadening conceptions of health and legal justice, from earliest times to the present, were companions in the sinuous course of medical progress. The practice of medicine was always, it seems to me, at least bifactorial, that is, its obligations were legal as well as medical.

The field under consideration is so broad and extensive that, within the limits provided for this lecture, I shall attempt to indicate how medicine developed within the legal atmosphere of the Babylonian *lex talionis*, the Roman *Justinian Code*, the Mediaeval *ecclesiastical* law, the English and earlier *common law*, and finally the modern *positive law*. It will be pointed out that juridical tradition and the differing ideas of the powers of the state, of sovereignty, and of administrative justice have left a bold impression on the growth of medicine.

At the outset, I would draw your attention to three generalizations: First, that medicine, in the practice of its art, always dealt with individuals as separate units, whereas law concerned itself not only with concrete cases but also with individuals as units constituting an aggregate. Secondly, that medicine and law alike control the life of man in terms of human conduct, human progress, and human welfare. Obviously there must be limitations upon individual human acts in considering the general welfare of the public and it is in this sense that law as an active process makes available to the public the contributions in technique and theory of medical advances. The third generalization is exemplified by the following two maxims: " Salus populi suprema lex est " (the welfare of the people is the supreme law) ; and " Lex est ratio summa, quae jubet, quae sunt utilia et necessaria, et contraria prohibet " [1] (Law is the highest reason which ordains what is useful and necessary and forbids the contrary.) Or to quote the Justinian Code,[2] " Jus is the art of what is good and fair." These generalizations point up the fact that medicine and law dovetail in any evaluation and interpretation of individuals as individuals and of individuals as units; also the control of human conduct in terms of human welfare, legally and medically considered, constitute the supreme law of a community. In others words, the function of the practice of medicine is modifiable and modified by the law.

Let us proceed to the consideration of the relation of medicine and law in the following four areas: 1. The Hammurabi Code; 2. Abortion; 3. Police Power, Inoculation, Vaccination, and Quarantine; 4. The Medical Practice Act.

I. *The Hammurabi Code and Medicine.*

This legal code [3] represents one of the earliest examples of the power to regulate the practice of physicians and surgeons; it embodies a concept of law as an imperative idea, an idea of a rule deriving its force from the authority of the sovereign.[4] Here we are dealing with law in its embryonic form as a series of isolated decrees for the settlement of specific issues.[5] This justly famous Hammurabi Code was a compilation of earlier customary law and royal ordinances. In issuing the law, the king claimed divine sanction and the state enforced and punished violations in accord-

---

[1] Roscoe Pound, *Introduction to the Philosophy of Law*, New Haven, 1922. Frederic J. Stimson, *Glossary of Technical Terms, Phrases, and Maxims of the Common Law*, Boston, 1881.

[2] *Digest of Justinian*, I, l. i. Tr. Charles H. Monro. Cambridge, Eng., 1904.

[3] C. A. Johns, *Babylonian and Assyrian Laws, Contracts, and Letters*, New York, 1904, pp. 62-63, s. 218-220.

[4] Roscoe Pound, More About the Nature of Law, in: *Legal Essays in Tribute to Orren Kip McMurray*, Berkeley, Calif., 1935, p. 515.

[5] William A. Robson, *Civilization and the Growth of Law*, New York, 1935, p. 31.

ance with the principle known as the *lex talionis*. The sacred origin of the law imposed a certain immobility upon the practice of medicine; moreover, the Hammurabi laws were recorded on diorite, a material which did not lend itself easily to change! Now, exactly what was the governing principle of the Hammurabi Code with reference to the practice of medicine? Clearly it was the operation of the lex talionis in *qualitative* terms, that is to say, it was a form of " mirror punishment," the operation of a principle of appropriateness.[6] For example, when a physician altered the details of customary treatment and the patient died, or when the physician in treatment destroyed an organ like an eye, a tooth, or a bone, the penalty was *in kind*, for it must be remembered that the *quantitative* compensation in the form of money was not, as in our day, part of the lex talionis. The penalty was made to fit, not the amount of damage inflicted but the nature of the damage. A doctor who treated a slave had merely to replace him if that slave died; however, if the doctor treated a freeman who died, then the surgeon's hands or head were cut off.[7] Is it any wonder that the physician in the time of Hammurabi, when punishment was meted out according to the social status of a patient, found it necessary to exercise caution or even to resolve not to treat patients for fear of being minus some significant part of his own anatomy? The lex talionis in the qualitative sense referred to was never in all cases an adequate or permanent rule of punishment. However, to achieve a more just functioning of the lex talionis Plato advocated both qualitative and quantitative penalties. Thus, a slave killed may be replaced by another slave or his owner may be paid twice his value. Furthermore, a practicing physician may be threatened with death if he injures a person by the use of magic charms. Aristotle [8] pointed out that " In Egypt it is permissible for doctors to alter the rules of their treatment after the first four days though a doctor who alters them earlier does so at his own risk." Here we are confronted with a time limiting factor regarding the treatment of disease. A risk was involved in violation of the written rule. Aristotle believed that a physician should be free to serve a patient unhampered by written rules, the infraction of which might subject the doctor to the risk of physical harm. The purpose, then, of the incurred risk was not to punish so much as to hold the physician

[6] H. F. Jolowicz, The Assessment of Penalties in Preventive Law, in: *Cambridge Legal Essays*, Cambridge, Eng., 1926, p. 204.

[7] E. S. Horgan, Medicine and Surgery in Ancient East—Babylonia and Egypt, *Sudan Notes and Records*, vol. 30, 1949.

[8] Aristotle, *Politics*, Bk. III, c. XV; 1286a, 12-14.

to a fixed rule of medical conduct. The main obligations performed by the Hammurabi Code lay in the avenging of wrong rather than in its prevention. The line of legal tradition in relation to medical practice as set down by Hammurabi was continued into the Roman period and incorporated in the great Justinian Code. For example, Ulpianus [9] remarks: "What has pleased the emperor has the vigor of law (Quod principi placuit, habet legis vigorem) because the lex regia which was passed concerning his rule, the people confided to him, and conferred upon him all his sway and power." This power controlled the actions of physicians as well as other artisans. Medicine in this early time was essentially sacerdotal; the supernatural concept of disease was dominant and medicine was practiced according to a fixed pattern.[10]

The compensation received by a physician in the time of King Hammurabi was apparently predicated upon the results achieved. Besides, in antiquity, the practice of surgery and medicine was never disconnected by educated physicians. For example, under the lex Aquilia, a plebiscite of the Roman Republic, if a surgeon operated on a slave unskilfully there was a good right of action by the slave on the contract. The same rule applied where a doctor made a wrong use of a drug (medicine); in fact where a man operated properly, but omitted further treatment, he would not get off free, but was held guilty of negligence. The lex Cornelia, for example, ordered the arrest of the doctor if the patient died through his negligence.[11] Several centuries later, in the records of the corporation of Beccles in Suffolk, it is ordered that a surgeon is to have a handsome fee if he can cure a certain girl of the disease under which she labors, but only half is to be paid if she dies under his hands.[12]

II. *Abortion.*

The judicial law of Moses enunciated in Exodus XXI, 22, 23, is as follows: "If men strive, and hurt a woman with child, so that her fruit depart from her, and yet no mischief follow: he shall be surely punished according as the woman's husband will lay upon him; and he shall pay as the judges *determine*. And if any mischief follow, then thou shalt give

[9] Charles Henry Monro, *The Digest of Justinian*, Cambridge, 1904-1909, vol. 1, Bk. I, tit. IV. 1.

[10] Henry E. Sigerist, *A History of Medicine*, vol. 1: Primitive and Archaic Medicine, New York, 1951.

[11] Charles Henry Monro (see reference 9), vol. 2, Bk. IX, tit. II, 7, 8.

[12] R. J. Mitchell and M. D. R. Leys, *A History of the English People*, London-New York, 1950, p. 273 et seq.

life for life." The death penalty noted here indicates that law was not a vast undifferentiated continuum unrelated to malpractice in medicine. As we come to the Greek period we are faced with a comparatively highly developed system of primitive law having apparently little in common with primitive custom and sacerdotal usage. The outlook on medicine is now more fluid and is based upon a body of principles containing the power of growth and variation. The citizen is not regarded as belonging just to himself but rather as belonging to the State and the provision made for each individual is naturally adjusted to the provisions made for the whole. Yet, curiously enough, this political outlook was quite consistent with a large measure of personal freedom in what was a comparatively highly developed system of private laws.[13] There was, no doubt, an unwritten law but it must be noted that the aristocracies, who were the custodians of the customary law, administered the law so partially for those of the nobility that a demand arose for the laws to be written and made accessible to the public.[14] The law in ancient Greece passed from the stage of traditional custom to a body of written enactments, individualized in its application. Euripides (480-406)[15] makes Theseus declare: " No curse is greater to a city than a king. For first, where'er no laws exist which bind the whole community, and one man rules, upon his arbitrary will alone depend the laws, and all their rights are lost. But under *written* laws the poor and rich an equal justice find." A case in point is the example of the Hippocratic Oath. You will recall the sentence in this oath which reads, " I will neither give a deadly poison to anybody if asked for it, nor will I make a suggestion to this effect. Similarly I will not give to a woman an abortive remedy." Edelstein [16] points out that poison is a drug and so is the pessary and that only in the capacity as his own apothecary and not as a healer of diseases does the Hippocratic physician agree to give either one of them to a patient. Edelstein also points out that the Oath is not a legal engagement. It seems to me that the law underlying the Hippocratic Oath is that of a rational or ethical idea, an idea of a rule of right and justice deriving its authority from its intrinsic reasonableness or conformity to ideals of

[13] M. Rostovtzeff, *The Social and Economic History of the Hellenistic World*, Oxford, 1941, vol. 2, p. 1088.

[14] A. E. R. Boak, A. Hyma, P. Slosson, *The Growth of European Civilization*, New York, 1938, p. 44.

[15] Euripides, *The Suppliants*, Everyman's Library, No. 271, Vol. 2, p. 296.

[16] L. Edelstein, *The Hippocratic Oath*, Text, Translation, and Interpretation, Supplements to the Bulletin of the History of Medicine, No. 1, Baltimore, 1943.

right and merely recognized, not made, by the sovereign.[17] This point of view is quite different than the one we observed in operation in the Hammurabi Code. It appears that abortion was commonly practiced in Greek and Roman times with reasonable public approval as a legitimate safeguard against excessive population. This was so because law was not regarded as a primary factor in Greek political life but secondary to the Constitution. Infanticide, for example, of defective children was practiced in Sparta and was allowable because there was no adequate distinction between public and private law. It was quite proper for any father to expose a new born child to death either because the child's paternity was doubtful or because the child was weak and deformed.[18] Thus, if infanticide was for the best interest of the life of the State then the law took on a protective character for those who, like physicians, engaged in this practice.[18a] To the Greeks, the conception of the natural right of man remained as strange as that of an acquired right. It was sound opinion, for example, to hold a midwife for murder if she administered a drug which killed a patient; however, if she gave a drug to a woman for her to take, then an action in factum was allowed since she furnished the cause of death rather than killed.[19] Legally considered the individual was swallowed up in the citizen and the citizen in the state. The Greeks did not, as we saw in the case of the Hammurabi Code, fall back upon a personal sovereign for legal sanctions and rarely gave these a direct Divine origin; laws were enforced by, but were in no sense a product of the government. Aristotle [20] remarks, " we do not allow a *man* to rule, but *rational principle*, because a man behaves thus in his own interests and becomes a tyrant." The State cannot give the right to a physician to perform an abortion for it has not itself the right to put an innocent person to death.[21]

With respect to the practice of abortion, a physician was bound by

[17] Roscoe Pound (see reference 4), p. 515.

[18] Plato, *Republic*, Bk. V, 459-460. Aristotle, *Politics*, Bk. VII, c. 16, 1335b 20 ff. Edelstein, *ubi supra*.

[18a] Infanticide, broadly viewed, consists in the destruction of the fetus in utero or of the child after it is born. The definition includes abortion and, inasmuch as doctors performed abortions, they too may be said to have engaged in the practice of infanticide. See, however, p. 507.

[19] *Digest of Justinian*, Bk. IX, tit. 11, 9. J. Walter Jones, Acquired and Guaranteed Rights, in: *Cambridge Legal Essays*, Cambridge, Eng., 1926, p. 223.

[20] Aristotle, *Nicomachean Ethics*, Bk. V, c. 6, 1134a, 35, Translated by W. D. Ross, Oxford, 1925 (*The Works of Aristotle*, ed. W. D. Ross, vol. IX).

[21] P. Vinogradoff, *Outlines of Historical Jurisprudence*, vol. 2: The Jurisprudence of the Greek City, London, 1922.

many laws. There was the divine law, Exodus 20:13, "Thou shalt not kill." There was the natural law which forbade any attempt at destroying fetal life. The conception of natural rights was based on the view that man as such has a sphere of action which is independent of the state and of his standing as a citizen. Aristotle [22] declared that law should sanction miscarriage induced before sense and life had begun in the embryo in all states where the system is opposed to unrestricted increase, in order to limit the size of each family. In the middle ages there was Canon Law which was international Christian law and therefore universal. The phrase "Extra ecclesiam nulla salus" (There is no welfare outside the Church) was universally accepted. The marriage law, for instance, was considered by the Church as her exclusive and absolute domain. Canon law was a great civilizing and humanizing factor to guide those who practiced medicine. The Council of Eliberis, in the 4th Century, refused Holy Communion all the rest of her life to an adultress who had procured the abortion of her child. The sixth Oecumenical Council declared that anyone who procured abortion should bear all the punishments inflicted on murderers. The Bull of Pius IX, (Apostolicae Sedis) decreed excommunication, that is, the deprivation of the sacraments and of the prayers of the Church, against all who seek to procure abortion. Gregory XIV had enacted the penalty of excommunication for abortion of a "quickened" child but as we shall presently see our present day laws make no such distinction.[23] These ecclesiastical laws gave a significant moral aspect to the practice of medicine and further, they emphasized the conception of natural law as a body of principles. In modern times, Blackstone [24] states the law thus: "Life is the immediate gift of God, a right *inherent* by nature in every individual; and it begins in contemplation of law, as soon as the infant is able to stir in its mother's womb." The influence of Blackstone on American medico-legal thinking is strikingly seen when it is recalled that nearly twenty-five hundred copies of Blackstone's *Commentaries* were absorbed by the colonies on the Atlantic seaboard before they declared their independence.[25] At this point in our discussion, let us keep clear in mind the distinction in medical practice between infanticide and feticide. Infanticide is the intentional destruction of a child

[22] Ernest Barker, *The Politics of Aristotle*, Oxford, 1946, Bk. VII, 1335b.
[23] C. Coppens, Art. "Abortion" in: *Catholic Encyclopedia*, New York, 1907, vol. 1, pp. 46-49.
[24] William Blackstone, *Commentaries on the Laws of England*, Oxford, 1765, vol. 1, p. 129.
[25] Frederic William Maitland, *English Law and the Renaissance*, The Rede Lecture for 1901, Cambridge, Eng., 1901, p. 32.

on the point of being born, at birth, or immediately after birth; feticide, on the other hand, is the intentional production of abortion. Legally, infanticide is restricted to the killing of a child *after* birth; feticide, the felonius killing of an *unborn* child. As far as the physician was concerned, the Greek and Roman law did not protect the *unborn* child for " the unborn child was not *homo*, not even *infans*, but merely a *spes animantis* " regarded as a part of the mother.[26] Greek thinking was mainly in the abstract; they did not think of the law of evidence or of the question of reasonable doubt. One must await the coming of the Christian era to see the idea established that a living being is that which is placed in the uterus ("An animal sit id quod in utero est."). The state of medicine during the mediaeval period was not sufficiently advanced to allow a doctor to tell whether a child in utero was alive. Indictments were usually quashed because of the difficulty of proving whether the unborn child was killed naturally or murdered. Indeed there might be various hypotheses other than that of murder of the unborn child to explain the facts.

Let us pass now from the divine law, the natural law, and the canon law to the common law. The principle of stare decisis was not in effect, for one finds almost no citations. Decisions were based on the ground of natural reason. At common law,[27] a child " en ventre sa mere " (in the womb of the mother) is *not* considered a person, the killing of whom is murder. If a woman be quick or great with child, if she takes or another gives her any potion to effect an abortion, whereby the child within her is killed, it is not murder nor manslaughter, by the law of England, because it is not yet in *rerum naturae*. It is, however, a great *misprision*, that is, a neglect or contempt.[28] If, however, a woman be with child and any person gives her a potion to destroy the child within her and she takes it and it works so strongly that it kills her, this is murder for the potion was not given to cure her of any disease, but unlawfully to destroy her child within her, and therefore he (the physician, perhaps) that gives a potion to this end must take the hazard and if it kills the mother, it is murder.[29] Later, in the reign of George IV [30] (1820-31), the doctor was

[26] A. E. Crawley, Art. "Foeticide" in: *Encyclopaedia of Religion and Ethics*, ed. J. Hastings, New York, 1922, vol. 6, p. 56.

[27] Hale's Pleas of the Crown, 433. Fitzherbert, *La Graunde Abridgement Collect*, London, 1565, 22 Edw. III Coron, 263; 8 Edw. II. Coron. 418; 3 Edw. III. Coron 163.

[28] *Ibid.*

[29] 1 Hale's P. C. 429.

[30] 9 George IV, c. 31, s. 13.

faced with two types of punishment if he attempted abortion, either a misdemeanor (before " quickening ") or a capital crime (after " quickening "). The law now read:

If any person, with intent to procure the miscarriage of any woman *being quick with child* (between 16 and 20 weeks) unlawfully and maliciously shall administer to her or cause to be taken by her any poison or other noxious thing, or shall use any instruments or other means whatever with the like intent, every such offender and every person counselling, aiding, or abetting such offender, shall be guilty of felony and being convicted thereof, shall suffer death as a felon. In any woman being NOT quick with child such offender shall be guilty of felony and being convicted thereof shall be liable at the discretion of the court to be transported beyond the Seas for any term not exceeding 14 years, not less than 7 years, or to be imprisoned with or without hard labor in the Common Goal or House of Correction for any term not exceeding 3 years, or if a male to be twice or thrice publicly or privately whipped (if the court shall so think it) in addition to such imprisonment.

This distinction in the English law which made the degree of punishment dependent upon the discovery of whether or not the child had quickened at the time the means to destroy it were adopted, had been condemned by all jurists and medical authorities. So broad a condemnation of a law respecting abortion set a new high standard for the practice of medicine.

In the United States, as recently as 1812,[31] the common law was quoted to the effect that it was no offense to perform an operation upon a pregnant woman *by her consent* for the purpose of procuring an abortion, unless the woman was *quick with child*. Subsequently, in 1851,[32] a statute was passed declaring that the procuring of an abortion is an offense whether the child had quickened or not and whether with or without the consent of the mother. Later still,[33] an opinion was rendered to the effect that it is not the murder of a living child which constitutes the offense, but the destruction of gestation by wicked means and against nature. In other words, the crime of abortion may be committed at any state of pregnancy. The moment the womb is instinct with embryo life and gestation has begun, the crime may be perpetrated. These later rulings of the Court are part of the positive law of the land. Positive or legal rights represent advantages accruing to man as a *social being* which are recognized and protected by the state as an organized body. A doctor was bound within the meaning of this law. In modern times, the assumption that equality and liberty are qualities inherent in man's nature as a

[31] Commonwealth v. Bangs, 9 Mass. 387. 1812.
[32] Smith v. The State, 33 Me. 48. 1851.
[33] State v. Slagle, 83 N. C. 632. 1880.

rational being gives way to the claim that they are inviolable fundamental rights which, being sanctioned by the law of nature, demand the recognition and protection of positive law. The advances in anatomy during the Renaissance under such men as Berengario de Carpi, Vesalius, and later, De Graaf, Albinus, and William Hunter, the increased knowledge of physiology and pathology, and the invention of the obstetrical forceps by Peter Chamberlen influenced the judicial opinion handed down by the courts in cases of malpractice.

III. *Police Power and Inoculation, Vaccination, Quarantine.*

There can be few matters more clearly within the police power of the state government than the conservation of the public health. On this power rests all the doctrine of quarantine, of compulsory vaccination, of sanitary sewerage, and the prevention of many forms of public nuisance. A learned and qualified membership of the medical profession is a sine qua non agency in protecting the public against the dangers of ignorance, quackery, and charlatanism. The police power is a branch of the law which is of the greatest importance and interest to medicine in making available for the public good the advances in preventive medicine. Freund defines the term " police power " as meaning the power of promoting the public welfare by restraining and regulating the use of liberty and property.[34] Justice Holmes [35] wrote an opinion in which he said, " It may be said in a general way that the police power extends to all the great public needs. . . . It may be put forth in aid of what is sanctioned by *usage* or held by the *prevailing morality* or strong and preponderant opinion to be greatly and immediately necessary to the public welfare." This appears to be a wide use of power by the state but in matters of public health it is accepted as good common sense. It is indeed more incisive power than despotic governments would have dared to claim in former times. For example, sanitary measures have been resented in India as interfering with the sanctity of private life by a population which tolerated for centuries the grossest forms of governmental oppression and spoliation. In a court ruling in 1925 [36] it was stated that " the police power includes *any* regulations for the protection of life and death. The State in the exercise of the police power, has the right to regulate any

[34] Ernst Freund, *The Police Power*, Chicago, 1904. George W. Wickersham, The Police Power, A Product of the Rule of Reason, *Harvard Law Review*, vol. 27, p. 297-316. 1914.
[35] Noble State Bank v. Haskell, 219 U. S. 104. 1910.
[36] People v. Witts, 315 Ill. 282. 1925.

and all occupations for the protection of the lives and rights and health of the people and may adopt any measures and regulations for that purpose, provided they do not infringe upon constitutional rights." We see that there are at least two main attributes of police power: first, to secure and promote public welfare toward which end the physician must play his part, and second, to exercise police power through restraint and compulsion which it is the obligation of the law to further. It may almost be said that this power is in accordance with the Bentham utilitarian philosophy of the greatest good for the greatest number.

The police power was, of course, unknown in ancient times. The establishment of a sanitary practice under ecclesiastical rule may be seen in the account of leprosy as recorded in Leviticus.[37] The priest ordered the cleansing of infected clothes, bodies, and houses where the leper was unclean. Also, the XII tables of the Roman law contain a sanitary regulation regarding the prohibition of burials in the city. Coming down to modern times, we find objections raised to the practice of inoculation under the *Common Law* as an infringement of the legal fundamental principle, " Sic utere tuo ut alienum non laedes." [38] (Use your own property in such a manner as not to injure that of another.) With the passage, in 1840, of "An Act to extend the Practice of Vaccination," it had been made in England and Wales and Ireland an indictable offense to produce or attempt to produce, by inoculation with variolous matter, the disease of smallpox.[39] In the United States, the state by virtue of its police power could compel the vaccination of children atending public schools.[40] Also, the right of physicians to exclude pupils from schools who refuse to be vaccinated during a smallpox scare was upheld.[41] In some states, pupils may be denied admission to public schools.[42] Public officers, who may be physicians, may establish sanitary cordons and preventive regulations under the right of preventing more serious injuries, provided they do not interfere with the natural right of the individual. Law makes possible the carrying out of mutual obligations of the medical profession and the public. Let us recall that natural law deals with the

[37] Old Testament, Leviticus c. XIII.
[38] Newsholme, Sir Arthur, *Evolution of Preventive Medicine*, London, 1927, p. 171. 1 BL. Comm. 306. 9 Coke Inst. 59.
[39] *The Statutes of the United Kingdom of Great Britain and Ireland*, 3 and 4 Victoria, 1840, c. 29, s. 8. Chronological Table and Index of the Statutes, 1235-1944, 1945, vol. 1, p. 317.
[40] Potts v. Breen, 167 Ill. 67. 1897.
[41] Duffield v. Williamsport School District, 162 Pa. 476. 1894.
[42] Jacobson v. Mass., 197 U. S. 11. 1905. 32 N. Y. Supp. 322 1895. 179 N. Y. 235. 1904.

284

rights and duties which follow from the first principle, " do good and avoid evil," and from the simple fact that man is man, nothing else being taken into account. This law may be traced back to the heritage of Classical and Christian thought in such exponents as Grotius, de Victoria, St. Thomas Aquinas, St. Augustine, Cicero, and the Stoics.[43] The aim of society in a legal sense is its own common good, the good of the social body, a common good for human persons; and to further this aim the doctor must contribute from his growing knowledge and discoveries. The physician must see that the maxim, " Obsta principiis " [44] applies to his field of work as it does in law. He must combat the first encroachments of a contagious disease, although in doing this, he will somehow interfere with the natural rights of individuals. One infected with contagion must be instantly removed beyond the reach of contact.[45] Society has every reason to expect the physician and the legal authority which goes with his action to prevent any injury which may threaten that society by an individual infected with a contagious disease. No one will dispute the right of the legislature to enact such measures as will give the medical profession the right to protect all persons from the impending calamity of a pestilence and to vest in local authorities such comprehensive powers as will enable them to act competently and effectively. However, the officials responsible must exercise their powers only when justified by the facts of the case and such facts must frequently be supplied by the doctor. A brief word about Quarantine. The importance of public health in the United States attracted the attention of the national legislature when Congress, in 1799, passed "An Act respecting Quarantine and Health Laws." [46] This Act clearly recognized the quarantine laws of the states. A system of quarantine laws established by a state is a rightful exercise of the police power for the protection of health which is not forbidden by the Constitution.[47] By the Act of 1878, certain powers in this direction were conferred on the Surgeon-General of the Marine Hospital Service in preventing the importation of disease; it was provided that " there shall be no interference in any manner with any quarantine laws or regulations as they now exist or may hereafter be adopted under *state* laws," [48] showing very clearly the intention of Congress to place the power for quarantine regulations in the hands of the individual states. Since that

[43] Jacques Maritain, *The Rights of Man and Natural Law*, New York, 1943, p 8.
[44] Spaulding v. Preston, 21 Vt. 13. 1848. Hazen v. Strong, 2 Vt. 427. 1830.
[45] *Ibid.*
[46] *U. S. Statutes at Large*, 1861, vol. 1, p. 474, 619. 118 U. S. 455, 464. 1886.
[47] *Ibid.*
[48] *Ibid.*

time, Congress had passed no quarantine law nor any other law to protect the inhabitants of the United States against the invasion of contagious diseases from abroad; and yet, during the late 18th and early 19th centuries, for many years the cities of the Atlantic Coast, from Boston to New York to Charleston, were devastated by the yellow fever. During all this time the Congress of the United States never attempted to exercise this or any other power to protect the people from the ravages of dreadful, contagious diseases. No doubt they believed that the power to do this belonged to the states; believed that what ought to be done could be better and more wisely done by the authority of the states who were familiar with the matter. Again may I point out that if the states were the proper agencies to deal with diseases, then the only source from which they could obtain the facts upon which to act for the welfare of the people was the medical profession and when they did so, then and only then could the growing knowledge of medicine guide the legislators.

IV. *The Medical Practice Act.*

In ancient times, the care and treatment of ill persons was carried out in accordance with what may be called the consuetudo, the custom, which placed the physician in the same position as the carpenter, the shoemaker, or other artisan. The so-called right to follow the healing art in medicine or surgery was a fundamental right of citizenship. Medicine was a regular part of general culture.[49] There were two kinds of doctors in Greece; the slave's doctor, who hurried from one patient to another prescribing treatment quickly and dictatorially without giving reasons or making a complete diagnosis; and the free man's doctor, who looked like a philosopher and talked with his patients as if they were pupils. The growing tendency in medicine was to regard not the sick, but the healthy people as the proper object of its care. The emphasis in medical practice had come to be on diet in its more meaningful sense of the general pattern of the life to be followed by a healthy person. This preventive point of view, as it may be called, captured the attention of the legislator too, for in the highest sense he too was a teacher of the citizen and wished to see wrongs prevented, rather than avenged. The Hippocratic physician strove to practice medicine by close adherence to theory and justice. The physician, for example, considered it just to advise the use of drugs to commit suicide in diseases in which pain had become intolerable. The

---

[49] Werner Jaeger, *Paideia, the Ideals of Greek Culture*, vol. 3, New York, 1944, p. 216. Plato, *Laws*, 720a-e; 957d-e; 857c-e.

concept of justice as derived from the Greeks postulated jural freedom, that is, equality before the laws. The Digest of Justinian [50] as formulated in Rome declared that jus is the art of what is good and fair and that its aim was to make men good not only by putting them in fear of penalties, but also by appealing to them through rewards. This proposition was a guidepost to physicians. Plato [51] referring to the problem of euthanasia, remarks, " Physicians and judges will look after those citizens whose bodies and souls are constitutionally sound. The physically unsound they will leave to die; and they will actually put to death those who are incurably corrupt." Our present law shrinks from any abbreviation of the span of life by a physician.

Common law is the basic law in almost every state and territory in the Union. This fact is of vast importance inasmuch as common law is a most powerful agency in promoting the application of advances in medical science. Under common law the practice of medicine was open to all who desired to follow it in any of its branches subject only to liability for damages in a case of lack of skill on the part of the practitioner and the right of government to proceed by quo warranto to prevent incompetents from following the profession.[52] One of the difficulties lay in the definition of the word " medicine." In the generic sense, the word " medicine " is the science and art of dealing with the prevention, care, and alleviation of disease: in its broader sense it refers to anyone who practices the art of healing disease and preserving health, a prescriber of remedies for sickness and disease. Legally, the term is a technical one, denoting a science or art which comprehends not only therapeutics but also the art of understanding the nature of diseases, the causes that produce them, as well as the art of cure and prevention of disease. With this background it was beyond the power of the state to prohibit the practice of medicine and surgery or any of its limited systems in the absence of any showing of injury or tendency of injury to the public health, safety, or morals.

Ecclesiastic law is exemplified by the action of the Fourth Lateran Council which, in 993, prohibited the regular clergy from performing any surgical operation involving the shedding of blood, thus leaving such operation to seculars and clerks. However, the priest-physicians were not prohibited from practicing medicine until 1131, at which time the Seventh Lateran Council forbade the monks and regular canons from pursuing

[50] Charles H. Monro (see reference 9), vol. 2, Bk. IX, tit. II, 7, 8.
[51] F. M. Cornford (translator), *The Republic of Plato*, New York-Oxford, 1945, p. 97 (Bk. III, 409-410).
[52] State v. Borah, 51 Ariz. 318. 1938.

the study of medicine. Later still, in 1163, the Council of Tours positively interdicted all surgical operations by the clergy.[53]

Statute law resulted in regulations which removed the clergy from the practice of medicine and surgery and brought into prominence barber-surgeons and apothecaries as the healers of the sick.

A chronologic survey of the early statutes passed in England is of interest at this point.[54] Until 1511 there was no distinctive law in Great Britain to distinguish the different branches of the profession of medicine. In 1511-12, third year of the reign of Henry VIII (1491-1547) a law was passed by Parliament "that no person within the city of London nor within seven miles of the same shall take upon him to exercise and occupy as a physician or surgeon except he be first examined and approved by the Bishop of London or the Dean of St. Paul or the Bishop of the Diocese outside the city provided this Act be not prejudicial to the Universities of Oxford and Cantebrigge." This Episcopal license to practice medicine or surgery remained in the hands of the Bishops who acted as delegates of the Pope and, in 1534, the licensing functions were transferred to the Archbishop of Canterbury acting for the King of England. Since this plan did not work well, the Royal College of Physicians in London was chartered in 1518 as a licensing body to regulate the practice of medicine, although this move was violently opposed by the Universities and by the Church. In 1523, the 14th and 15th years of Henry the VIII, the physicians of London became a Body Corporate. In 1540, the 32nd year of Henry VIII by Act of Parliament, "four physicians of the Fellowship of Physicians shall be chosen to enter into the house or houses of all and every Potecary within the said city only to search, view, and see such Potecary wares, drugs, and stuffs as the said Potecaries have." By this same Act of Parliament, it was declared legal that "any of the fellowship of Physicians may practice and exercise the said science of Phisick in all branches." In 1542-3, the 34th and 35th years of Henry VIII, in order to encourage all persons skilled in the nature of herbs, roots, and waters, an Act was passed "permitting persons being no surgeons to minister medicines outwards, to cure sores by herbs and ointments, or stone or ague by drinks, without being sued by surgeons for

[53] Joseph M. Toner, *Contributions to the Annals of Medical Progress and Medical Education in the United States*, Washington, 1874.

[54] C. Wall, *The History of the Surgeon's Company, 1745-1800*, London, 1937. J. B. Hurry, *The Ideals and Organization of a Medical Society*, London, 1913. *The Statutes of the Realm*, Printed by Command of His Majesty, King George the Third, From Original Records and Authentic Manuscripts, vol. 3, 1817. 3 Henry VIII, c. 11; 14-15 Henry VIII, c. 5; 32 Henry VIII, c. 40; 23 Henry VIII, c. 5; 1 M, sess. 2, c. 9.

so treating the sick." This was the so-called Quack's Charter. In 1549, Edward VI began his visitation of the University of Oxford. The existing statutes were discounted as being "antiquated, semibarbarous, and obscure," and the visitors were given sweeping powers in drawing up new statutes, including the right to assign one college solely to the study of medicine. The new statutes laid down that the medical student had to study six years, to dispute twice, to respond once, and to see two anatomical dissections before obtaining his B. A. He had to perform two dissections and to prove that he had effected at least three cures before he was admitted to practice. He had to see two or three more dissections, and to dispute and respond twice, before his D. M. This brief survey clearly shows the impact of the letter of the law on the practice of medicine.

In 1532, the first criminal code in Europe was enacted that contained statutory provisions directing the taking of medical testimony in all cases where death was occasioned by violent means. This code laid the foundation for legalized autopsies in criminal cases. In this same year, Henry VIII gave evidence of an enlightened public health policy by supporting an Act of Parliament which established Commissioners of Sewers in all parts of the Kingdom. In 1553, in the reign of Mary I (1516-1558), Parliament enacted a law that all Justices, . . . upon request of the President of the College of Physicians, shall aid and assist him in the execution of acts or statutes. As we glance back again at the remarkable reforms concerning the growth of medicine and the letter of the law in the reign of Henry VIII, they may be said to be due in great measure to the influence upon Henry VIII of men like Sir Thomas More, John Chambre, Thomas Linacre, and Ferdinand de Victoria [55]—all trained minds, sensitized to the nascent spirit of the Renaissance, and all aware of the evils practiced upon the sick by empirics, quacks, and illiterate monks.

Tudor England was not a time of building but of laying the foundation in medicine, surgery, public health, and laws related to them. To Henry VIII must go a salute for his vision in regulating the practice of medicine by reasonable laws and perhaps especially for grasping the opportunity to work at first through the Church, since its arm reached everywhere and was efficient. Henry VIII not only relied on the authority of the Church in religion, upon the aristocracy in politics, and upon Aristotle and Galen in science, but also rested his support upon the common people of the middle classes.

In the United States no one has a natural, absolute, or vested right to

[55] Sir Arthur Salisbury MacNalty, *The Renaissance and Its Influence on English Medicine, Surgery, and Public Health*, London, 1946.

practice medicine or surgery or any of their branches or systems.[56] It is
a conditional right subject to approval by an incorporated medical society,
or a diploma from a medical faculty of a university, and a license from a
board of medical registration. These legal factors make rights subordinate
to the public power to preserve and protect the public health. Where a
license is required, the practice of medicine without it is forbidden and
punished and it becomes important, therefore, to determine what is meant
by the practice of medicine. The question may arise in connection with
the administration of domestic remedies, emergency services, treatment
by massage, mental or spiritual treatment.

The practice of medicine embraces the following:[57] First, the understanding of the nature, character, and symptoms of a disease; second, the
proper remedy for a disease; and third, the giving or prescribing of a
remedy for a disease.

Practicing medicine without a license is never a crime but only a misdemeanor and is legally in the same class as running an automobile without a license, or exceeding the prescribed speed limit.

For the protection of the public two legal methods are employed: one,
the restrictive method, that is, compliance with certain legal regulations;
the other, the definitive method, which permits the public to choose
qualified or unqualified persons to treat them in case of illness. The
definitive method is the principle upon which the English medical practice act is based; in the United States the restrictive method obtains.

The preamble of the British Act of 1858[58] which created the General
Council of Medical Education and Registration of the United Kingdom
reads in part: " Whereas, it is expedient that persons requiring medical
aid shall be enabled to distinguish qualified from unqualified practitioners,
be it therefore enacted " etc. This first comprehensive act brought to a
close the loose period of medical practice so ably presented by Huxley.[59]
It did away with laissez faire in British medicine. A new test basis for
legislative standard was provided.

Violation of the act does not consist in practicing medicine and surgery
without a license, but in claiming to be a legally qualified practitioner of

[56] 50 La. 2 Ann. 1358. 1898. Louisiana State Board Examiners v. Fife et al., 162 La.
681. 1926.
[57] *Words and Phrases*, Permanent Edition, 1658 to Date, St. Paul, Minn., 1940, vol.
26, pp. 935-48. Underwood v. Scott, 43 Kan. 714. 1890.
[58] G. K. Richards, *The Statutes of the United Kingdom, Great Britain, and Ireland*,
London, 1858. 21-22 Victoria, c. 90, ss. 15, 47-52, sch. A.
[59] T. H. Huxley, The State and the Medical Profession, *The Nineteenth Century*,
1884, No. 84, pp. 228-238.

medicine when one is not. Punishment falls only on the man who *pretends* to be legally qualified when he is not.

In England any person who desires may engage in the treatment of the sick by any means whatsoever without incurring the slightest penalty, provided he does not claim to be legally qualified and licensed when he is not, the assumption being that any person who goes to an unqualified person for treatment does so at his own risk and that the object of a medical practice act is not to prevent the treatment of the sick by unlicensed persons, but to enable the public to discriminate between those who are qualified and those who are not.

The legal effect of this law is not the creation of a new misdemeanor, namely, the practice of medicine without a license, but is an application of the old common law principle of the illegality of obtaining money under false pretenses. The violator of the law is prosecuted and punished, not for the technical violation of a license law, but for claiming to be what he is not and for being a fraud and a cheat.

In the U. S. the medical practice legislation has been along restrictive laws and has endeavored by the establishment of certain standards to restrict the treatment of the sick to those possessing such qualifications and to prevent all others from engaging in it.

The growth of the practice of medicine is peculiarly correlated with two special aspects of law; first, with the precise definition of the medical practice act and second, with the police power of the state. Governments were the agencies that exercised control over the content and the standards of medical education.[60] In Germany, for example, it was direct government control; in England, the government prescribed qualifications either by royal edicts, parliamentary acts, common or statute laws; in the United States the control was left to the individual states. The problem of the medical practice act in the United States is so vast that I shall, in the main, limit this discussion to some features which pertain to the state of Massachusetts.

The first regulation of medical practice in Massachusetts was an Ordinance passed by the General Court in 1649 [61] to the effect,

Forasmuch as the law of God allows no man to impair the life or limbs of any other, but in a judicial way,—It is therefore ordered that no person or persons whatsoever, employed at any time about the bodies of men, women, and children,

---

[60] Helen R. Wright, Art. "Medical Education" in: *Encyclopaedia of the Social Sciences*, New York, 1933, vol. 10, p. 289.

[61] R. H. Fitz, The Rise and Fall of the Licensed Physician in Massachusetts, 1781-1860, *Trans. Assoc. Amer. Physicians*, vol. 9, 1894, pp. 1-18. Old Colony Laws, p. 28.

for the preservation of life or health, as surgeons, midwives, physicians, and others, presume to exercise or put forth any act contrary to the known approved rules of the art . . . without the advice and consent of such as are skillful in the same art, or at least of some of the wisest and gravest there present, and consent of the patient or patients. Which law, nevertheless, is not intended to discourage any from all lawful use of their skill, but rather to encourage and direct them in the right use thereof; and inhibit and restrain the presumptuous arrogancy of such as through perfidence of their own skill, or any other sinister respects, dare boldly to attempt to exercise any violence upon or towards the bodies of young or old.

Here was the basis for the practice of medicine in the colonial and pre-revolutionary period. It was not required that one be licensed nor was a felony involved if a patient died under the hand of an unlicensed physician. This opinion stems back to a declaration of the learned Lord Chief Justice Hale in the sixteenth century who declared " that since slaves and physic were before licensed physicians and chirurgeons that therefore unlicensed physicians be not subject to the penalties of statute law; also that it is not a felony if one dies under the hand of an unlicensed physician." [62] It was contended that any other point of view would be apocryphal and serve merely to gratify and flatter doctors of physic. This opinion was not in the best interests of the public.

From this unrestricted period of medical practice we come to the early nineteenth century when every state in the Union except North Carolina, Pennsylvania, and Virginia enacted laws which left the examination of physicians in the hands of physicians. It was hoped that these legislative acts would exclude quacks and unqualified practitioners of medicine. It was not a felony, for example, to treat the sick with their consent and with honest intention no matter how ignorant one was of the quality of the remedies used.[63] Such Court opinion gave considerable impetus to the quacks to continue their nefarious work. It was not until nine years later, in 1818, that the legislature passed "An Act regulating the Practice of Physicians and Surgeons." [64] This Act provided, " that no person entering the practice of physic or surgery shall be entitled to the benefit of law, for the recovery of any debt or fee accruing for his professional services unless he shall have been licensed by the officers of the Massachu-setts Medical Society or shall have graduated a doctor in medicine in Harvard University." Prior to this act any one who came up to the published standard was entitled to examination and to be licensed. The

[62] 1 Hale's Pleas of the Crown, 429.
[63] Commonwealth v. Thompson, 6 Mass. 134. 1809.
[64] Gen Laws, Mass. vol. 2, 1823. St. 1818 c. 113, s. 1.

constitutionality of the above cited act of 1818 was challenged but it was ruled that, " The Court are all of opinion, that the law in question was not repugnant to the 6th article of the Bill of Rights and further that its validity could not be impeached on the ground that it was a violation of any principle of the Constitution." [65] By this positive legislation, the Commonwealth of Massachusetts set the mandate that before one could engage in the practice of medicine, it was necessary to obtain good professional education and the sanction and permission of the Massachusetts Medical Society or the customary sanction of a degree from a university known to have a medical faculty. This was a direct attack against ignorant, careless, unskillful practitioners of medicine. It further emphasized the fact that physicians and surgeons are responsible not only for due care and diligence but also for that degree of skill and capacity which ordinarily belong to those who practice medicine within the limits of the state of science and the means of education available at any particular period. In 1884, Justice Holmes declared that " good intentions constitute no ground for the privilege of endangering human life." [66] This ruling undermined an earlier court opinion that " there is no law which prohibits any man from prescribing for a sick person with his consent if he honestly intends to cure him by his prescription, however gross his ignorance of the quality of the remedy or the nature of the disease or both." It now became clear that if a person, publicly practicing as a physician, with foolhardy presumption or gross negligence, prescribed a course of treatment which caused death, he might be found guilty of manslaughter although he acted with the consent of the patient and with no evil intent. However there were many who still argued before the members of the Legislature that it was impossible to regulate the practice of medicine as an art in which there were no standards: that anyone had the right to practice the healing art at his own peril and regardless of his ignorance, liable only to civil damages.

The medical practice act which affected a separation between the educational qualifications of physicians and the licensing board was argued as being in conflict with the Constitution of the United States. The Court, however, rendered the opinion that statutes of exclusion of unlicensed persons are not designed to confer on those who are licensed an exclusive benefit, privilege, or right and where that result does follow it is merely the collateral and incidental effect of provisions enacted solely with a

[65] Hewitt v. Charier, 16 Pick. 353. 1835.
[66] Commonwealth v. Pierce, 138 Mass. 165. 1884.

view to secure the welfare of the community. Further, the protection of the public from those who undertake to treat or manipulate the human body without that degree of education, training, and skill which the Legislature has prescribed as necessary to the general safety of the people is within the police power of the state.[67]

The Board of Registration in Medicine in The Commonwealth of Massachusetts was established in 1894. The legislative act required that, " on and after the first day of January 1895, the Board shall examine all applicants for registration as licensed physicians and surgeons and that this act would not apply to clairvoyants, or to persons practicing hypnotism, magnetic healing, mind cure, massage methods, christian science, cosmopathic or any other method of healing; provided such persons do not violate any of the provisions of section 10 of the act." [68] Although the Massachusetts Medical Society desired as early as 1884 to put on the statute books of the state a Medical Practice Act, it was not until ten years later, 1894, that a draft of the bill was drawn. In Massachusetts before the passage of the Medical Practice Act, the educated and the uneducated were rated as equals as far as medical standards went and one man was as good as another in the eyes of the law with the result that Massachusetts was one of the last states in the Union to adopt a Medical Practice Act. From our present vantage point of view, one may see the injustice and inadvisability of permitting a diploma from a medical school to serve at the same time as a license to practice. The Legislature now sets the standards of medical education and the Board of Registration sees that they are fulfilled by qualified candidates. The doctrine of stare decisis applies to the practice of medicine. This doctrine expresses the policy of the Courts to stand by precedents, and when a court has once laid down a principle of law as applicable to a certain state of facts, it will adhere to that principle and apply it to all future cases where the facts are substantially the same. It is on this doctrinal basis that the practice of medicine and the letter of the law protect the health of the public.

Concluding Remarks:

Although our attention is rarely called to the influence of the letter of the law upon the growth of medicine except when a violation is committed,

---

[67] Commonwealth v. Porn, 196 Mass. 326, 1907. Dent v. West Va. 129 U. S. 114. 1888. Hewitt v Charier, *ubi supra*; Commonwealth v Zimmerman, 221 Mass. 184. 1915.

[68] *First Annual Report of the Board of Registration*, Boston, 1895. Public Document No. 56. W. L. Burrage, *A History of the Massachusetts Medical Society, 1781-1922*, Norwood, Mass., 1923.

yet, from the survey made here, one may argue that law pervades the science of medicine like air pervades our lungs. Medicine like law concerns itself with duty, right, property, and crime; law, in fact, binds together the tissues of medicine. Our discussion clearly indicates that neither medicine nor law exists in isolation or in vacuo; on the contrary, down through the centuries, they react one upon another for the general welfare of the public.

Medicine enunciated by a man-god such as Imhotep, or based upon an ethical standard as in Hippocratic medicine, or dictated by a natural instinct as in primitive man and functionally expressed in the king-priest-physician relationship, or modern medicine developed within society by its own vitality—all these forms of medicine are practically affected by legal procedure. In broad perspective, then, Primitive, Greek, Mediaeval, Renaissance, and Modern medicine are paralleled respectively by lex talionis, idea of justice, ecclesiastic, natural, and positive law. This essay highlights the fact that law is not peripheral to but rather central in the growth of medicine.

APPENDIX

AN ACT CONCERNING PHESICIONS & SURGEONS *

3° Hen. VIII. c. 11, A.D. 1511-12

Forasmoche as the science and connyng of Physyke (and Surgie) to the pfecte knowledge wherof bee requisite bothe grete lernyng and ripe expience ys daily within this Royalme exccised by a grete multitude of ignoraunt psones of whom the grete partie have no mañ of insight in the same nor in any other kynde of lernyng some also (can 3) no tres on the boke soofarfurth that comon Artifics as Smythes Wevers and Women boldely and custumably take upon theim grete curis and thyngys of great difficultie in the which they partely use socery and which crafte partely applie such (medicyne 1) unto the disease as be verey noyous and nothyng metely therfore to the high displeasoure of God great infamye to the faculties and the grevous hurte damage and distruccion of many of the Kyng's liege people most spally of them that cannot descerne the uncunyng from the cunnyng; Be it therfore to the suertie and comfort of all man people by the auctoritie of thys psent parliament enacted that noo pson within the Citie of London nor within vij myles of the same take upon hym to exccise and occupie as a Phisicion (or Surgion) except he be first examined approved and admitted by the Bisshop of London or by the Dean of Poules for the tyme beyng callyng to hym or them iiij Doctours of Phisyk (and for Surgie other expt psones in that facultie) And for the first examynacion such as they shall thynk convenient; and aftward alway iiij of them that have been soo approved upon the payn of forfeytour for evy moneth that they doo occupie as Phisicions (or Surgeons) not admitted nor examined after the tenour of thys Acte of vii to be employed the oon half therof to thuse of our Sovaign Lord the Kyng and the other half therof to any pson that wyll sue for it by accion of dette in which no Wageour of Lawe nor pteccion shalbe allowed. And ov thys that noo pson out of the seid Citie and Pcinete of vij myles of the same except he have been as is seid before approved in the same take upon hym to excise and occupie as a Phisicion (or Surgeon) in any Diocesse within thys Royalme but if he be first examined and approved by the Bisshop of the same Diocese or he beyng out of the Diocesse by hys Vicar genall either of them callyng to them such expert psons in the seid faculties as there discrecion shall thynk convenyent and gyffying ther letts testimonials under ther sealle to hym that they shall soo approve upon like payn to them that occupie (the 2) contarie to thys acte as is above seid to be levyed and employd after the fourme before expssed Provided alway that thys acte nor any thyng therin conteyned be pjudiciall to the Univsities of Oxford and Cantebrigge or either of them or to any privilegys gaunted to them.

---

* *Note:* To the Original Act a small Schedule is attached containing the following Words: " Memorand that Sowrgeons be comprised in this Acte like as Phisicons for like mischief of ignorant psones psumyng to exercise Sowrgerie."

AN ACTE CONCNING PHISICONS.

14° & 15° Hen. VIII. c. 5, A. D. 1523

In the moost humble wyse Sheweth unto Your Highnes your true and faithfull Subjects & Liegemen, John Chamber, Thomas Linacre, Fernandus de Victoria your Phisicions and Nicholas Halswell, John Fraunces and Robt Yaxley and all oder Men of the same faculte withyn the Cities of London and sevyn myles about; that where Your Highnes by Your moost gracious tres patentes beryng date at Westm the xxiij daye of Septembr the tenth yere of your moost noble reign, for the coen Welth of this your Realme in due exccising and practising of the facultie of Phisike and the good ministracion of medecyns to be had, have incorporate and made of us and of our cumpanye aforesaid one Bodie and ppetuall Coialtie or Felisship of the Facultie of Phisik and to have ppetual succession and coen Scale and to chose yerely a psident of the same Felisship and Coialtie to ovse rule and govern the said Felisship and Coialtie and all Men of the same facultie, with dyvs oder libties and privileges by your Highnes to us graunted for the coen Welth of this your Realme as in your said moost gacious tres patentes more at large is specified and conteigned the Tenour whereof foloweth in thies wordes: And forsomoch that the makyng of the said Corporacion is meritorious and very good for the coen Welth of this your Realme, It is therfor expedient and necesarie to pvde that no pson of the said Polytyk bodie and Coialtie aforesaid be suffred to exccyse and practyse physyk but oonly thise psonnes that be pfounde sad and discrete groundlie lerned and deplie studied in physyk; In consideracion wherof and for the further auctorysyng of the same tres patents and also enlargyng of further articles for the said Coen Welth to be had and made; Pleasith it your Highnes with the Assent of your Lordes Spuall and Temporall and the Comons in this psent parliament assembled to enacte ordeign and establish that the said Corporacion of the said Coialtie and Felisship of the Facultie of Physyk aforesaid, And all and evy Graunte Articles and other thyng conteigned and specified in the said tres patentes be approved graunted ratefied and confermed in this present parliament and clerely auctorised and admytted by the same, good laufull and avaylable to your said bodie corporate and their Successours for ev in as ample and large mann as may be taken thought and construed by the same.

And where that in Diocesys of Englond oute of London it is not light to fynde alwey Men hable to sufficiauntly examyn after the Stature such as shalbe admytted to excersyse Physyk in them, that it may be enacted in this psent parliament, that noo pson fromhensforth be suffred to excercyse or practyse in Physyk through Englond untill such tyme that he be examined at London by the said President and three of the said Electys; And to have frome the said President or Electys tres testimonialx of their approvyng and examinacion, except he be a Graduat of Oxforde or Cantebrygge which hath accomplisshed all thyng for his fourme without any grace.

CONCNING PHISICIANS.

32 Hen. VIII. c. 40., A. D. 1540

And that it may please your moste Roiall Majestie by thauctoritie aforesaid that it may be further enacted ordeynid and established for the comon welth and suertie of your loving subjectis of this your Realme in and for thadministration of medecynes to suche of your said subjectis as shalhave neede of the same, that from hensfurth the said President for the tyme being comons and fellowes and their successours may yerely, at suche tyme as they shall thincke moste mete and convenient for the same, electe and chuse foure psons of the said comons and fellowes of the best larned wisest and mooste discrete suche as they shall thincke convenient and have experience in the said facultie of Fisicke; And that the saide foure psonnes so elected and chosen, aftre a corporall othe to them ministred by the said psident or his deputie, shall and may by vertue of this psent acte have full auctoritie and power, as often as they shall thinke mete and convenient, to entre into the house or houses of all and evy Poticary nowe or any tyme herafter using the myterie or crafte of a Poticary within the said Cittie onely to serche viewe and see suche Poticary wares druggs and stuffes as the said poticaries or any of them have or at any tyme heraftre shalhave in their house or houses; and all such wares drugges and stuffes as the said foure psonnes shall then fynde defective corruptid and not mete nor convenient to be mstrid in any medicynes for the helth of mens body the same iiij psonnes, calling to them the warden of the said mystery of Poticaries within the said cittie for that tyme being or one of them, shall cause to be brent or otherwise destroye the same as they shall thincke mete by their discretion:

And forasmuche as the science of phisicke dothe comprehend include and conteyne the knowledge of surgery as a speciall membre and parte of the same, therefore be it enacted that anny of the said company or felawiship of Phisitions, being hable chosen and admitted by the said psident and feliship of Physicians may from tyme to tyme aswell within the Citie of London as elswhere within this Realme practise and exercise the said science of Phisick in all and evy his membres and partes, any acte statute or provision made to the contrarie notwithstanding.

AN ACTE THAT PERSONES BEING NO COEN SURGEONS MAIE MYNISTRE MEDICINES OUTWARDE.

34° and 35° Hen. VIII. c. 8, 1542-3

Where in the parliament holden at Westm in the thirde yere of the Kings moste gracious reigne, amongst other things for the advoyding of sorceryes witchcrafte and other inconvenences, it was enacted that no psone within the Citie of London, nor within seven myles of the same, shoulde take upon him to exercyse and occupie as Phisician or Surgeon, except he be first examyned approved and admytted of the Bisshopp of London and other, undre and upon certaine peynes and penalties in the same acte mencioned; *Sithens* the making of which said acte the companie and Felowship of Surgeons of London, mynding oonlie thyre own lucres, and nothing the profits or ease of the diseased or patient, have sued troubled and vexed divers honest psones as well men as woomen, whome God hathe endued with the knowledge of the nature kind and operacon of certeyne herbes, rotes and waters, and the using and mynistering of them to suche as been pained with customable diseases, as Womens brested being sore, a Pyn the Web in the eye, uncoomes of hands, scaldings, burnings, sore mouthes, the stone strangurye soucelin and morfew and such other lyke diseases, and yet the saide psojes have not takin any thing for theyre peynes and cooninng, but have myinistered the same for the poore people oonelie for neighbourhode and Goddes sake and of pitie and charytie and it is nowe well knowen that the surgeons admytted wooll doo no cure to any psone, but where they shall knowe to be rewarded with a greater soome or rewarde than the cure extendeth unto, for in cace they woulde mynistre theyre coonning to sore people unrewarded, there shoulde not so many rotte and perishe to deathe for lacke of helpe or surgerye as dailie doo, but the greatest parte of surgeons admytted been muche more to be blamed than those psones that they trouble, for althoughe the most parte of the psones of the saide crafe surgeons have small cooning, yet they wooll take great soomes of money and doo little therfore, and by reasone thereof they doo often tymes impaire and hurte theyre patients rather thenne do them good: In consideracon whereof and for the ease comforte socour helpe relief and healthe of the Kings poore Subjects inhabytaunts of this his Realme, nowe peyned or deseased, or that hereafter shallbe payned or deseased, Be it ordeyred established and enacted by thauctorytie of this pnt paliament, that at all tymes from hensforthe, it shalbe legull to every psone being the Kings Subjects having knowledge and experience of the nature of herbes, rotes and waters or of the operacon of the same by speculation or practyse, within any parte of the Realme of Englande, or within any other the Kings Domynons, to practyse use and mynistre in and to any outward sore uncoom wounde ap ostemacons outwarde swelling or disease, any herbe or herbes oyntementes, bathes, pultes and emplasters, according to theyre cooning experience and knowledge in any of the diseases sores and maladies aforesaide and all otherlyke to the same, or drunken for the stone strangurye or agues, without suite vexacon trouble penalties or losse of theyre goods. The foresaide Statute in the foresaide thirde yere of the Kings most gracous reigne, or any other acte ordinance or statute to the contrarye hereof heretofore made in any wise notwithstanding.

PROFESSIONAL ETHICS AND THE DEVELOPMENT OF AMERICAN LAW AS APPLIED TO MEDICINE*

CHESTER R. BURNS

Various historical interpretations can be offered about the development of American law as applied to medicine. Mine emerges from a special interest in the history of professional ethics in American medicine. I am fully aware of the tentative nature of my conclusions and that I shall be raising more questions than I can answer. If my analysis is too simplistic, I know that lawyers will correct my errors about the law, that physicians will correct my errors about medicine, and that fellow historians will rush to my defense by responding to those corrections.

Since the beginning of civilization, individuals and groups have developed a variety of ways to order their judgments about ideal human behavior. These ideals have been expressed in myriad religious, philosophical, and scholastic traditions. Some ancient Greek physicians delineated certain professional ideals and distinguished them from more general ones so important to the priests, philosophers, and teachers of ancient Greece. Although they may have reflected personal and social ideals, the ancient Greek doctors sought patterns of specifically professional ethics, patterns which have framed the Western quest for professional standards.[1]

For the sake of brevity, I shall pass over many centuries and use only examples that belong to the story of the evolution of professional ethics in the United States.[2] It is helpful to arrange the professional ethics of American physicians in terms of three categories of human relationships: those involving the interactions of students and teachers, those occurring during the transactions of an individual physician with his individual patients, and those emerging from the relationships of a physician with a variety of governing and non-governing groups in a community. Although there are other categories of professional relationships, I shall limit this discussion to an examination of some ways in which American law has developed in relation to these three areas of medical ethics. I shall attempt to demonstrate some important connections between the creation of ethical standards in American medicine and the legal responses of American citizens and law professionals.

Laws may refer to rules established by an authoritative individual or group in a society. These laws are specific acts of will created by politically sanctioned powers. These laws become behavioral directives about interpersonal actions. Legal systems, thus, are instruments for social ordering and may be juxtaposed to the ethical systems that are used as intramural instruments for ordering professional groups. I now offer some juxtapositions within four

*Adapted from a lecture given at The Johns Hopkins University School of Medicine, October 15, 1974.

major areas of medico-legal relationships: licensure, malpractice, public health legislation, and forensic medicine.

Licensure

How are credentials established in medicine? How do citizens in a community recognize and sanction a person qualified to render health care services? How can these credentials be recognized and accepted by all citizens? How does a given citizen distinguish between the qualified health care professional and the unqualified one, or between the qualified one and the quack, or between the qualified professional and the unethical one?

The principal methods for dealing with the problems posed by these questions are licensure, certification, and accreditation—all are examples of credentials, of awarding badges. As mechanisms for intramural evaluation and recognition, certification and accreditation are voluntary activities on the part of a given health profession. Licensure is a combined extramural-intramural process by which a governmental agency, usually staffed by peer professionals, grants qualified persons permission to engage in a given occupation or profession.

The history of medical licensure in America affords a provocative example of the transactional nature of relationships between professional ethics and legal responses. Although a state may establish boards of medical examiners and licensure procedures, they have little meaning unless there are reputable schools producing qualified individuals who are worthy of being licensed, worthy of displaying their diplomas (badges).

During the early years of the American republic, there was considerable interest in the development of medical schools with high standards even though these early schools were seen as supplements to the preceptorial system. Many of the early schools were associated with universities, and their curricula were patterned after Old World models.[3] In response to these circumstances, thirteen states had constituted medical licensing boards by 1832. In states with reputable medical schools, however, a medical degree was usually considered a license to practice. No further examinations by a medical society or a licensure board were required. In nearly all states, candidates were required to pass some form of examination given by either a school, board, or society. Unexamined practitioners who professed to be doctors and who charged fees for their services could be penalized with fines permitted by the licensing statutes. There is little evidence, however, that the licensing boards enforced these statutes. Said Daniel Drake in 1832, "More than half of the states of the Union have laws to regulate the practice of medicine, but I am by no means convinced, that they have ever done any real good to the profession or society."[4]

The licensure laws had not prevented the widespread growth of unorthodox medical practice. Some physicians recommended more legislative actions against the unorthodox practitioners. Astounded at the legislators' apathy, one Vermont physician exclaimed: "Venerable legislators, if ye have no regard for the dead, have mercy on the living."[5] The legislators were not apathetic in granting state charters to orthodox practitioners who were establishing proprietary schools in many parts of the country, although these charters imposed no uniformity on the policies of these schools. Nor did the legislators cease to charter unorthodox practitioners.

Consequently, between 1832 and 1870, state legislators upheld Drake's viewpoint and either repealed laws that sanctioned the orthodox practitioners or did not enact any new licensure laws. The overall effect of these legislative actions should not be misinterpreted. Either the penalty clauses of existing statutes were abolished, or no legal restrictions were placed on unlicensed or unexamined practitioners. The charters of existing medical societies were usually not repealed. Moreover, the regular procedures for licensing remained intact in some states, for example, in New York, South Carolina, Louisiana, and Indiana. There were simply no penalties for practicing without a license. This did not prevent graduates from obtaining a license if they desired one, at least in the states that still had licensing boards. Furthermore, both orthodox and unorthodox practitioners were still subject to the processes of common law decisions about malpractice.

Each citizen had a right to decide freely if he would be treated by an orthodox or an unorthodox practitioner. With faith in the common sense of doctors, legislators believed that the diplomas of all medical schools could serve as licenses or societal badges. Unfortunately, however, there was an enormous variation in the value of these badges before 1870. The situation changed afterwards.

Between 1870 and 1910, the ideals of many medical educators led to numerous institutional reforms in American medical education, reforms that established a basis for licenses of uniform and superior value. In addition to establishing much higher entrance requirements, medical schools created a graded curriculum with longer and more numerous terms required for graduation. By acknowledging the importance of the basic sciences and by developing avenues of clinical training during and after formal medical schooling, some medical schools developed curricular patterns which served as models for twentieth-century changes, models championed so vigorously by Abraham Flexner in 1910.[6]

Concurrent with these reforms in medical education, licensing policies were rejuvenated and state boards of medical examiners were established throughout the United States.[7] By 1898, only the Alaska territory had no legal regulation. Six states required only the registration of diplomas. Eleven accepted either an approved diploma or a board exam. Twenty-two states required both diplomas from qualified medical schools and satisfactory completion of examinations given by their state boards, an approach that became the model for the future. After the newly formed Council on Medical Education of the American Medical Association surveyed medical schools in 1904, it recommended examination of all candidates by state boards. By 1912, a federation of state medical boards was organized. Without reviewing the details of twentieth-century events, medical practice acts have been enacted separately in some fifty-five jurisdictions of the United States.

In these acts, none of the following is uniform: standards required for eligibility, types of examinations, methods of examination, criteria for passing grades on these examinations, costs of licensure, interstate endorsement policies, qualifications of members of the boards, grounds for disciplinary action and revocation of licenses, the nature of separate boards of basic science examiners, and policies toward foreign medical graduates. With the development of the FLEX examination, greater uniformity is now assured for types and methods of examination and interstate endorsement policies. Also, at least half of the separate boards of basic science examiners have become inactive. Even with the variations, inconsistencies, and changes, these medical practice acts have been enforced in some states.

By examining the files of the Federation of State Medical Boards of the United States, Derbyshire found a total of 938 actions that had been taken against physicians by Boards of Medical Examiners between 1963 and 1967: 68 reprimands, 161 suspensions, 334 revocations, and 375 probations. The causes of these actions included narcotic addiction, mental incompetence, fraud and deceit in practice, felony conviction, criminal abortion, alcoholism, unprofessional conduct, moral turpitude, gross malpractice, fraud in application, gross immorality, fee splitting, and gross misconduct.[8]

From a societal point of view, the purpose of these laws and their administration is to prevent harm from occurring to patients by the acts of unqualified practitioners and to prevent acts done by persons who, for whatever reason, are no longer qualified to be professional physicians. Professional competence and incompetence is the underlying concern of the entire licensure process. How ironic that until very recently professional incompetence has seldom been listed as a cause for disciplinary action under a medical practice act. Yet, the main purpose of licensure policies is to secure competent and qualified physicians and to inhibit the actions of the unqualified or incompetent.

With its examination policies a medical school grants the moral right of practice to a qualified graduate. Upon successful completion of its examinations, a state board converts this moral right into a legal one. The right to practice medicine as a physician is a societal privilege, not a natural right. Knowledge and skills are the bases for both rights. The medical licensing system is a way of identifying and acknowledging certain ideals of the medical profession. The license becomes a political sanction of those values championed by the profession and professed by the individual members desiring the sanction.

A physician's moral rights, thus, are those claims by him that are in accordance with what is good, proper, and just in medical science and practice. His legal rights are those same claims that have been guaranteed or sanctioned by the legal system. Although there are many similarities between moral and legal rights, there are important differences, especially as these rights are converted into responsibilities. Some of these differences are examined in the next section on medical malpractice.

Malpractice

Although physicians have been sued for malpractice since the beginning of this country, the problem has not received very serious attention until quite recently, as signified by the 1,060 page report issued by Senator Ribicoff's Sub-committee in 1969 and the report of the HEW Commission on Malpractice published in 1973. One of the fascinating aspects of the problem involves the relationship between professional ethics and legal precedents established by common law decisions about medical malpractice. The similarities and differences between moral and legal responsibilities can be illustrated by examining some of the recurring precedents offered by judges adjudicating malpractice accusations, even before the Civil War.[9] Four examples are offered.

A physician is legally responsible for professing certain kinds of knowledge and certain skills. A physician should be appropriately educated and trained. Evidence of a suitable education, although necessary, however, is not sufficient in disproving malpractice in a particular case. Reciprocally, patients should select a properly educated doctor. But, selecting one does not guarantee a verdict for the patient in a malpractice suit against that doctor. Nevertheless, this legal precedent upholds the value judgments of physicians who believe that uneducated physicians are immoral. When state legislators ignored or repealed regulations about medical education between 1830 and 1870, the state supreme court justices—in contrast—usually acknowledged the superiority of an orthodox medical education.

The second maxim: A physician is legally responsible for utilizing ordinary skills in rendering ordinary and reasonable care. But how is the nature of ordinary skill and ordinary care to be determined? Who determines the spectrum of extraordinary–ordinary–subordinary skill and care? Should there not be uniform standards of good care everywhere? The ethical problem is to determine the nature of these criteria and standards. Ordinary skill and care constitute the legal maximum and the ethical minimum: A physician who claims to adhere to the ethical maximum, i.e., professing extraordinary skill and care, usually forfeits his rights to legal protection in cases of malpractice accusation. Furthermore, most thoughtful persons would want physicians to utilize extraordinary skill and care in managing their particular problems.

The third precedent: A physician is not responsible for errors of judgment. When there are reasonable grounds for therapeutic differences of opinion, a physician who exercises his best judgment is not responsible for mistakes in that judgment. Ethically, however, are not mistakes in treatment among the most serious errors of physicians? Choosing the best of several ways of managing a problem is fundamental to therapeutics and professional ethics. A physician, however, is not liable—not legally responsible—for so-called "honest" mistakes in selecting a management approach that is not effective or produces an undesired effect.

The fourth example: A physician is not legally required to guarantee a cure. From the point of view of professional ethics, restoration to sound health—cure—is desired by both physician and patient. This ideal, however, is not legally sanctioned. Moreover, legal responsibility is not measured by the result of therapeutic efforts, even though this is clearly a principal criterion in determining the right and wrong of medical practices. In fact, the consequences of treatment are the chief reasons for malpractice accusations altogether and the end result of treatment is a fundamental ethical concern of both doctor and patient. Yet, patients cannot legally expect a cure, and a physician has little legal backing if he promises one.

If the American society, via its common law decisions about malpractice accusations, does not hold physicians liable for cure, for extraordinary skills and care, or for mistakes, then why should physicians really worry about the ultimate outcome of their care; why should they do their best? The legal precedents derived from malpractice adjudications seem to have a levelling influence on the professional ideals of physicians. Or, they offer a different, even contradictory and inconsistent, set of values from those developed within the profession itself. If this claim is valid, it may not be correct to assert unequivocally that medical malpractice accusations would be decreased if physicians would adhere strictly to professional ethics. Relationships between legal and ethical norms must be analyzed more carefully.

The HEW Commission asserted that "the genesis of virtually every malpractice claim or suit is a physical or mental injury or other adverse result of treatment sustained by the patient. This does not mean that every malpractice claim or suit is founded on negligent conduct by physicians or other health-care providers."[10] The available statistics suggested that most of the alleged injuries were not caused by negligence. Even so, the Commission concluded, "every study produced to date indicates that there are many times more medical injuries than there are claims, and while most of these injuries are not due to negligence, many of them can be prevented, if this is the area which we believe deserves major attention." Whatever language you wish to use— provider proficiency, performance efficiency, quality professional care—the basic concern is professional competence: Establishing it, maintaining it, and improving it. And, in any discussion of competence, we are concerned with professional values, ethics, and ideals.

Public Health Legislation

Throughout the history of professional ethics in Western medicine, a premium has always been placed on knowledge and on the application of that knowledge in the care of individual patients. For ancient and medieval physicians, however, professional responsibilities toward a community *qua* community were not important features of professional standards. As national states evolved during the modern era and as communities became more concerned about health care, especially during epidemics, the medical profession was challenged with an increasing number of public claims and a corresponding increase in attempts to secure legally the professional services that were regarded as necessary or desirable.

Numerous authors have presented details of the history of public health in the United States.[11] Recall the following: establishment of city health boards (Baltimore in 1793); reports of McCready, Griscom, and Shattuck; surveys of the American Medical Association; the National Quarantine and Sanitary Conventions; establishment of the Metropolitan Board of Health for the State of New York in 1866; founding of the American Public Health Association in 1872; the creation of a National Board of Health between 1879 and 1883; and the organization of the Department of Health, Education, and Welfare in 1953. It is noteworthy that the state governments which revitalized or established state health boards and departments between 1870 and 1900 were also involved in reviving or creating new licensure laws during the same period.

The multiple kinds of health care legislation enacted in this country during the past 200 years have afforded physicians new and, at times, difficult obligations as professionals. I submit three generalizations about the relationship between public health legislation and professional ethics, realizing fully that each needs more elaboration than that afforded in this essay.

(1) American physicians have always had difficulty in circumscribing the nature of their public responsibilities, either as citizens or professionals. (2) In persistently opposing or minimizing the role of governmental activity in medicine, American physicians have attempted to free themselves of political responsibilities. (3) American physicians can no longer deny the implications of a fundamental addition to their obligations as professional persons: They have obligations to communities that extend beyond the care of individual patients.

In 1847, Charles Lee, a highly regarded New York practitioner, delivered a commencement address in which he reviewed a physician's obligations towards society. Physicians, said Lee, were not only "conservators of the public health," but they should also "advance the great cause of intellectual and moral progress, and of civilization and happiness." Physicians, however, should choose medical, not political, means in attempting to achieve these great ends. They should be patriots, but not partisan politicians. "There is, indeed, something in the noisy pursuits of politics, which seems to me utterly incompatible with the character of a man of science, and wholly ruinous to the professional advancement, and even mental improvement, of the medical practitioner. . . . Shun politics, Gentlemen, as you would the poisonous upas; and whoever tempts you to enter the political field, set him down as your worst enemy."[12]

Yet, Lee exhorted the graduating students to disseminate knowledge that pertained to matters of public health and to instruct judges and lawyers about all questions of forensic medicine. Physicians were expected to shun politics, but not politicians. They were expected to avoid the vicissitudes of political office, but not the issues of health and disease that affected the body politic. In my judgment, this fundamentally schizoid posture has been present in the attitudes of many American physicians ever since. How many physicians have demonstrated a sense of participation, even vicariously, in the activities of their governments, city, state, or federal? In dealing with certain aspects of health legislation, American physicians have been innovative and creative. In dealing with others, the hallmark of physician behavior has been non-involvement or resistance. I suggest that a major reason for this resistance is the attempt of physicians to rid themselves of the burdens and challenges of dealing with the political, economic, and social implications of their professional actions.

In realizing that physicians (and other health care professionals) can no longer free themselves of such political and social responsibilities, it is important to understand that these responsibilities, *qua* professional persons, represent a very recent addition to the spectrum of professional ethics. Prior to 1700, roughly, most physicians believed that they were discharging their obligations to society by administering adequate medical care directly to individual patients. There were no generally accepted obligations to a community *qua* professional person. But by the middle of the nineteenth century, even in the *laissez-faire* Jacksonian democracy of the American republic, these obligations were being codified in the first code of ethics adopted by the American Medical Association (1847).[13] Henceforth, physicians had obligations to use their knowledge and skills in solving the health problems and meeting the health needs of communities. In dealing with the day-to-day problems of health care legislation, we must not forget that this set of professional obligations is very young, indeed, and has not been accepted by numerous conscientious practitioners devoted to the care of their individual patients.

Forensic Medicine

A special portion of the new responsibilities of physicians toward communities involves their obligations toward the judiciary branches of American government. This is the realm of forensic medicine and pathology. From the very beginning of our country, physicians have been asked to testify at coroner's inquests and at various judicial proceedings. In the early part of the nineteenth century, several professors in medical schools accepted the importance of these duties and began to provide their students with lectures on various aspects of forensic medicine. In 1810, Benjamin Rush lectured on the subject, and in 1813 James Stringham was appointed Professor of Medical Jurisprudence at Columbia's College of Physicians and Surgeons in New York City. The most important event in this early history was the publication in 1823 of Theodric Romeyn Beck's two volumes entitled *Elements of Medical Jurisprudence*. By the time of Beck's death in 1855, there had been four British, one German, and five American editions of his book.

Since that time, many textbooks of forensic medicine and forensic pathology have been published, specialized societies and journals have been established, and courses have been taught in medical and law schools.[14] Physicians and health care professionals have become involved extensively in providing medical opinions needed at a large number of judicial occasions. Testimony has involved personal injury claims after auto or industrial accidents, workman's compensation claims after occupational injury, causes of death in accidental or criminal situations, the mental capacities of individuals who initiate contracts or wills and the mental conditions of the criminally accused to name only a few circumstances.

Although it has had a relatively low profile in both medicine and law, the concern with forensic medicine has been a relative constant throughout American history. If understood as the use of medical knowledge in courts, it should not be threatening to competent physicians. It simply involves a claim by the legal system on the medical profession, one that is strikingly different from the other legal claims that I have discussed. Historically, it can be understood best as the development of American medicine as applied to law, and, as such, deserves a separate analysis in another essay.

In summary, I have analyzed some relationships between professional ethics and legal maxims. In licensure, the ultimate source of moral authority resides in the profession, whereas the ultimate source of legal authority resides in the legislatures. Presumably, the state boards have the responsibility of informing both the profession and the public about the provisions of the medical practice acts that they administer. The total spectrum of licensure laws involves more than fifty distinct statutes, although there are important similarities between them. Ostensibly, these acts sanction qualified practitioners and protect the public from unqualified ones. The validity of these acts is directly dependent upon the scientific and educational standards adopted by schools of medicine in the various jurisdictions.

Is a physician competent because he knows and obeys the laws of a given medical practice act? The answer must be an unqualified no. The nature of the physician's competence—his professional goodness—is not determined by the law. It is determined by the nature and extent of the knowledge and skills that he professes to possess. The laws of a medical practice act are primarily procedural, not substantive. Licensure laws acknowledge that a given person possesses the knowledge and skill requisite for being a member of a profession and allow that person to receive remuneration for applying that knowledge and skill in the care of individual patients. Licensure laws do not determine the nature of that knowledge and skill, nor the validity of its central role in professional ethics.

The source of ultimate moral authority in malpractice proceedings must also lie with the medical profession, whereas the source of legal authority resides in the legislative and judicial branches of government. Although decisions may be made on the basis of legal desiderata, the ultimate problem is one of determining whether or not a physician performed a bad practice. In the final analysis, this is a medical, not a legal judgment. The precedents that are established by the courts adjudicating particular cases become the legal rules, although statutory laws may also have some bearing. The function seems to be one of redressing wrongs committed on individual patients, and, indirectly, sanctioning certain right ways of behaving as physicians. The values implicit in these judgments pertain to those that involve individual patient care, that is, those about transactions between an individual physician and an individual patient.

In reviewing legal maxims emerging from adjudications of medical malpractice accusations, a curious paradox emerges. Contrary to popular opinion, it almost seems as if attending to the highest ethical standards in professional medical care is actually un-American, legally speaking, and if successful, traps health care professionals in a web of significantly increasing malpractice claims. Regardless, the basic problem in malpractice, as with licensure regulations, is one of professional competence and incompetence.

It is no accident that the HEW Commission on Medical Malpractice offered several recommendations about licensing and certification.[15] The Commission believed that most state medical practice acts did not have adequate provisions for disciplining physicians who were found to be incompetent. The Commission recommended that state boards be authorized to issue disciplinary actions such as remedial education requirements, in addition to reprimand, suspension, or revocation of licenses. The Commission also believed that state licensure laws should require periodic re-registration of health care professionals, registration that would be dependent upon demonstration of regular participation in approved continuing medical education programs. Again, the basic problem is maintaining the scientific, technical, and interpersonal skills of physicians at high levels.

As far as health legislation is concerned, the ultimate source of moral and legal authority is the network of publicly elected representatives and their appointed officials. Legislatures and government agencies are responsible for creating health-related laws at multiple levels of political organization: city, county, state, or federal. Presumably, these laws secure the community's demands for preserving health and preventing disease.

A review of the history of health care legislation suggests that American physicians have had extensive difficulties in incorporating new societal obligations into their patterns of professional norms. Today, American physicians, with greater frequency than ever before, are re-examining the political, economic, and social consequences of their professional obligations.

In forensic medicine, the sources of legal authority are our judicial institutions, with ultimate moral authority resting in the public. The decisions of the courts become common law maxims, although various legislative statutes may also bear on these decisions. The function is one of utilizing medical knowledge in adjudicating specific civil and criminal cases. The values involve all of those pertaining to civil and criminal justice. As in the past, American physicians will be expected to continue honoring those values as a component of their community obligations.

In 1690, one North American colonial, Gabriel Thomas, wrote: "Of lawyers and physicians I shall say nothing, because this country is very peaceable and healthy: Long may it so continue and never have occasion for the tongue of the one or the pen of the other—both equally destructive of men's estates and lives."[16] In the past two centuries, much has come from the tongues and the pens of both lawyers and physicians. I have described some of their interactions, with the hope that my comments will help in understanding better the development of American law as applied to medicine. It is also my hope that the future words, either spoken or written, of American lawyers and

American physicians will be more constructive than destructive in the subsequent developments of American law as applied to medicine.

Acknowledgments: I am indebted to Robert Derbyshire, M.D. for his suggestions and comments.

Notes

1. Ludwig Edelstein, "The Professional Ethics of the Greek Physician," in *Ancient Medicine Selected Papers of Ludwig Edelstein,* edited by Owsei Temkin and C. Lilian Temkin. Baltimore: The Johns Hopkins Press, 1967, pp. 319–348.
2. For other details, see Chester R. Burns, "Comparative Ethics of the Medical Profession Outside of the United States," *Tex. Rep. Biol. Med.,* 1974, *32*:181–187; and "Reciprocity in the Development of Anglo-American Medical Ethics, 1765–1865," *Proceedings of the XXIII International Congress of the History of Medicine,* London: Wellcome Institute of the History of Medicine, 1974, Vol. 1, pp. 813–819.
3. William Frederick Norwood, "American Medical Education from the Revolutionary War to the Civil War," *J. Med. Educ.,* 1957, *32*:433–447.
4. Daniel Drake. *Practical Essays on Medical Education and the Medical Profession in the United States.* Reprint of the 1832 edition. Baltimore: The Johns Hopkins Press, 1952, p. 91.
5. John Putnam Batchelder. *On the Causes Which Degrade the Profession of Physick; an Oration Delivered Before the Western District of the N.H. Medical Society, at its Annual Meeting in May, 1818.* Bellow Falls, Vermont: B. Blake, 1818, p. 8. For further details and different interpretations about the period before 1860, see Joseph F. Kett, *The Formation of the American Medical Profession, The Role of Institutions 1780–1860.* New Haven: Yale University Press, 1968.
6. Robert P. Hudson, "Abraham Flexner in Perspective: American Medical Education, 1865–1910," *Bull. Hist. Med.,* 1972, *46*:545–561; Chester R. Burns, "The Forms and Reforms of American Medical Education, 1875–1910," unpublished MS.
7. Richard H. Shryock. *Medical Licensing in America, 1650–1965.* Baltimore: The Johns Hopkins Press, 1967.
8. Robert C. Derbyshire. *Medical Licensure and Discipline in the United States.* Baltimore: The Johns Hopkins Press, 1969, pp. 77–79.
9. Chester R. Burns, "Malpractice Suits in American Medicine Before the Civil War," *Bull. Hist. Med.,* 1969, *43*:41–56.
10. Department of Health, Education, and Welfare. *Medical Malpractice. Report of the Secretary's Commission on Medical Malpractice.* Washington, D.C., 1973, p. 22.
11. For a recent study, see John Duffy's *A History of Public Health in New York City, 1625–1866,* and *A History of Public Health in New York City, 1866–1966.* Both were published in New York by the Russell Sage Foundation, the former in 1968 and the latter in 1974.
12. Charles A. Lee. *Address to the Graduates of Geneva Medical College, Delivered in the Presbyterian Church, Geneva, January 26, 1847.* New York: Benedict, pp. 12–13.
13. *Proceedings of the National Medical Conventions, held in New York, May, 1846 and in Philadelphia, May, 1847,* pp. 83–106. See especially Chapter III.

14. Chester R. Burns, "The Teaching of Medical Ethics and Jurisprudence in American Medical Schools," in *The Education of American Physicians Historical Essays in Honor of William Frederick Norwood.* Edited by Ronald L. Numbers. University of California Press. In press.
15. *Medical Malpractice, op. cit.,* pp. 51 ff.
16. Charles Warren. *A History of the American Bar.* Boston: Little, Brown, and Co., 1911, p. 107.